Biochemical Correlates
of
Brain Structure and Function

Biochemical Correlates
of
Brain Structure and Function

Edited by

A. N. DAVISON

*Institute of Neurology, The National Hospital,
London, England*

1977

ACADEMIC PRESS

LONDON · NEW YORK · SAN FRANCISCO

A Subsidiary of Harcourt Brace Jovanovich, Publishers

ACADEMIC PRESS INC. (LONDON) LTD
24/28 Oval Road
London NW1

United States Edition published by
ACADEMIC PRESS INC.
111 Fifth Avenue
New York, New York 10003

Library of Congress Catalog Card Number: 76 53112
ISBN: 0 12 206650 2

PRINTED IN GREAT BRITAIN BY
WILLIAM CLOWES & SONS LIMITED
LONDON, BECCLES AND COLCHESTER

List of Contributors

R. BALÁZS, MRC Developmental Neurobiology Unit, Medical Research Council Laboratories, Woodmansterne Road, Carshalton, Surrey SM5 4EF, England

T. J. CROW, Division of Psychiatry, Clinical Research Centre, Watford Road, Harrow, Middx HA1 3UJ and Division of Physiology and Pharmacology, National Institute for Medical Research, The Ridgeway, Mill Hill, London NW7 1AA, England

A. N. DAVISON, Miriam Marks Department of Neurochemistry, Institute of Neurology, The National Hospital, Queen Square, London WC1N 3BG, England

D. DE WIED, Rudolf Magnus Institute for Pharmacology, Medical Faculty, University of Utrecht, Vondellaan 6, Utrecht, The Netherlands

DEBORA B. FARBER, Department of Anatomy, University of California School of Medicine, Los Angeles, California 90024, U.S.A.

ANTONIO GIUDITTA, International Institute of Genetics and Biophysics, via G. Marconi 10, 80125 Naples, Italy

JEFF HAYWOOD, Department of Biochemistry, University of Leeds, Woodhouse Lane, Leeds, Yorks LS2 9JT, England

P. D. LEWIS, Department of Histopathology, Royal Postgraduate Medical School, Hammersmith Hospital, London W12 0HS, England

L. LIM, Miriam Marks Department of Neurochemistry, Institute of Neurology, The National Hospital, Queen Square, London WC1N 3BG, England

RICHARD N. LOLLEY, Development Neurology Laboratory, Veterans Administration Hospital, Sepulveda, California 91343, U.S.A.

A. J. PATEL, MRC Developmental Neurobiology Unit, Medical Research Council Laboratories, Woodmansterne Road, Carshalton, Surrey SM5 4EF, England

STEVEN P. R. ROSE, Brain Research Group, Open University, Milton Keynes, Bucks. MK7 6AA, England.

B. K. SIESJÖ, Research Department 4, E-Blocket, University Hospital, S-221 85 Lund, Sweden

Tj. B. VAN WIMERSMA GREIDANUS, Rudolf Magnus Institute for Pharmacology, Medical Faculty, University of Utrecht, Vondellaan 6, Utrecht, The Netherlands

Preface

With the delineation of the broad principles of intermediary metabolism of the brain and the identification of specific brain constituents it has been possible to begin the important task of correlating structure and function of the nervous system with its biochemistry. Such studies as those of Oliver Lowry and his group in St. Louis on the biochemical basis of cellular architecture, the changes in macromolecular metabolism, associated with learning, or the attempts to isolate and study the properties of neurone and neuropil, have thrown light on both the utility and drawbacks of such research.

In this book we have reviewed some examples of contemporary work interrelating structure with function of the nervous system. The developing brain provides a novel system for this kind of study but, as is indicated in the first chapter, at least broad correlates can be drawn between changing biochemistry and increasing physiological activity. Unfortunately few indications of precise structural and biochemical parameters are available, and this is particularly true in relation to higher mental activity. There is welcome progress in our understanding of the underlying molecular basis of nerve differentiation and growth of the developing brain, which is dealt with by Lim, and the equally important concept of the cell cycle and its control is the subject of the contribution by Balázs, Patel and Lewis.

Perhaps the clearest biochemical and physiological correlations are those concerning sensory functions. For example, the finding by Margolis of a unique protein in the olfactory system and the concentration of the dipeptide carnosine in the olfactory epithelium raises new and stimulating possibilities of functional significance. Although the exact role of the pigments in photoreceptor excitation remains uncertain there is a relationship between the visual cycle and the electroretinogram β-wave. The properties of the developing retina and its functional biochemistry with specific reference to the cyclic nucleotides are discussed by Lolley and Farber in their chapter.

Considerable success has been achieved in the key problem of nervous transmission. The concepts of transmitter release, storage and re-uptake are well established. Individual transmitters have been ascribed to specific neurones and their tracts, using the methods of selective lesioning. This technique has been particularly useful in delineating GABA-ergic and cholinergic tracts and, as Crow shows in Chapter 5, the method is valuable also for the catecholamine pathways and hence potentially of special relevance to psychiatric and neurological problems. One of the most interesting developments of recent years has been the demonstration by Ingvar and his group of cerebral blood flow alteration in concert with mental activity. At the biochemical level the same principle is illustrated by Sokoloff's use of ^{14}C-deoxyglucose to map the regions in brain with altered glucose utilization in response to changes in local functional activity. Siesjö reviews the physiologically important factors regulating the supply of oxygen and glucose and the relation of metabolic rate to the metabolic state of the brain.

The final three chapters deal with varying aspects of behavioural neurochemistry. The remarkable activity of the pituitary hormone peptides is described by van Wimersma Greidanus and de Wied. This is followed by Rose and Haywood's critical account of the neurochemist's contribution to the problem of learning. The authors are cautious—"biochemistry can at best provide a description of learning in molecular terms not, it is emphasized, its prediction or control". The recent association of sleep with memory processes links the previous and the final chapter. Giuditta describes the extensive work reported on the biochemistry of sleep, including the extraordinary finding of the sleep-inducing peptides.

Despite the controversial nature of the subject, as shown even in the limited scope of this book, there is real progress to report and stimulating and meaningful new lines of enquiry need to be pursued.

November 1976   A. N. Davison

Contents

Chapter 3
Metabolic influences on cell proliferation in the brain

Chapter 4
Cyclic nucleotides and neuronal function: cyclic-GMP-dependent photoreceptor degeneration in inherited retinal diseases

Chapter 5
Neurotransmitter-related pathways: the structure and function of central monoamine neurones

Chapter 6
Physiological aspects of brain energy metabolism

Chapter 9

The biochemistry of sleep

Chapter 1

Biochemical, Morphological and Functional Changes in the Developing Brain

A. N. DAVISON

Miriam Marks Department of Neurochemistry, Institute of Neurology, The National Hospital, Queen Square, London, England

I. Introduction

Comparison of the biochemistry of the developing nervous system with its changing morphology and function offers one way of establishing possible general biological correlates. Relatively little information is available about the chemistry of events immediately following conception and embryological development of the neural crest. We shall, therefore, concentrate on the period following establishment of adult neuronal populations, when dendritic growth and increase in synaptic connectivity overlaps with development of glia and myelination. Study of this period of the brain "growth spurt" is particularly rewarding, since at this time functional change is accompanied by a transient period of most rapid growth of the brain. Besides being a unique period of critical physiological importance, it is also recognized as a *vulnerable* period in development. Minor restrictions in supply of substrate imbalance of hormones or nutritional intake may, at this time only, lead to permanent distortion of the normal developmental pattern (Dobbing, 1974). The experimental studies of Dobbing and Smart (1974) indicate that early nutritional deprivation may have a lasting effect on motor coordination and possibly behaviour. These animals appear to over-react to unpleasant situations or show heightened excitability even in relatively unstressful situations. The mature brain seems to be much less affected by such stress (e.g. hypothyroidism, p. 53).

A. *"The Growth Spurt"*

As judged by the rate of increase in brain wet weight, the sequence of developmental events appears to be common to all species, but the timing of the process varies. The human "growth spurt" is perinatal, beginning in mid-pregnancy and ending approximately two years after birth. When the acute period is over, there is small increase in overall weight with no significant change in the mature nervous system. Amongst the elderly there may even be a diminution in brain weight, probably associated with loss of nerve cells in those over sixty years of age. In contrast, the rat brain wet weight increases to a maximum rate at about ten days after birth; only slow increase in weight takes place after six months. The guinea-pig lies between these two species, since its brain develops mainly before birth.

These considerations are clearly of considerable importance when attempting to relate events in the developing nervous system of experimental animals with changes in man. For example, the newborn rat or rabbit may be regarded as equivalent in brain development terms to that of say an 18-week-old human foetus and a newborn guinea-pig to a 2–3-year-old human child. One has, therefore, to be careful in extrapolating between species, especially in relation to birth.

Besides timing, another and major complication is the changing morphology of the developing tissue. After early embryological development the central nervous system undergoes a series of interrelated and exceedingly complex morphological and biochemical changes. Multiplication of neuroblasts leads to an early achievement of adult cell numbers. This is overlapped and followed by multiplication of spongioblasts with resultant formation of glia. In the human brain it would seem that there is some temporal separation in the formation of neurones and glia. Thus, the rate of accumulation of DNA follows two maxima, one presumably due to neuroblast formation and the other to glia. During development cell migration occurs finally leading to the elaborate adult pattern of neurones and glial cells (Sidman and Rakic, 1974). The situation is further complicated for various parts of the nervous system undergo

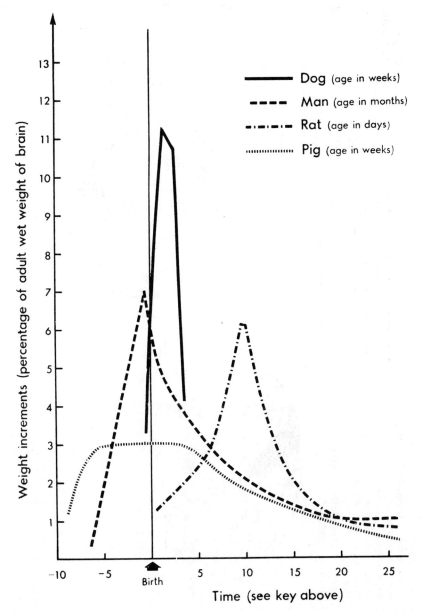

Fig. 1. The timing of brain growth in different species in relation to growth. Curves of the rate of brain growth in different species are expressed as weight increments (percentage of adult wet weight of brain) per unit period of time. (From Davison and Dobbing, 1965—with permission.)

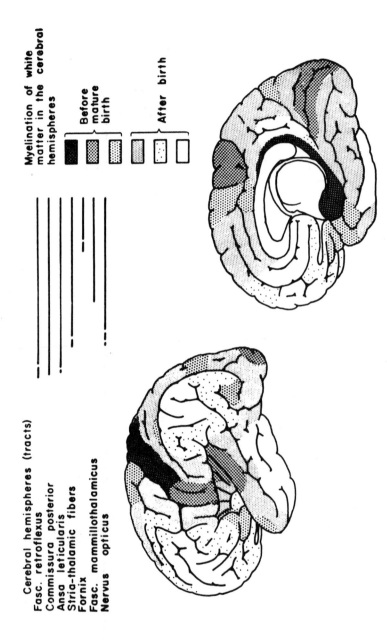

Fig. 2. Schedule of myelination in various fibre systems of human brain (Lucas *et al.* 1931; Flechsig, 1876). (After Friede, 1966—with permission.)

development at different times. This is clearly seen for myelination, which begins in the phylogenetically older regions of the brain (e.g. brain stem) with quite different times of onset and duration in each part. Certain processes, in specific areas may, therefore, appear to be differently susceptible at any one time to a retarding stress. Thus in the newborn cerebellum neuronal multiplication is more vulnerable than that of spinal-cord neurones.

Table 1

Biochemical correlates of brain structure

Subcellular component	Biochemical "marker"	Cellular component	Biochemical "marker"
Nucleus	DNA polymerase I	Myelin	Cerebrosides
Mitochondria:		Oligodendroglia	Carbonic anhydrase
Outer membrane	Monoamine oxidase		Pseudo cholinesterase
Inner membrane	Succinic dehydrogenase		S-100 protein
Presynaptic terminal	Glutamate decarboxylase	Astrocytes	β-glucuronidase Glial fibrillar protein
Postsynaptic region	Cholinergic receptor protein Adenyl cyclase Guanyl cyclase?	Neurones	Protein 14:3:2 β-galactosidase
External synaptic membranes	$\left\{\begin{array}{l}\text{Gangliosides}\\ \text{AChe}\end{array}\right.$	Axons	Tubulin
Microsomes	RNA Cytochrome NAD reductase	Macrophages	Cathepsin A
Plasma membrane	5′-nucleotidase	Capillaries	γ-Glutamyl transpeptidase
Lysosomes	Acid hydrolases		
Peroxisomes	Catalase D-Amino acid oxidase		

It is difficult to quantify these various processes by morphological techniques and neurochemists have sought, with some success, for biochemical correlates of these anatomical changes. Since myelin can be identified histologically, is easily isolatable and contains characteristic components (galactolipid, basic protein and cyclic nucleotide phosphohydrolase) analysis of this abundant membrane from adult nervous tissue is relatively easy. Determination of DNA has been used as an index of total cell numbers (Friede, 1966; Balázs,

1973). The analysis of DNA for this purpose depends on the constant amount of the nucleic acid in stable diploid nuclei, and in some respects this does not fully apply even to predominantly non-dividing nervous tissue (e.g. extranuclear DNA; see Davison and Dobbing, 1968). Other biochemical correlates are even less certain. The gangliosides for nerve endings, S-100 protein for glia etc. and changes in membrane or organelle composition may even occur during maturation. Thus although analysis of subcellular fractions has been of considerable value (Maccioni and Caputto, 1968) it should be noted that there is increasing evidence of synaptosomal preparations, separated by centrifugation, being contaminated by glial fragments (Henn *et al.*, 1976). Nevertheless, with these reservations, biochemical analysis permits a more quantitative assessment of structural change than was possible by histology. Consideration of changes in the whole rat brain serves as an illustration of these general principles.

B. *The Developing Rat Brain*

1. *Cellular changes*

The rate of change in DNA content of the rat brain suggests that cellular multiplication is maximal at about the tenth postnatal day. Most of the neurones are formed at birth in the forebrain but cell division is most active postnatally in the cerebellum, where 97% of the final number of cells is acquired during the first three weeks (Balázs and Richter, 1973). Brizzee and his colleagues (1964) showed that 145 000 nerve cells.mm^{-3} were present in the ten-day-old rat cerebral cortex (area 2) and this number of neurones decreased to 110 000 at 20 and 50 days with a slow decrease in density to 85–90 000 in the mature brain (100 days). Neuroglial packing density increased from 30 000 cells.mm^{-3} at ten days to 50 000 at 50–100 days, slowly increasing to 85 000 cells.mm^{-3} in two-year-old animals. Thus, the glial/neuronal index increases during the first two years of life from about 0·2 to 0·95. Clearly, the overall process is much more complex than this for the effects of cell migration, the loss of redundant cells, as well as the question of each cell type and its localization need to be considered.

2. *Subcellular changes*

Histological examination of various areas of the developing rat brain shows that the increase of dendrite aborization and formation of

Table 2

Changes in glycolipids, succinic dehydrogenase activity and brain organelles of rat cerebrum during development

	3–5 days	%	15 days	%	20 days	%	25 days	%	Adult
Mitochondria (mg/g wet wt)	7·2 ± 2·0	39	15·9 ± 6·9	85	17·7 ± 8·5	95	18·7 ± 2·4	100	18·7 ± 2·4
Synaptosomes (mg/g wet wt)	8·1 ± 2·1	46	15·1 ± 5·8	85	17·6 ± 7·4	100	20·4 ± 1·7	115	17·7 ± 2·0
Gangliosides (mg/NANA.g wet wt^{-1})	450 ± 30	33	1100 ± 200	80	—	—	1400 ± 260	106	1320 ± 250

Percentage changes are of normal adult values. (After Maccioni and Caputto, 1968.)

synaptic contacts occurs at about the same time as the onset but not the duration of myelination. These changes are reflected in age-related alterations in the yield of subcellular particles obtained by the differential and gradient density fractionation of brain homogenates.

3. Synaptosomes

The increased weight of synaptosomes obtained from 5 to 15 days after birth correlates with the observed increase in number of nerve terminals. For example, in the rat lateral geniculate nucleus synaptic density increases from the fifth postnatal day to the adult level at day 13 (Karlsson, 1967). In other areas of the central nervous system synaptogenesis extends much longer so that by the 20th postnatal day 80% of adult synapses are found in the striatum, 70% in the cerebellum but only about 40% in the hippocampus (Cragg, 1974). Some synapses form in the superior colliculus before opening of the eyes (two weeks after birth) but a later stage of synapse formation by collicular axons 25–40 days after birth is dependent on visual stimulation within a defined period (Lund and Lund, 1972). Cragg (1969) found that in the lateral geniculate nucleus synapses are formed in animals reared in the dark but, again, that the number increases after visual experience.

4. Mitochondria

In the rat, apparent increase in the number of cerebral mitochondria extends to about 25 days after birth (Table 2). Although mitochondria are present in the newborn rat brain there is the interesting possibility that they are biochemically immature (Gregson and Williams, 1969). Mourek et al. (1975) have found in the five-day-old rat that although the specific activity of rotenone-insensitive NADH cytochrome c-reductase in the outer membrane of the organelle is comparable to that of mature mitochondria, the succinate cytochrome c-reductase of the inner membrane of the immature is six times less active than in the adult. During development Barnard and Lindberg (1969) and Pigareva (1972) found denser mitochondrial cristae and, similarly Chepelinsky and Rodrigues de Lorez Arnaiz (1970) observed an increase in the content of cytochrome which may have resulted from a higher organization of the inner membrane. In the developing chick brain Barberis and Gayet (1973) have observed relative increase in specific activity of mitochondrial cytochrome oxidase (inner) and decrease in the monoamine oxidase (outer) membrane specific activity.

5. Myelination

The lipid composition of the foetal rat brain resembles that of other tissues, but just prior to the onset of myelination there is accumulation of lipid droplets around nerve axons and a dramatic change in composition follows as myelination begins. The process is heralded by the migration of interfascicular oligodendrocytes and the plasma membrane of the reactive glial cell encircles suitable-sized axons. At first the membrane appears to be loosely wound around the nerve fibre, but it soon becomes compact with apparently only traces of cytoplasm between the lamellae. A myelin-like fraction can be isolated by centrifugal procedures from the brain at an early stage of myelination (Davison, 1971). The composition of the fraction resembles that of a modified plasma membrane with a relative abundance of phospholipid and high molecular weight proteins, a small amount of the typical myelin basic protein is present. A similar purified membrane fraction (SN4—prepared by Waehneldt, 1975) contains more of the marker enzyme 2', 3'-cyclic nucleotide 3'-phosphohydrolase than the parent myelin.

6. Intermediary metabolism

During postnatal development of the rat brain there is a major shift from anaerobic glycolysis and activity of the pentose phosphate pathway to respiration. Thus the adult brain is dependent on oxygen and utilization substrate (primarily glucose) for energy metabolism, whereas the neonate rat is remarkably resistant to an anaerobic atmosphere (Himwich et al., 1942). The high activity of the glucose-6-phosphate shunt in the infant rat supplies ribose and deoxyribose for nucleotide synthesis in addition to NADPH for sterol and fatty acid biosynthesis. The latter requirement is also supplemented by NADPH from cytoplasmic isocitric acid dehydrogenase activity which is high at birth and falls during postnatal development. In contrast, respiratory enzyme activity and that of most transmitter synthesizing enzymes does not start to increase until approximately five days after birth in the rat when there is a steady increase up to 20 days. At the same time, glucose derivatives are increasingly metabolized via the GABA-shunt (γ-aminobutyric acid-shunt) and dicarboxylic acids formed by transamination. These biochemical changes in energy metabolism and transmitter synthesis coincide with the onset of electrical activity and physiological maturation so that this time was designated the "Critical Period" by Flexner (1955). Enna *et al.* (1976) using a specific probe for muscarinic cholinergic receptor protein, measured increase of this protein in developing chicken brain. Comparison was made with changes in acetylcholinesterase and choline acetyltransferase activities, binding of GABA and glutamate decarboxylase activity. The greatest increase in enzyme activity and receptor binding takes place between the 14th and the 18th day of development. It is at this time in the chick that morphologically distinct synapses appear in largest numbers, together with mature electrical activity and motor coordination. Due to the complexities of the system and the gross level of analysis Enna *et al.* (1976) were unable to correlate physiological events with any specific neurochemical development. Early work had suggested that development of postsynaptic glycine-receptor binding in chick embryo spinal cord was preceded by presynaptic nerve terminal glycine marker activity, suggesting that they could induce development of the postsynaptic receptor.

Brain stem choline acetyltransferase activity is reduced in the undernourished postnatal rat (Eckhert *et al.*, 1976) indicating that the development of cholinergic nerve terminals may be affected. Neonatal hypothyroid rats have decreased activities of both choline acetyltransferase and acetylcholinesterase. These findings are of special interest in view of the proposal that cholinergic neurones are involved in higher mental activity (Drachman and Leavitt, 1974).

7. *Electrical activity*

Onset of clear electrocortical activity in the rat occurs from 5 to 6 days postpartum, although weak activity may be present earlier (Ellington and Rose, 1970). Adult EEG (electroencephalograph) patterns are attained during the third postpartum week. Cerebral electrical responses to stimuli begins from the onset of electrical activity but not consistently until the end of the second week. Deza and Eidelberg (1967) found first cortical action-potentials on day four, preceded by rhythmic membrane oscillations resembling postsynaptic potentials (see Fig. 3). In the visual cortex evoked potentials can be elicited in 12-day-old rats (Mourek *et al.*, 1967) and the adult picture is reached by about 20 days after birth. No action potentials were detected by Deza and Eidelberg (1967) in the cortex before the fourth postnatal day, although they were readily obtainable in the diencephala from

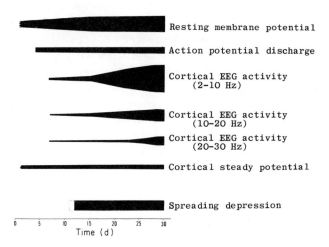

Fig. 3. Development of cortical electrical activity in the rat. Data indicating progressive changes in electrical activity as a function of age are shown. (After Deza and Eidelberg, 1967—with permission.)

Table 3

Chronological age at which mean score on behavioural test is attained

Behavioural test	Size of litters		
	Small	Intermediate	Large
Rooting	1·0 ± 0	1·0 ± 0	1·0 ± 0
Cliff aversion	2·5 ± 0·5	3·0 ± 0·5	3·0 ± 0·5
Hair growth	8·5 ± 1·0	9·0 ± 2·0	9·0 ± 0·5
Ears open	13·0 ± 1·0	15·0 ± 2·5	15·0 ± 3·0
Righting	3·0 ± 1·0	3·0 ± 0·5	6·5 ± 1·5
Forelimb placing	4·0 ± 0·5	5·0 ± 1·5	8·5 ± 2·0
Forelimb grasping	3·0 ± 0·5	11·0 ± 1·5	12·0 ± 3·5
Bar holding	10·0 ± 1·0	13·5 ± 1·5	14·5 ± 2·0
Vibrissae placing	3·0 ± 0·5	7·0 ± 0·5	14·0 ± 4·0
Eyes open	13·0 ± 0·5	15·5 ± 3·0	16·5 ± 4·0
Startle	15·0 ± 1·5	16·5 ± 3·0	17·0 ± 2·5

Ten mice from each litter size were tested. Some measures are grouped into a composite motor and others a sensory capacity score. Small litters consisted of 4, intermediate 8 and large groups 16 per mother from within 8h of birth. Mice were weaned at 20d on unlimited food. Deficits in body and brain weights were not restored on rehabilitation by 60d (i.e. mean brain weights 0·60 ± 0·08 small litters, 0·51 ± 0·05 and 0·41 ± 0·01 for intermediate and large litters at 60d). (After Castillano and Oliverio, 1976.)

birth (related to earlier morphological development). A resting steady potential could be detected between the cortical surface and a reference lead from the first postnatal data with little change with increasing age (for reviews see: Ellington and Rose, 1970; Myslivicek, 1970).

It is possible to demonstrate retardation in the maturation of reflex and electrical activity in mice subjected to malnutrition 12 hours to 17 days after birth (Castillano and Oliverio, 1976). Experimental findings of this type may eventually link up with observations on mentally retarded children. Such diverse conditions as perinatal galactosaemia, hormonal insufficiency, virus and bacterial infection as well as malnutrition (Hertzig et al., 1972) may permanently interfere with brain development (Davison, 1974; Dobbing, 1974). In order to understand the scientific basis of such retardation we must probe more closely into the molecular mechanisms controlling brain growth and differentiation.

References

Balázs, R. (1973). Biochem. Soc. Spec. Publ. 1, 39–57.
Balázs, R. and Richter, D. (1973). In "Biochemistry of the Developing Brain" (W. Himwich, ed.), Vol 1. Dekker, New York, pp. 253–286.
Barberis, C. and Gayet, J. (1973). J. Neurochem. 20, 1765–1769.
Barnard, T. and Lindberg, O. (1969). J. Ultrastruct. Res. 29, 239–310.
Brizzee, K. R., Vogt, J. and Kharetchko, X. (1974). Progr. Brain Res. 4, 136–146.
Castillano, C. and Oliverio, A. (1976). Brain Res. 101, 317–325.
Chepelinsky, A. B. and Rodriguez de Lorez Arnaiz, G. (1970). Biochim. Biophys. Acta 197, 321–323.
Cragg, B. G. (1969). Brain Res. 13, 53–67.
Cragg, B. G. (1974). Brit. Med. Bull. 30, 141–145.
Davison, A. N. (1971). In "Myelin" Neurosci. Res. Progr. Bull. 9, Part 4, 465–470.
Davison, A. N. (1974). In "Biochemistry of Mental Illness" (L. L. Iversen and S. P. R. Rose, eds) Proc. Conf. Mental Illness, Open University, Dec. 1972, Biochem. Soc. Spec. Publ.1, pp. 27–37.
Davison, A. N. and Dobbing, J. (1966). Brit. Med. Bull. 22, 40–44.
Davison, A. N. and Dobbing, J. (1968). In "Applied Neurochemistry" (A. N. Davison and J. Dobbing, eds). Blackwell Scientific Publications Ltd., Oxford, pp. 253–286.
Deza, L. and Eidelberg, E. (1967). Exper. Neurol. 17, 425–438.
Dobbing, J. (1974). In "Scientific Foundations of Paediatrics" (J. A. Davis and J. Dobbing, eds). Heinemann, London, pp. 565–577.
Dobbing, J. and Smart, J. L. (1974). Brit. Med. Bull. 30, 164–168.
Drachman, D. A. and Leavitt, J. (1974). Arch. Neurol. 30, 113–121.
Eckhert, C., Barnes, R. H. and Levitsky, D. A. (1976). Brain Res. 101, 372–377.

Ellington, R. J. and Rose, G. H. (1970). *In* "Developmental Neurobiology" (W. A. Himwich, ed.). C. C. Thomas, Springfield, Illinois, pp. 441–474.

Enna, S. J., Yamamura, H. I. and Snyder, S. H. (1976). *Brain Res.* **101**, 177–183.

Flexner, L. B. (1955). *In* "Biochemistry of the Developing Nervous System" Proc. 1st Int. Neurochem. Symp. Oxford 1954. Academic Press, New York and London, pp. 281–295.

Friede, R. L. (1966). "Topographical Brain Chemistry". Academic Press, New York and London, p. 418.

Gregson, N. A. and Williams, P. L. (1969). *J. Neurochem.* **16**, 617–626.

Henn, F. A., Anderson, D. J. and Rustad, D. G. (1976). *Brain Res.* **101**, 341–344.

Hertzig, M. E., Birch, H. G., Richardson, S. A. and Tizard, J. (1972). *Pediatrics*, **49**, 814–824.

Himwich, H. E., Bernstein, A. O., Herrligh, H., Chester, A. and Fazekas, J. F. (1942). *Amer. J. Physiol.* **135**, 387–391.

Karlsson, U. (1967). *J. Ultrastruct. Res.* **17**, 158–175.

Lund, J. S. and Lund, R. D. (1972). *Brain Res.* **42**, 21–32.

Maccioni, H. F. and Caputto, R. (1968). *J. Neurochem.* **15**, 1257–1264.

Mourek, J., Himwich, W. A., Mysliviček, J. and Callison, D. (1967). *Brain Res.* **6**, 241–251.

Mourek, J., Proukova, V., Svobodova, Z. and Kraml, J. (1975). *Develop. Psychobiol.* **8(5)**, 447–452.

Mysliviček, J. (1970). *In* "Developmental Neurobiology" (W. A. Himwich, ed.). C. C. Thomas, Springfield, Illinois, pp. 475–527.

Pigareva, Z. D. (1972). Moscow: Akademiia Med. Nauk. SSSR.

Sidman, R. L. and Rakic, P. (1974). *In* "Pre- and Postnatal Development of the Human Brain", (S. R. Berenberg, M. Caniaris and N. P. Masse, eds). Mod. Probl. Paediat. Vol. 13. Karger, Basel, pp. 13–43.

Waehneldt, T. V. (1975). *Biochem. J.* **151**, 435–437.

Chapter 2

Regulation of RNA Metabolism in the Developing Brain

L. LIM

Miriam Marks, Department of Neurochemistry, Institute of Neurology, Queen Square, London, England

I. Introduction

In the development and differentiation of the brain, as in other organs, regulated genetic expression results in the ordered appearance of protein macromolecules. Some of these proteins (e.g. receptors) specifically determine the functional characteristics of neural tissue, while others are found universally as, for example, enzymes or structural components like tubulin. It is obviously extremely difficult to analyse the regulated synthesis of each of these different proteins, since the developing brain contains changing populations of various cell types, each with its own particular protein composition. One approach has been to study synthesis of a characteristic cellular protein—such as the glial S-100 protein. Alternatively, the examination of gross changes in the metabolism of different nucleic acid components involved in protein synthesis provides invaluable information on the gross control of brain development. Consider the sequence of changes in the metabolism of ribosomal RNA (rRNA) observed during the "critical period". In the case of the developing rat brain the adult complement of rRNA is acquired by the second week after birth. This accumulation of rRNA ceases abruptly at the end of cellular division (Adams, 1966; Balázs *et al.*, 1968). The relationship of these changes in ribosomal RNA with that of messenger RNA (mRNA) which directs the activity of the polysomes or organized ribosomes on which proteins are synthesized may now be stated.

II. General Scheme of the Synthesis of Messenger RNA and Ribosomal RNA in Animals

RNA has been shown to be synthesized in separate compartments in the nucleus: rRNA in the nucleolus and mRNA in the nucleoplasm or non-particulate part of the nucleus. Two different polymerases, detected in most tissues examined including brain, are involved. They can be distinguished on the basis of their sensitivity towards α-amantine which inhibits the polymerase responsible for mRNA synthesis at concentrations not affecting rRNA synthesis. These DNA-dependent RNA polymerases are complex enzymes consisting of multiple and different subunits. Changes in RNA synthesis observed during growth and differentiation of mammalian cells may, it appears, be regulated either at the level of the interaction of these enzymes with chromatin (nuclear protein containing the DNA templates for the various proteins) or less likely by changes in the properties of the RNA polymerases themselves (Biswas *et al.*, 1975; Jacob, 1973). Changes in the activity of the polymerases in brain nuclei have been reported to occur during development (see Giuffrida *et al.*, 1975).

The mRNA and rRNAs are synthesized as large precursors and undergo certain modifications before they are transported into the cytoplasm (Fig. 1). The ribosomal RNA is transcribed as a 45S

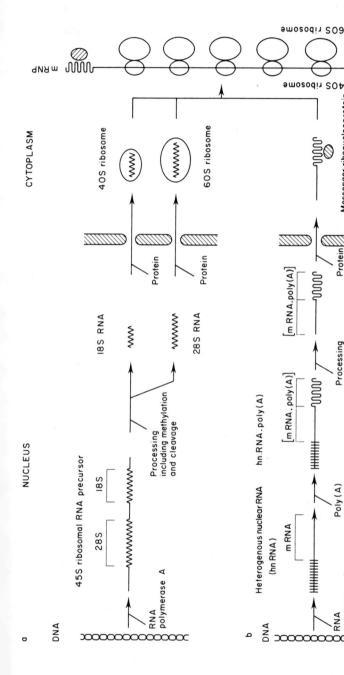

Fig. 1. General scheme of the synthesis of messenger and ribosomal RNA in animal cells. Ribosomal RNA and messenger RNA are synthesized from different sequences of DNA by RNA polymerase A and B respectively. The ribosomal RNA precursor (45S RNA) is processed to yield 28S and 18S rRNA. The RNA then complexes with protein to form the 60S and 40S ribosomal subunits. The messenger RNA is synthesized as a large precursor called heterogenous nuclear RNA (hnRNA). Poly(A) is added (usually 100–200 nucleotide residues) to the hnRNA by poly(A) polymerase. The RNA is cleaved to yield polyadenylated mRNA (poly(A)-RNA) which complexes with protein to form a messenger ribonucleoprotein (mRNP). Although in this scheme the mRNA is shown to be polyadenylated, mRNA can also be found without poly(A) segments. The ribosomal subunits and the mRNP are found associated in the cytoplasm as aggregates—the polysomes.

preribosomal RNA, which is approximately twice the molecular weight of the combined 28S and 18S RNA, both of which are present in the initial transcript (Darnell, 1968; Maden, 1971). Large RNA, after methylation of the rRNA components, is cleaved to yield the different precursors for both types of rRNA. The processing of 18S RNA occurs first and this RNA combined with protein is then transported into the cytoplasm as part of a 40S ribosomal subunit. The precursor of the larger rRNA is subsequently cleaved from the remaining RNA, undergoing successive reductions in size from 41S to 32S to 28S and this is then transported out, again complexed with protein, as a 60S ribosomal subunit.

Some aspects of mRNA synthesis have been clarified recently (Darnell *et al.*, 1973; Brawerman, 1974) following the original observation that reticulocyte haemoglobin mRNA contain a segment of poly(A) (Lim and Canellakis, 1970). With the notable exception of histone mRNA, most mammalian mRNAs contain poly(A) at the 3′–OH terminus. The presence of this homopolymer is a convenient tag and makes it possible to follow the synthesis of most mRNAs. As a result it is considered probable that mRNA is made as a rather large transcript (about $5-50 \times 10^3$ nucleotides) synthesized mostly from unique DNA sequences. Some of this heterogeneous nuclear RNA (hnRNA) is then polyadenylated at the 3′–OH terminus. Cleavage of polyadenylated RNA—poly(A)-RNA—occurs within the nucleus to give mRNA. The polyadenylated mRNA complexed with protein finally appears in the cytoplasm as messenger ribonucleoprotein (mRNP) normally associated with polyribosomes. It should be noted that the protein composition of the nuclear and cytoplasmic mRNP particles may be different.

III. Developmental Changes in the Metabolism of High Molecular Weight RNA in Rat Forebrain

A. *Nucleocytoplasmic Relationships: Synthesis and Transport of RNA*

Berthold and Lim (1976a, b) followed the metabolism of both mRNA and rRNA by measuring incorporation of $[^{32}P]$ Pi into high molecular weight RNA (HMW RNA) purified from other nucleic acids by precipitation with LiCl. The labelling pattern of the RNA was examined both in the nucleus, where it is made, and in the cytoplasm, where it functions. A complicating factor is the changing composition of the rat brain during development, especially with regard to membrane-containing elements, e.g. myelin, which accumulate from the second week of birth. The different degrees of cytoplasmic contamination of nuclear fractions separated by centrifugation interferes with accurate assessment of changes in the nucleocytoplasmic relationship of HMW RNA during development. This problem was overcome by using the method of Georgiev (1967) involving a mild phenol treatment of crude nuclear fractions to release all cytoplasmic contaminants, and to prepare purified nuclear fractions. Analysis of the specific radioactivity of the synthesized HMW RNA in both cellular compartments makes it clear that the accumulation of rRNA in the forebrains of neonatal rats is due to a free flow of newly-synthesized RNA from the nucleus to the cytoplasm. In contrast, in the adult forebrain there is restricted movement of RNA from nucleus to cytoplasm (Fig. 2). This is seen in the young rat brain as a continuous relatively rapid increase in the ratio of the specific radioactivity of RNA in the cytoplasm to that in the nucleus (the ratio C/N being a measure of the transfer of RNA) over the 48 h period of labelling. The final high value at the 48 h

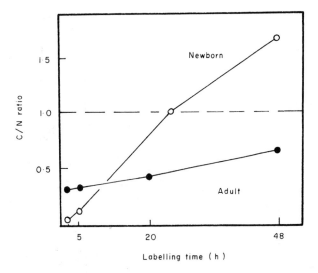

Fig. 2. Nucleocytoplasmic relationships of HMW RNA in adult- and newborn-rat forebrain. Adult rats (150 days old) and 3-day-old rats were each injected intracranially with 1 mCi of [^{32}P] Pi/g of brain. HMW RNA was isolated by phenol extraction and precipitation with 2·0 MLiCl from cytoplasmic and purified nuclear fractions of forebrains of rats killed at various times after the injection. Data are plotted as a ratio of the specific radioactivity of the ^{32}P-labelled RNA in the cytoplasm (C) to that in the nucleus (N) at the various times indicated. (From Berthold and Lim, 1976b.)

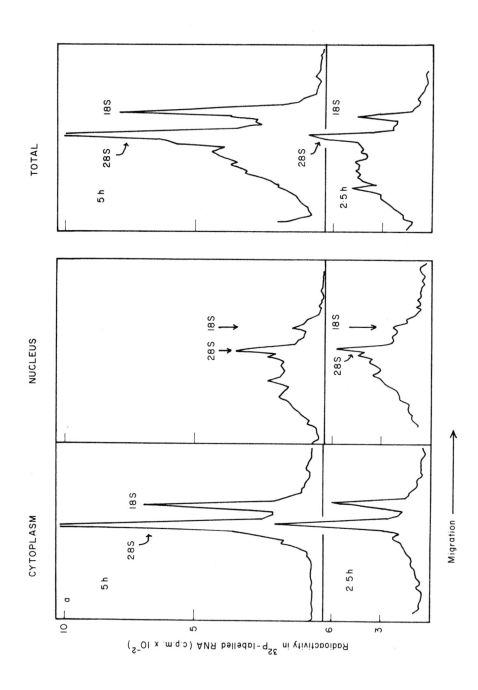

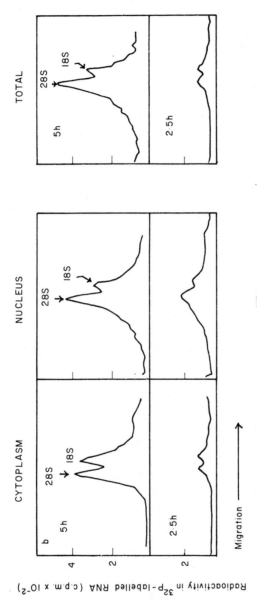

Fig. 3. a. *above* and b. *below*. Processing of ribosomal RNA. ^{32}P-labelled HMW RNA was isolated from the nuclear and cytoplasmic fractions of a. newborn- and b. adult-rat brains 2·5 h and 5 h after the injection of [^{32}P]Pi. Electrophoresis was performed on 2% polyacrylamide gels at 5 mA for 1·5 h. (From Berthold and Lim, 1976b.)

period indicated that continuous transfer of RNA to the cytoplasm has depleted the nucleus of much of its content of radioactive RNA. In contrast, in the adult forebrain, the C/N ratio is not substantially increased over a 48 h period. The correspondingly low C/N ratio at 48 h shows that only a fraction of the RNA is transferred into the cytoplasm and that most of the HMW RNA remains within the nucleus. These results are in keeping with the current view that much of the RNA in the nucleus of differentiated or adult tissues undergoes intranuclear turnover (Harris, 1974).

B. *Processing of Ribosomal RNA*

Other changes in the metabolism of the RNA during development can be detected by electrophoretic characterization. At early periods of labelling, 28S and 18S RNA represent a smaller proportion of the radioactive HMW RNA in the immature brain nuclei than in adult brain nuclei. At both ages the 28S and 18S rRNA are major components of the radioactive HMW RNA in the cytoplasm (Fig. 3). It appears that in the young brain, transfer of rRNA into the cytoplasm is coupled to the processing of the rRNA precursor, so that processed 28S and 18S rRNA accumulates not within the nucleus but in the cytoplasm. In contrast, in the adult continued processing of rRNA precursor without a high level of transport of rRNA into the cytoplasm leads to accumulation of the 28S and 18S RNA within the nucleus. This RNA is then subjected to further "processing", i.e. degradation, as part of the general pattern of RNA turnover within the nucleus. This turnover of RNA in crude nuclear preparations of adult rat brain has previously been reported (Adams, 1966). In proliferating cells it has been demonstrated that cytoplasmic rRNA is stable, while in differentiated cells cytoplasmic rRNA turns over with a half-life of several hours (Green, 1974). Thus in the older rat brain, the small proportion of rRNA transported out is necessary for replacement of that which undergoes cytoplasmic turnover.

C. *Characterization of Brain Polyadenylated RNA*

In the brain polyadenylated RNA can be found within the nucleus and cytoplasm (Lim *et al.*, 1974; DeLarco *et al.*, 1975). Microsomal poly(A)-RNA has the informational properties of mRNA since it can direct the synthesis of the brain specific myelin encephalitogenic protein when injected into *Xenopus* oocytes (Fig. 4). Brain microsomal poly(A)-RNA is also active in directing the synthesis of tubulin and actin in the wheat germ *in vitro* system (Gozes *et al.*, 1975). Thus in brain, as in other tissues, polyadenylated RNA corresponds to mRNA. Brain mRNA appears to have some form of secondary structure to which the poly(A) in the mRNA contributes (White *et al.*, 1975). This involvement of poly(A) in the secondary structure has also recently been observed in other mammilian mRNAs (Jeffrey and Brawerman, 1975).

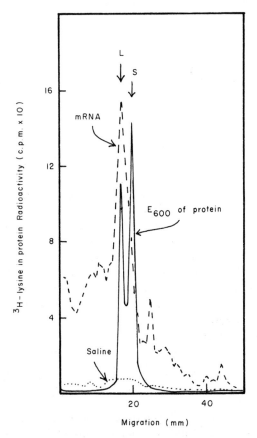

Fig. 4. Synthesis of the myelin encephalitogenic protein directed by brain poly(A)-RNA. Rat brain microsomal poly(A) was injected into *Xenopus* oocytes which were incubated in medium containing ³H-lysine for 18 h. Basic proteins were extracted and the ³H-labelled encephalitogenic protein was selectively immunoprecipitated with specific antiserum to myelin basic proteins. The radioactivity of immunoprecipitates from RNA-injected, as well as buffer-injected control, oocytes are superimposed on the pattern of rat myelin basic proteins electrophoresed concurrently on a different gel. L: large myelin basic protein (only this was immunoprecipitated). S: small myelin basic protein. (From Lim *et al.*, 1974.)

Early work based on hybridizing excess RNA to radioactive unique DNA sequences (the presumptive template for mRNAs) indicated that a greater variety of presumptive mRNAs was made in adult mouse brain than in other tissues (Hahn and Laird, 1971). The complexity of this brain mRNA was found to increase with age, i.e. more kinds of mRNAs were made in adult brain than in the juvenile or embryonic brain (Grouse et al., 1972). More recently, newer techniques involving hybridization of poly (A)-RNA to radioactive complementary DNA were used to confirm that more varieties of mRNA are made in the mouse brain than in non-neural tissue (Ryffel and McCarthy, 1975). The radioactive specific complementary DNA sequences were synthesized by reverse transcriptase from templates of poly(A)-RNA isolated either from mouse brain, liver or L-cells. It was demonstrated that there are at least 11 000 extra messenger RNA sequences specific for the brain.

D. Progressive Decrease in the Synthesis of Polyadenylated RNA

Although there may be more varieties of poly(A)-RNA in the adult brain, a greater amount is synthesized in the immature brain than in the adult. The progressive decrease in animals of different ages in synthesis of poly(A)-RNA during development was demonstrated by measuring the contribution of poly(A)-RNA to HMW RNA synthesized over an appropriate 5 h labelling period (Berthold and Lim, 1976a). The proportion of cortical poly(A)-RNA synthesized falls from a value of 35% in the three-day-old rat to 22–23% in the 40-day-old or 150-day-old adults. The corresponding values for the brain stem RNA remained at 27–30% from the sixth day after birth (Table 1). These results also depicted in Fig. 5 are in accord with the observation that the vertebrate brain develops in a caudal–rostral direction and that the brain stem is in a much more developed state than the cortex in the period immediately following birth (Schade and Ford, 1973).

In the forebrain of the young animal, poly(A)-RNA is transported into the cytoplasm equally as efficiently as rRNA, whose synthesis and export occur in a coordinated fashion. In the adult the restricted flow of macromolecular information results in high intranuclear turnover of not only rRNA but also poly(A)-RNA (Berthold and Lim, 1976b). Intranuclear turnover of poly(A) has previously been shown in liver (Lim et al., 1969; 1970) and recently kinetic studies on L-cells have clearly demonstrated that not all poly(A) leaves the

Table 1

Developmental changes in synthesis of polyadenylated RNA in cortex and brain stem

Age (d)	Brain region		Radioactivity in polyadenylated RNA	Relative difference $[(A - B)/B \times 100]$
3	Cortex	(A)	34·5	+29·7
	Brain stem	(B)	26·7	
5	Cortex	(A)	34·3	+16·7
	Brain stem	(B)	29·4	
8	Cortex	(A)	31·9	+ 7·8
	Brain stem	(B)	29·4	
40	Cortex	(A)	22·2	− 22·2
	Brain stem	(B)	28·6	
150	Cortex	(A)	23·5	− 22·9
	Brain stem	(B)	30·6	

Rats of different ages were killed 5 h after the intracranial administration of [^{32}P] Pi. HMW RNA was isolated from the cerebral cortex and brain stem and the polyadenylated RNA fractionated by affinity chromatography on oligo (dT) cellulose (from Berthold and Lim, 1976a).

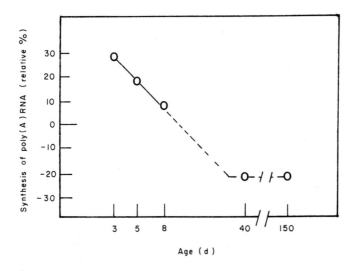

Fig. 5. Developmental changes in the synthesis of polyadenylated RNA in cerebral cortex (A) and brain stem (B). Data from Table 1 (last column) are plotted as the relative percentage $[(A - B)/B \times 100]$ versus age of the animals. (From Berthold and Lim, 1976a.)

nucleus (Perry *et al.*, 1974). These studies on liver and mouse L-cells can be taken to show that in other tissues, as in adult brain, not all the poly(A)-RNA leaves the nucleus. In the brain at all ages there is turnover of cytoplasmic poly(A)-RNA (Berthold and Lim, 1976b). Because of the difficulties in interpreting kinetic experiments when knowledge of the nucleotide precursor pools is limited, it is not at present possible to give values for the half-life of the brain mRNA.

E. *Molecular Weight Distribution of Polyadenylated RNA*

The mean size distribution of poly(A)-RNA species in the nucleus and cytoplasm of the forebrain of young rats (Fig. 6) is larger than

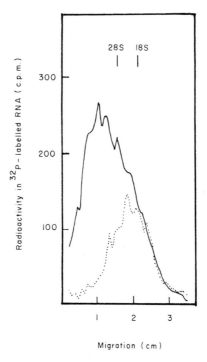

Fig. 6. Molecular weight distribution of ^{32}P-labelled polyadenylated RNA isolated from newborn-rat forebrain. Polyadenylated RNA was isolated from 3-day-old rat forebrains at 2·5 h after the intracranial administration of [^{32}P] Pi. Electrophoresis was performed on 2% polyacrylamide gels at 5 mA for 1·5 h. The positions of marker 28S and 18S RNA are shown. The mean molecular weight of the nuclear RNA was estimated to be 2·5 × 10^6 while that of the cytoplasmic RNA was 0·8 × 10^6. Cytoplasm ....; nucleus ———. (From Berthold and Lim, 1976b.)

corresponding adult values (Fig. 7). There are additional indications that in development different populations of mRNA are made. Within each age group the poly(A)-RNA has a higher mean molecular weight in the nucleus than in the cytoplasm. This is explainable on the basis of a precursor–product relationship between the two. A decrease in the size of the adult brain mRNA (i.e. cytoplasmic poly(A)-RNA) which occurs over the 3–48 h period may well be the result of a decrease in the size of the poly(A) segments, indicating further processing (Lim and Cancellakis, 1970). The changes in size of the mRNA, as detected by polyacrylamide gel

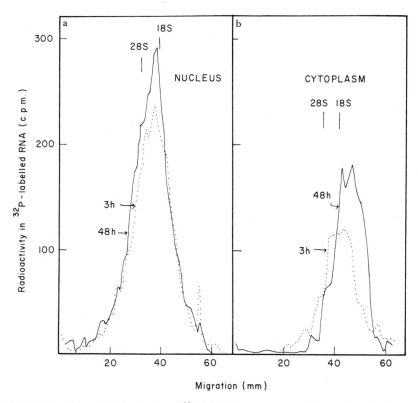

Fig. 7. Molecular weight distribution of ^{32}P-labelled polyadenylated RNA isolated from adult rat forebrain. Polyadenylated RNA was isolated from a. nuclear and b. cytoplasmic fractions of the brains of 150-day-old rats. The rats had previously been injected with [^{32}P] Pi either 3 h or 48 h before killing. Conditions for electrophoresis are as in Fig. 6. The mean molecular weight of the nuclear RNA was estimated to be 1·3 × 10^6 at both times of labelling. The mean molecular weight of the cytoplasmic polyadenylated RNA was 0·6 × 10^6 after 3 h and 0·5 × 10^6 after 48 h of labelling. 3 h labelling ....; 48 h labelling ———. (From Berthold and Lim, 1976b.)

electrophoresis, may appear too large to be explained by changes in the length of poly(A) segments (which consist of 100–200 adenine residues). These apparently large changes can occur as a result of anomalous migration of poly(A) containing RNA species (Pinder *et al.*, 1974). The original observation on the progressive shortening of the poly(A) segments of haemoglobin mRNA led to the suggestion that poly(A) was involved in the regulation of translation. It was proposed that the length of the poly(A) in the mRNA decreased as a result of successive rounds of translation and that it determined the stability of the mRNA. More recent evidence on a stabilizing role of the poly(A) segment has come from studies using haemoglobin mRNA from which the poly(A) segment has been enzymically excised. This mRNA is functionally less stable than intact mRNA when assayed either in *Xenopus laevis* oocytes or in the ascites cell free system (Huez *et al.*, 1974).

F. *Content of Poly(A)*

Throughout development of the rat forebrain, the poly(A) content of the cellular and of the cytoplasmic HMW RNA remains constant (Table 2). The cytoplasmic fraction accounts for 75–80% of the HMW RNA. Since the unchanging poly(A) content presumably relates to a constant mRNA content, these studies reveal a finely regulated relationship between the cellular concentration of mRNA and rRNA throughout development. Thus, although mRNA represents a greater proportion of the high molecular weight RNA synthesized in the young than in adult brain, the young brain does

Table 2

Poly(A) content of HMW RNA during postnatal development of rat forebrain

Age	(ng poly(A)/µg HMW RNA)	
(d)	Total cellular	Cytoplasm
4	1·31	1·37
14	1·44	1·35
30	1·36	1·30

HMW RNA was purified from total homogenates and cytoplasmic fractions of forebrains of rats of different ages. The poly(A) content was estimated by an assay method involving hybridization to ^{3}H-poly(U) (from Berthold, 1975).

not acquire a higher mRNA concentration. This maintenance of a constant mRNA content, despite differences in the proportion of mRNA synthesized, can be explained by developmental changes in the metabolic properties of the rRNA which forms the bulk of HMW RNA. The rRNA is stable in the young, but not in the adult brain. In both young and adult brains mRNA is being degraded constantly. In the adult, newly synthesized rRNA and mRNA are exported to the cytoplasm to replace both forms which have undergone turnover. While rRNA tends to be stable and to accumulate in the young brain, mRNA is degraded and proportionately more mRNA synthesis is required. This is to provide mRNA for ribosomes which are constantly being exported from the nucleus, and to provide mRNA for existing ribosomes present in the cytoplasm whose mRNA complement has been degraded.

G. Interactions of Ribosomal Subunits and of mRNA on Polyribosomes

In the brain, as in other mammalian tissues, mRNA-protein complexes interact with ribosomal subunits to form polyribosomes on which protein synthesis is carried out. Each polyribosome is an aggregate of 80S ribosomes, consisting of 40S and 60S subunits attached to a single mRNA molecule. During the course of protein synthesis each 80S ribosome traverses the length of the mRNA and at the end of each round of translation (i.e. upon completed synthesis of the polypeptide chain) the 80S ribosome dissociates into the constituent subunits. These subunits then bind sequentially to the mRNAs to begin another round of translation. The 40S binds first in a step requiring the participation of initiation factors. There are different numbers of ribosomes per mRNA molecule depending on the nature of the mRNA (e.g. in reticulocytes the average is five ribosomes per haemoglobin mRNA whereas in muscle tissue there may be up to five dozen ribosomes attached to myosin mRNA). In the brain, the population of polyribosomes present at different stages of development will contain different populations of mRNA. The changes in the metabolic properties of mRNA during brain development discussed previously, are also accompanied by changes in the properties of cerebral polyribosomes.

Polyribosomes can be partially dissociated *in vitro* into 60S and 40S subunits by treatment with 0·5 M KCl. This salt treatment reduces interactions between the two subunits of each ribosome. There is a proportion of 80S monoribosomes which remain undissociated by

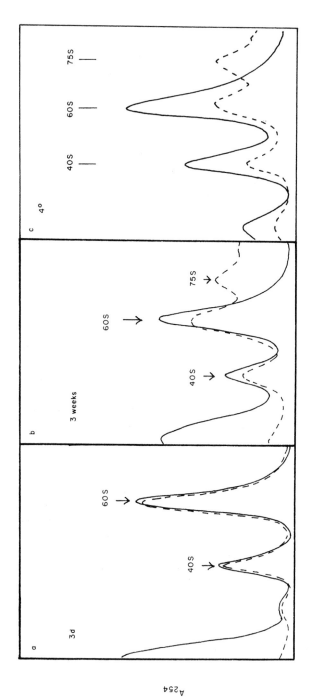

Direction of sedimentation ⟶

Fig. 8. Differences in the dissociability of cerebral polyribosomes from neonatal and older rats. Cerebral polyribosomes from a. 3-day-old and b. 3-week-old rats were resuspended in dissociation medium (0·5 M KCl, 5 mM MgCl₂, 50 mM Tris-HCl pH 7·6). These polysomes were incubated, with or without 1 mM puromycin in the medium at 4° for 15 min and then at 37° for 10 min. Dissociated polysomes were analysed at 25° on 5–20% sucrose density gradients containing the medium. Direction of sedimentation is from left to right. a. Dissociated polysomes from 3-day-old brains, b. dissociated polysomes from 3-week-old brain. With puromycin ———, without puromycin – – – –, c. the polysomes were resuspended in medium without puromycin and incubated and analysed on sucrose density gradients at 4°. 3-day-old brains ———, 3-week-old brains – – – –. (From Lim and White, 1974.)

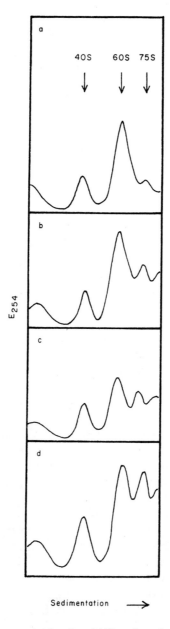

Fig. 9. Developmental changes in the dissociability of cerebral polysomes. Free cerebral polysomes isolated from the brains of rats of a. 6 days, b. 9 days, c. 12 days, d. 18 days were subjected to dissociation conditions without puromycin at 4° and then analysed on sucrose density gradients. (From Lim and White, 1974.)

this treatment because of the presence of newly-synthesized peptides and, or mRNA-proteins. This population of 80S ribosomes is presumably at the beginning of each mRNA since only short segments of nascent peptides are effective in conferring stability towards 0·5 M KCl treatment. These ribosomes can be dissociated by incubating at 37° with puromycin, which discharges the stabilizing nascent peptide from the mRNA-protein ribosome complex (Blobel, 1971; Martin *et al.*, 1971). Alternatively, complete dissociation can be accomplished by using 0·5 M KCl at pH 9·0. This latter treatment will reduce interactions between mRNA-proteins and ribosomes (Lim and White, 1974).

The cerebral polyribosomes of newborn rats are completely dissociated into 60S and 40S subunits by treatment with 0·5 M KCl, without using puromycin, either at 37° or at 4°. This behaviour is in sharp contrast to that of cerebral polyribosomes of much older rats (Fig. 8). Complete dissociation of the latter requires incubation with puromycin. The ease of dissociability is unique to neonatal cerebral polyribosomes. Polyribosomes from neonatal liver have similar properties to either those from liver or cerebrum of the adult rat. There is always a proportion of 80S ribosomes resistant to the action of 0·5 M KCl. The unique dissociability of cerebral polyribosomes, exhibited in very young rats, gradually decreased with age. By the 18th day after birth, cerebral polyribosomes are dissociated by 0·5 M KCl to the same extent as those of the adult (Fig. 9). These results suggest that there are changes in the composition of cerebral polyribosomes with age, possibly accounting for the difference in stability of cerebral polyribosomes of neonatal and adult rats.

"Hybrid" polyribosomes can be formed *in vitro* by incubating ribosomal subunits from the young in a protein synthetic system derived from the adult. This system contains adult cerebral polyribosomes as well as other components, including initiation factors. Our preliminary results indicate that ^{32}P-labelled subunits from neonatal polyribosomes can contribute to the formation of 80S ribosomes which resist the dissociating action of 0·5 M KCl (Elliott, R. and Lim, L. unpublished observations). Thus, the changes in the properties of cerebral polysomes during development appear to be due to changes in components other than the constituent subunits, for example, the proteins binding to mRNA.

IV. Summary of Changes in the Nucleocytoplasmic Relationship of High Molecular Weight RNA During Development of Rat Forebrain

The changes in the metabolism of mRNA and rRNA during development are considered in terms of alterations in the nucleocytoplasmic relationship. Where possible, these changes are shown in Fig. 10. In the neonatal brain, most of the HMW RNA synthesized within the nucleus is exported into the cytoplasm to meet the needs of growing cells. Considering the poly(A)-RNA component, proportionately more is synthesized by the young compared with the adult in order to maintain a constant mRNA to rRNA ratio. This additional mRNA synthesis is required in the young because of the accumulation of stable rRNA (1). The rRNA precursor (the other component being synthesized) is processed so that there is accumulation of 28S and 18S rRNA in the cytoplasm but not in the nucleus (2). In contrast, in the adult brain (3 and 4) there is intranuclear turnover of poly(A)-RNA as well as 28S and 18S rRNA.

In the cytoplasm throughout development, mRNAs interact with the subunits containing the 28S and 18S RNA to form polyribosomes. In neonatal brain rRNA is not degraded, whereas mRNA turns over rapidly (5). In order to accommodate the influx of new and changing populations of mRNA, polyribosomes have to be able to dissociate readily into required subunits for the formation of newer populations. In the adult brain both rRNA and mRNA in the adult cytoplasm turn over, i.e. they are degraded and replaced by new rRNA and mRNA from the nucleus (6). The polyribosomes from adult brains compared with those from the young contain components which do not have such a wide disparity in their metabolism. This is reflected in the relative stability of adult polyribosomes compared with juvenile polyribosomes.

V. The Effects of Amino Acid Imbalance on Polyribosomes During the Vulnerable Period of Their Development

The relative metabolic instability of polyribosomes in the developing rat forebrain can be viewed as a consequence of the need to separate two major components (mRNA, rRNA) with widely disparate

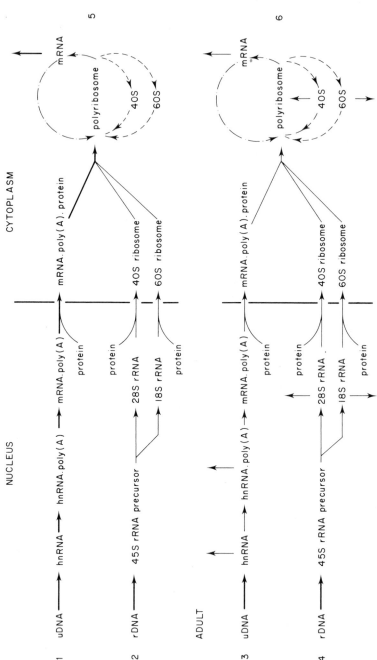

Fig. 10. Developmental changes in the nucleocytoplasmic relationships of HMW RNA in the rat forebrain. Horizontal arrows represent synthesis and processing of RNA. Vertical arrows represent degradation. Dashed lines indicate reutilization of components in the ribosome–mRNA–polyribosome cycle. In all cases the thickness of the lines and arrows is an indication of the relative rate of metabolism. In the young brain any intranuclear turnover of RNA will be obscured by the pattern of RNA metabolism and geared towards accumulation of rRNA in the cytoplasm. Only mRNA containing poly(A) is considered for clarity. uDNA: unique DNA (with some repetitive DNA); rDNA: ribosomal DNA. Details of the scheme will be found in the text.

turnover rates. This instability may be a contributory factor to the vulnerability of the developing brain. At early periods in its development the brain is extremely susceptible to amino acid and hormonal imbalance as well as to undernutrition. Some effects of these are seen particularly in the development of the cerebellum (Balázs 1968). In man, a metabolic disorder such as phenylketonuria, can lead to impairment of intellectual performance. The alterations in the makeup of the brain include a decreased content of myelin. In experiments with the rat the administration of phenylalanine to immature animals can cause inhibition of myelin protein synthesis in the forebrain (Agrawal et al., 1970). This inhibition probably results from decreased uptake of other essential amino acids sharing the same transport system as phenylalanine and interference with the organization of polyribosomes (Appel, 1966; Davison, 1973). This inhibition of protein synthesis brought about by a decreased availability of amino acids has been shown previously to occur in isolated mammalian cells, e.g. ascites cells (Hogan and Korner, 1968). There is an accompanying increase in the level of monoribosomes. In the normal course of protein synthesis subunits are released from polyribosome complexes after each complete round of translation. The 40S subunit then reattaches to the mRNA and is in turn joined by a 60S subunit to initiate another round of protein synthesis. An accumulation of inactive monoribosomes is an indication of decreased rates of initiation since these monoribosomes are formed from subunits which would otherwise become part of the polyribosome complex (Henshaw et al., 1973). This accumulation of inactive monoribosomes at the expense of polyribosomal formation can also be seen in the hyperphenylalaninaemic immature rat brain (Fig. 11). A similar effect has previously been demonstrated in brains of foetal rats whose mothers were given phenylalanine (Wong et al., 1971) and much more recently in brains of phenylalanine-treated immature mice (Taub and Johnson, 1975).

The phenylalanine-induced effect can also be demonstrated as a decrease in the free polyribosome content of forebrains from treated and control rats (Johnson et al., 1975). The majority of brain cytoplasmic polyribosomes are free, i.e. not attached to membranes of the endoplasmic reticulum. These polyribosomes can be isolated by centrifuging the cytoplasmic extract over a cushion of 2·0 M sucrose. Monoribosomes and diribosomes are retarded by the viscosity barrier imposed by the cushion of sucrose, so that they do not sediment with the polysomes (Noll, 1969). An increased level of monoribosomes such as that seen in Fig. 11 therefore leads to a decreased recovery of

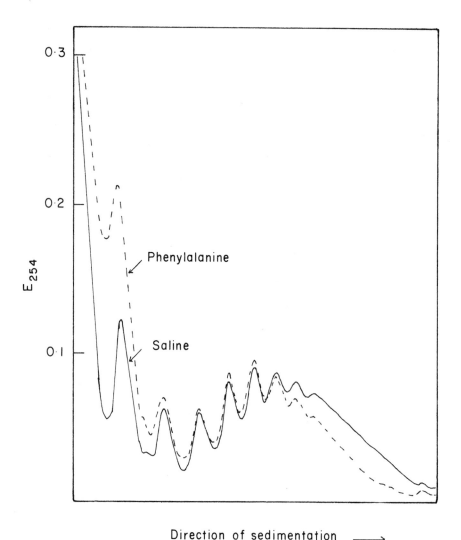

Direction of sedimentation ⟶

Fig. 11. The effect of phenylalanine administration on polyribosomes of the immature rat forebrain. Rats (17-day-old) of both sexes were injected intraperitoneally with a 1 g/kg body wt of L-phenylalanine 20% (w/v) in 0·09% (w/v) NaCl solution containing 2% (w/v) Tween 80 or with saline-Tween injections alone (Agrawal *et al.*, 1970). The forebrains of rats killed 30 min later where homogenized in 0·25 M sucrose containing Tris buffer (50 mm Tris-HCl, pH 7·6, 25 mM KCl and 12 mM $MgCl_2$). There was a fourfold increase in the brain level of phenylalanine in the treated animals. The postmitochondrial supernatant was obtained by centrifugation of the homogenate at 15 000 g/10 min and analysed on 12–35% sucrose density gradients in Tris buffer after centrifugation at 80 000 g/2·5 h at 4°.

polyribosomes. This decrease in the polyribosome content can be estimated on the basis of protein measurements (Table 3). There is a significant loss of 10%. Alternatively, this loss can be demonstrated upon sucrose gradient analysis (Fig. 12). The gradient analyses are important in showing that this loss in content of polyribosomes is due to accumulation of monoribosomes which do not pellet with the polyribosomes and not to increased ribonuclease activity.

Table 3

Decrease in brain content of free polyribosomes upon phenylalanine administration

	µg polyribosomal protein/mg protein in postmitochondrial supernatant
(a) Control	17·43 ± 0·83 (3)
(b) Hyperphenylalaninaemic	15·72 ± 0·64 (4)

Postmitochondrial supernatants were obtained from the brains of 14-day-old (a) control and (b) phenylalanine-treated rats, as described in Fig. 12. Aliquots were removed for protein estimation. Free polyribosomes were isolated by centrifuging the postmitochondrial supernatant over a cushion of 2·0 M sucrose in the Tris buffer in the MSE 65 Ti rotor at 240 000g/2·3 h. The polysomal pellets were dissolved in 0·05 M NaOH and protein estimated by the Lowry method. The results shown include the number of rats and S.D.s $p < 0.05$.

Noll (1969) has demonstrated that ribonuclease causes random breaks in the mRNA and the size distribution of polyribosomes therefore shifts to the lighter region. The polyribosomes recovered from all the brains had the same size distribution with a mean size of about 8–9 ribosomes, ruling out a ribonuclease-mediated loss. The simultaneous administration of amino acids which share the same transport system with phenylalanine, e.g. valine, tryptophan, led to normal recovery of polyribosomes. This would imply restoration of normal rates of protein synthesis. Other amino acids, e.g. arginine and lysine were not effective. This observation suggests that the lowering of brain phenylalanine levels by administration of other appropriate amino acids could be an effective therapy for phenylketonuriacs and prove to be much less expensive than a phenylalanine-free diet.

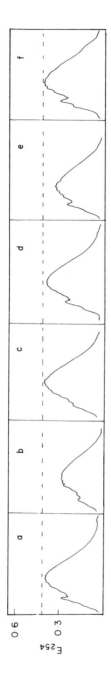

Direction of sedimentation ⟶

Fig. 12. Analysis of polyribosomes isolated from rats injected with phenylalanine and combinations of other amino acids. 17-day-old rats were injected with saline or with different amino acids and killed 30 min later. Free polyribosomes isolated from these homogenates, as described in Table 3, were analysed as shown in Fig. 11. The different amino acids, injected in amounts calculated to give equivalent increases in the serum concentrations of these amino acids relative to that of phenylalanine, were (g/kg body wt): phenylalanine (1·0), valine (2·11), tryptophan (1·03), arginine (3·93), lysine (5·22). Each analysis is of equivalent weights of brain and the u.v. absorbance thus represents relative recoveries of intact polyribosomes. The dotted line gives an indication of the control values as depicted by the peak absorbance: a. saline alone; b. phenylalanine; c. phenylalanine, valine, tryptophan; d. valine and tryptophan; e. phenylalanine, arginine, lysine; f. arginine, lysine.

VI. Concluding Remarks Including an Hypothesis for the Regulation of mRNA Synthesis

The gross changes in RNA metabolism that occur must be viewed not only in the context of maturing and differentiating cells but also in terms of the changing population of cellular types within the brain. Further complexities are introduced when regional specificity of the brain has to be considered. The studies discussed in the previous sections however have proved useful in indicating the general trend of changes that occur in the synthesis of the various types of RNA as well in the cellular interaction of the RNA-containing components. An intriguing observation which has emerged from these studies is that the content of mRNA (as measured by the content of poly(A)) is maintained at a constant level throughout development. Additional evidence that this content remains constant has come from our studies on the effects of hypothyroidism on the developing rat forebrain (L. Lim, W. Berthold and A. J. Patel, unpublished

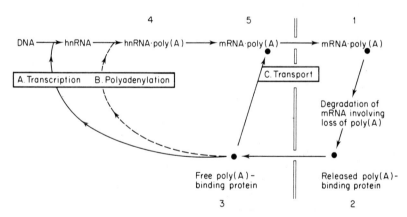

Fig. 13. Regulation of mRNA synthesis: proposed cyclic role of protein binding to poly(A). 1. Cytoplasmic mRNA contains a poly(A) segment to which a protein(s) binds. 2. Upon degradation of the mRNA, involving a loss of the poly(A) segment, this protein is released. 3. The protein is translocated into the nucleus (cf. histones). Here it can either stimulate A. transcription (by acting like a σ factor e.g. *E.Coli* RNA polymerase (Biswas *et al.*, 1975) or as a derepressor) or B. polyadenylation of hn RNA by activating the poly(A) polymerase. 4. Either of these actions will result in the formation of increased amounts of poly(A)-RNA. 5. The binding protein, having a preferential specificity for the poly(A) segment of the mRNA, reverts to being part of the mRNA-protein complex which is then transported out, thus completing the cycle. C. Alternatively, the free protein may be required only for the "transport" of poly(A)-RNA from the nucleus to the cytoplasm. It could also be required for this purpose in addition to being required in A. and B. In all three schemes the poly(A) segment of the cytoplasmic mRNA serves to regulate the availability of a binding protein which has nuclear function(s).

observations). There are obviously different mechanisms operating to regulate mRNA synthesis during development, when the cell is accumulating RNA within the cytoplasm, and in the adult when no net synthesis is obtained. We hypothesize, that in the adult, the synthesis of mRNA could be regulated by proteins binding to poly(A) regions of intact mRNA which shuttle between nucleus and cytoplasm as part of a monitoring system which couples degradation and synthesis of mRNA (details in Fig. 13). Whether this mechanism is restricted to the brain or whether it applies generally remains to be established.

Acknowledgements

The counsel and support of Professor Alan Davison is gratefully acknowledged. I thank Wolfgang Berthold, John White, Christine Hall and Dave Johnson for their contributions to the work. Support was provided by the Nuffield Foundation, the Medical Research Council and the Brain Research Trust.

References

Adams, D. H. (1966). *Biochem. J.* **98**, 636–640.
Agrawal, H. C., Bone, A. H. and Davison, A. N. (1970). *Biochem J.* **117**, 325–331.
Appel, S. H. (1966). *Trans. N.Y. Acad. Sci.* **29**, 63–70.
Balázs, R. (1973). *Biochem. Soc. Spec. Publ.* , 39–57.
Balázs, R., Kovacs, S., Teichgraber, P., Cocks, W. A. and Eayrs, J. T. (1968). *J. Neurochem.* **15**, 1335–1349.
Berthold, W. (1975). Ph.D. Thesis, University of London.
Berthold, W. and Lim, L. (1976a). *Biochem. J.* **154**, 517–527.
Berthold, W. and Lim, L. (1976b). *Biochem J.* **154**, 529–539.
Biswas, B. B., Ganguly, A. and Das, A. (1975). *Progr. Nucl. Acid Res. Mol. Biol.* **15**, 145–184.
Blobel, G. (1971). *Proc. Nat. Acad. Sci. U.S.A.* **68**, 832–835.
Brawerman, G. (1974). *Annu. Rev. Biochem.* **43**, 621–642.
Darnell, J. E. (1968). *Bacteriol. Rev.* **32**, 262–290.
Darnell, J. E., Jelinek, W. K. and Molloy, G. R. (1973). *Science* **181**, 1215–1221.
Davison, A. N. (1973). *Biochem. Soc. Spec. Publ.* **1**, 27–37.
DeLarco, J., Abramovitz, A., Bromwell, K. and Guroff, G. (1975). *J. Neurochem.* **24**, 215–222.
Georgiev, G. (1970). *Progr. Nucl. Acid Res.* **6**, 259–351.
Giuffrida, A. M., Cox, D. and Mathias, A. P. (1975). *J. Neurochem.* **24**, 749–755.
Gozes, I., Schmitt, H. and Littauer, U. Z. (1975). *Proc. Nat. Acad. Sci. U.S.A.* **72**, 701–705.

Green, H. (1974). *In* "Control of Proliferation in Animal Cells" (B. Clarkson and R. Baserga, eds). Cold Spring Harbor Laboratory, pp. 743–755.

Grouse, L., Chilton, M. D. and McCarthy, B. J. (1972). *Biochemistry* **11**, 798–805.

Hahn, E. W. and Laird, C. D. (1971). *Science* **173**, 158–161.

Harris, H. (1974). "Nucleus and Cytoplasm". Clarendon Press, Oxford.

Henshaw, E. C., Guiney, D. G. and Hirsch, C. A. (1973). *J. Biol. Chem.* **248**, 4367–4376.

Hogan, B. L. M. and Korner, A. (1968). *Biochim. Biophys. Acta* **169**, 128–139.

Huez, G., Marbaix, G. *et al.* (1974). *Proc. Nat. Acad. Sci. U.S.A.* **71**, 3143–3146.

Jacob, S. T. (1973). *Progr. Nucl. Acid Res.* **13**, 93–126.

Jeffrey, W. R. and Brawerman, G. (1975). *Biochemistry* **14**, 3445–3451.

Johnson, D., White, J. O., Lim, L. and Davison, A. N. (1975). *Biochem. Soc. Trans.* **3**, 93–94.

Lim, L. and Canellakis, E. S. (1970). *Nature (London)* **227**, 710–712.

Lim, L. and White, J. O. (1974). *Biochim. Biophys. Acta* **366**, 358–363.

Lim, L., Canellakis, Z. N. and Canellakis, E. S. (1969). *Biochem. Biophys. Res. Commun.* **34**, 536–540.

Lim, L., Canellakis, Z. N. and Canellakis, E. S. (1970). *Biochim. Biophys. Acta* **209**, 112–127.

Lim, L., White, J. O., Hall, C., Berthold, W. and Davison, A. N. (1974). *Biochim. Biophys. Acta* **361**, 241–247.

Maden, B. E. H. (1971). *Progr. Biophys. Mol. Biol.* **22**, 127–177.

Martin, T. E., Wool, I. G. and Castle, J. J. (1971). *Methods Enzymol.* **20**, 417–429.

Noll, H. (1969). *In* "Techniques in Protein Biosynthesis" (P. N. Campbell and J. R. Sargent, eds), Vol. 2. Academic Press, London and New York, pp. 101–179.

Perry, R. P., Kelley, D. E. and La Torre, J. (1974). *J. Mol. Biol.* **82**, 315–331.

Pinder, J. C., Staynov, D. Z. and Gratzer, W. B. (1974). *Biochemistry* **13**, 5373–5378.

Ryffel, G. U. and McCarthy, B. J. (1975). *Biochemistry* **14**, 5373–5378.

Schade, J. P. and Ford, D. H. (1973). "Basic Neurology". Elsevier Press, Amsterdam.

Taub, F. and Johnson, T. C. (1975). *Biochem J.* **151**, 173–180.

White, J. O., Hall, C., Lim, L. and Davison, A. N. (1975). *Biochem. Soc. Trans.* **3**, 94–95.

Wong, P. W. K., Fresco, R. and Justice, P. (1972). *Metabolism* **21**, 875–881.

Chapter 3

Metabolic Influences on Cell Proliferation in the Brain

R. BALÁZS, A. J. PATEL AND *P. D. LEWIS

MRC Developmental Neurobiology Unit,
Medical Research Council Laboratories,
Woodmansterne Road, Carshalton, Surrey, England

I. Introduction

To a greater or lesser extent, cell division in the growing brain continues after birth in all mammals, including man. It is not only early in its development, but also after birth, that the brain is especially susceptible to adverse metabolic factors (see e.g. Balázs *et al.*, 1975a). One function of brain growth which is vulnerable during this period, often with long-term consequences, is cell proliferation. The

* Department of Histopathology, Royal Postgraduate Medical School, Hammersmith Hospital, London, England.

aim of this review is to examine the effects of various factors—hormonal, nutritional and pharmacological—on brain cell division, and to discuss, on the basis of available evidence, mechanisms of control of cell replication in the central nervous system. In the experimental situation, study of the postnatal animal is often expedient, and much of the work which will be examined has been carried out on such animals. However, since the nature of postnatal cell proliferation in the brain can best be understood in the context of the histogenesis and morphogenesis of the nervous system as a whole, we have felt it necessary to open this chapter with a brief survey of the early development of the brain. Comprehensive reviews of this rapidly growing field are readily available (e.g. Altman, 1969; Jacobson, 1970; Sidman, 1970; Berry, 1974; Phelps and Pfeiffer, 1975) and these can be consulted for more detailed information.

II. Brief Outline of the Histogenesis and Morphogenesis of the Vertebrate Nervous System

A. Early Development

The nervous system, which has the distinction of being the first organ to be formed in the embryo, originates from a longitudinal mid-dorsal thickening of the embryonic ectoderm called the neural plate. It has been shown that the anlage of the nervous system is induced by the underlying chordamesoderm (notochord) (Spemann, 1938). The inductive capacity of the notochord is present for a much longer period (from early blastula till the tailbud stage) than the ability of the overlying ectoderm to react, which is confined to the gastrula stage (for references, see Jacobson, 1970). It would appear that liberation of chemical substances is instrumental in the induction phenomenon which can take place even when direct contact between interacting tissues is prevented by a physical barrier such as a millipore filter. The neural plate consists of a layer of neuroepithelial germinal cells attached to each other at their outer margins by a basement membrane, but free at their inner margins. It is generally assumed that all types of neurones and neuroglia are derived ultimately from these common stem cells. However, it would appear that the germinal cells in the neural plate constitute a mosaic with different fates, although it is not known when and how this commitment arises (Jacobson, 1970).

As development continues, the borders of the neural plate elevate to form the neural folds, whose progressive elevation and medial bending result in the formation of the neural groove (Fig. 1). Later the edges of the neural folds meet forming the neural tube. The outer surface of the neural plate becomes the surface lining of the lumen of the neural tube, and the inner surface of the neural plate covers the outside of the neural tube. Recent results indicate that microtubules and microfilaments play an important role in the changes of cell shape underlying the formation of the neural tube (for review, see Karfunkel, 1974). During closure of the neural tube, some cells at the edges of the neural plate detach dorsally to form the neural crest. Cells originating from the neural crest form ultimately a number of

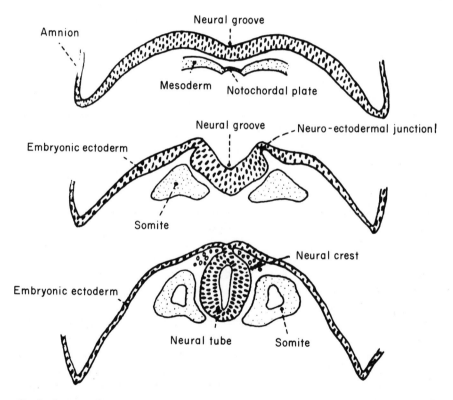

Fig. 1. Cross-sections through the nervous system at different stages of early development. A thickening of the embryonic ectoderm overlying the notochord forms the neural plate, which through further development gives rise to the neural groove and the neural tube. During the closure of the neural tube some cells at the lateral margins of the neural ectoderm detach to form the neural crest. (Illustration from Ford, 1975—with permission of the author and the publisher.)

structures in the cranium and trunk, such as some of the cranial nerve ganglia, the spinal sensory ganglia and constituents of the sympathetic nervous system. The cell lineages derived from the neural crest include besides neurones the chromaffin cells of the adrenal medulla, Schwann cells and melanocytes (Weston, 1971).

B. *Primary Germinal Sites*

The cranial portion of the neural tube gradually expands to form the brain vesicles in the 10–11-day-old rat embryo, while the caudal portion becomes the spinal cord. The cavities within the brain vesicles are called the ventricles and are continuous with the central canal of the spinal cord. At first, the wall of the brain vesicles is one or two cells deep and consists of a column of neuroepithelial (ventricular, germinal or matrix) cells. As the cells proliferate, the wall of the vesicles increases in thickness and its cells appear pseudostratified and palisaded. The neuroepithelial germinal cells are relatively homogeneous in terms of DNA synthesis, proliferation kinetics and ultrastructure (see also p. 60; for references see Jacobson, 1970). In spite of the increased width of the vesicle wall, cell proliferation is the same morphologically as at the earlier stage of columnar epithelium; premitotic cells are elongated and attached at their inner and outer ends to the ventricular and pial surfaces respectively. Before mitosis the nucleus migrates into the ventricular end of the cell and the basal end becomes detached and retracted so that the cell rounds up in a juxtaventricular position. After mitosis, the separated daughter cells again attach to the subpial basement membrane and the nuclei migrate away from the ventricle into the basal part of the process. DNA synthesis starts almost immediately and continues throughout the migration of the nucleus both towards the pial and, later, the ventricular surface. This cycle is then repeated (Sauer, 1935, 1936). Already at a very early stage from day 12–14 in the rat embryo some cells do not enter the replication cycle but move away from the ventricular surface and congregate under the basement membrane. Most of these cells will differentiate ultimately to become neurones (neuroblasts), but it seems that some glioblasts are also already formed at this stage (Phelps and Pfeiffer, 1975). Neuroblast formation accelerates, and by the 16th day of gestation in the rat a definitive lamina of cells has been formed below the pia dividing the brain vesicle, that will become the cerebral cortex, into five layers: marginal layer, cortical plate, intermediate zone, subventricular zone and ventricular zone (for nomenclature see Boulder Committee, 1970;

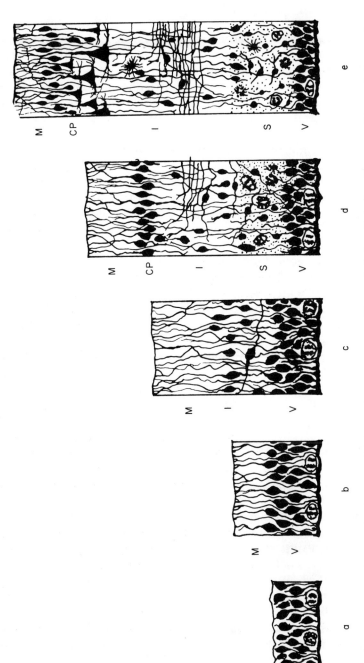

Fig. 2. Various stages (a–e) of the development of the central nervous system. CP: cortical plate, I: intermediate zone, M: marginal zone, S: subventricular zone, V: ventricular zone. (From Boulder Committee, 1970—by permission of Anat. Record.)

Fig. 2). The marginal layer and the intermediate zone become respectively layer I and the white matter of the definitive cortex, while cells of the cortical plate differentiate into neurones of all the other layers. Ultimately cells in the ventricular and subventricular zones differentiate into ependymal and subependymal cells. The latter cells constitute the secondary germinal pool in the forebrain (see below).

The time of origin of neurones in the mammalian cerebral cortex has been determined by autoradiographic studies (Angevine and Sidman, 1961; Berry et al., 1964). The rationale of these experiments is that labelled thymidine is rapidly incorporated into the DNA in replicating cells. The animals are killed a long time after a single pulse of [^{3}H]thymidine, when the histogenesis of the central nervous system has already been completed. The radioactivity of those cells which have undergone many divisions in the meantime will be so much diluted that autoradiography cannot detect labelling. On the other hand, cells which received [^{3}H]thymidine during their final replication will show heavily labelled nuclei. These studies have shown an "inside-out" sequence of arrival of neurones in the cerebral cortex (Angevine and Sidman, 1961). After their formation in the germinal zone, the neuroblasts migrate through the intermediate zone and the cortical plate, coming to rest in a position above this lamina. The next wave of neuroblasts migrates through the previously deposited cells. Thus, in the rat, neurones generated up to day 16 of gestation populate layer VI, while those formed at about days 17, 18 and 19–21 respectively are localized in layers V, IV and II–III (Berry et al., 1964; Fig. 3). The histogenesis of the cerebral cortex is completed prenatally in most mammalian species, including humans, but there are some species, such as the hamster, in which the last wave of cortical neurones is formed in the first few days after birth. The speed of migration is appreciable: estimates vary between 10 and 100 μm/h depending on species and developmental age (Hicks and D'Amato, 1968; Fujita et al., 1966; Altman, 1969). Thus cells formed early in the ventricular zone may reach the marginal layer in approximately 36 h, but as the migration path becomes longer with development those formed later may take as much as six days to arrive at their final destination.

The mechanism of cell migration is not yet understood (for the various hypotheses, see Berry, 1974). One of the more recent proposals is that cells migrate along the paths of central fibre tracts (Hicks and D'Amato, 1968). Afferent fibres reach the brain vesicles at relatively early stages in gestation (about day 16 in the rat), when central fibre tracts such as the thalamocortical fibres are also identifiable. However, the observations of Berry and Hollingworth (1973) do not support this hypothesis: these authors have shown that after unilateral transection of the internal capsule, the migration of the neuroblasts is normal although the thalamocortical fibres are absent. Rakic (1971a, b) has suggested that the neuroblasts are guided towards their final destination by glial processes which are attached to both the pial and the ventricular surfaces. Whether or not this hypothesis is valid (Bignami and Dahl, 1974; Sotelo and Changeux, 1974b), it implies that at least certain types of glial cells originate relatively early in the ontogenesis of the central nervous system.

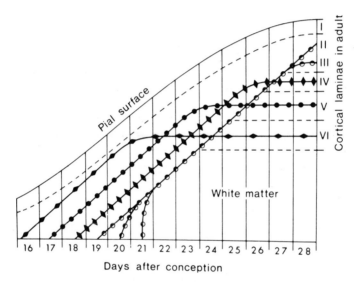

Fig. 3. The "birthdays" and the pattern of migration of neuroblasts in the developing neocortex of the rat. (From Berry *et al.*, 1964, as redrawn by Jacobson, 1970—by permission of the authors and the publisher.)

Evidence indicating that gliogenesis begins while neurogenesis is in progress is accumulating. Berry and Rogers (1966) have found, at the 18th day of gestation, cells in the ventricular zone which are destined to become glia in the cerebral cortex, and it seems that in the cerebellar cortex the Bergmann glia, as well as proliferating glial cells in the layer which will become the internal granular layer, originate from the primary ventricular germinal zone much earlier than the majority of nerve cells (Fujita *et al.*, 1966).

C. Secondary Germinal Sites

It is not yet known whether neurones and glia originate from the same germinal cells or there are different precursors of these major two cell lineages in the brain. However, it would appear that although some glioblasts are formed at early stages of development the great majority of the glial cells originate relatively late and (at least in the forebrain) from the secondary germinal matrix, the subependymal layer, which progressively replaces the ventricular zone as the major germinal matrix. In the mouse the subependymal layer is detectable from the 14th day of gestation: it is a truly stratified structure localized above the ependymal cells lining the forebrain ventricles, and it does not show the interkinetic nuclear movements characteristic of the primary neuroepithelial germinal zone. Other secondary germinal layers are the hippocampal germinal zone (Angevine, 1965), the external granular layer in the cerebellum (Ramon y Cajal, 1890) and an extensive zone in the hindbrain which gives rise to cells located in the medulla (Taber-Pierce, 1967).

The long-axoned neurones in the central nervous system originate exclusively from the primary germinal matrix, the ventricular zone, which however also forms some glioblasts. On the other hand, the secondary germinal zones produce the majority of the glial cells, but they also give rise to interneurones in certain regions.

1. Histogenesis of the cerebellum

A study of the cerebellum offers certain advantages in the investigation of cell proliferation in the central nervous system. At birth, the rat cerebellum contains only about 3% of its final cell number (Balázs et al., 1971). Thus the majority of nerve cells are formed in the postnatal period (the neurone to glia ratio in the adult is approximately 1:1, Lewis et al., 1976).* Factors influencing

* An approximate value of neurone to glia ratio can be derived from estimates on the rise of the cell population in the cerebellum (calculated from the DNA content), on the total number of Purkinje cells and on the ratios of Purkinje cells to the various interneurones from which the granule cells are the most abundant in the cerebellum; the other interneurones constitute approximately one tenth of the granule cell number, thus here for the sake of simplicity only the Purkinje cell to granule cell ratio will be mentioned. The variation of the latter two estimates is considerable in the literature, and accordingly the neurone to glia ratio varies depending on the values considered in the calculation: e.g. on the basis of Purkinje cell to granule cell ratio of 1:200 in adult rats (Altman and Anderson, 1971) and total Purkinje cell number of 320 000 (Armstrong and Schild, 1970) a neurone to glia ratio of 1:2 can be obtained (Balázs et al., 1974). However, by using respective values of 1:250 (Smolyaninov, 1971) and 400 000 (a mean of the estimates of Armstrong and Schild, 1970 and Smolyaninov, 1971) the computed ratio is 1:1 (Lewis et al., 1976).

neurogenesis can therefore be studied with relative ease. The cerebellar cortex is a clearly stratified structure and our knowledge about the time of origin (for reviews, see Fujita, 1969; Altman, 1969) as well as the role and interconnections of the different types of nerve cells in the cerebellar neuronal circuits is well advanced (Eccles *et al.*, 1967; Palay and Chan-Palay, 1974). Further, behavioural studies are becoming increasingly important in the elucidation of the functions of the nervous system, and methods are particularly well developed for the evaluation of motor skills, in which the cerebellum plays an important role.

The only efferent neurones in the cerebellar cortex are the Purkinje cells, and they are formed on day 11–13 in the mouse embryo (Miale and Sidman, 1961). These cells migrate into the superficial part of the mantle zone by the 17th day of gestation. Other cells derived from the ventricular germinal zone include not only nerve cells, such as the Golgi II cells (formed perinatally) and the neurones of the roof nuclei, but also glial cells (Bergmann glia and dispersed glial precursors in the parenchyma). All interneurones, with the exception of the Golgi II cells, are generated from the secondary germinal matrix, the external granular layer. This is formed from germinal cells produced at the rhombic lip in the roof of the fourth ventricle at about day 11 in the mouse foetus, before day 17 in the rat embryo and at 60–80 days gestation in man (Addison, 1911; Raaf and Kernohan, 1944; Woodard, 1960; Miale and Sidman, 1961). The cells migrate outwards to cover the whole surface of the cerebellum. Cell replication at first results in an increase in the numbers of germinal cells. However, by a few days after birth, some of the daughter cells migrate out from the external granular layer, whose total area changes during development depending on the balance of cells emigrating from and remaining in this layer. In the rat both the total area of the external granular layer and cell replication in terms of DNA synthesis rate, reach their maxima at about day 13. At this age the fractional increase in cell numbers was calculated to be 15·2% per day (Patel *et al.*, 1973). After the second postnatal week, both the area of the external granular layer and cell proliferation, in terms of DNA synthesis, are progressively diminishing (see Fig. 5). By 21–24 days of age this germinal zone disappears and active DNA synthesis comes to an end, while DNA content in the cerebellum reaches the adult level (Altman, 1969; Patel *et al.*, 1976) (see Fig. 5).

The "birthdays" of the various interneurones in the rat cerebellum have been established by Altman (1969). The basket cells are formed in the first week, the stellate cells towards the end of the second week,

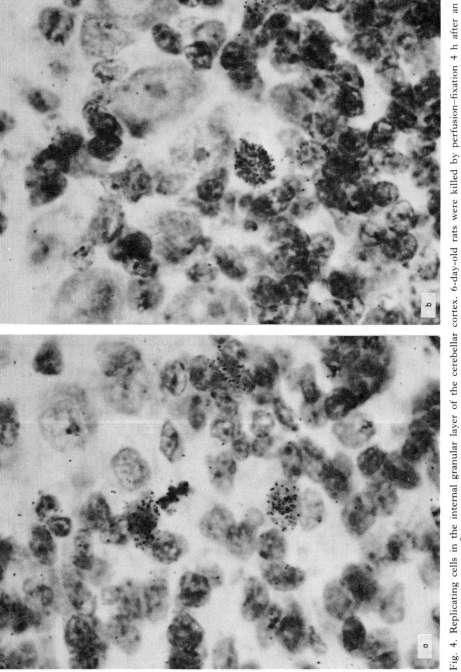

Fig. 4. Replicating cells in the internal granular layer of the cerebellar cortex. 6-day-old rats were killed by perfusion–fixation 4 h after an intraperitoneal injection of [³H]thymidine. Labelled cells can be seen in metaphase (a) and prophase (b). (Mayer's haemalum. × 1500.)

while approximately 50% of the granule cells are generated during the third week after birth. In the first few postnatal days, replicating cells can be detected in the site of the future internal granular layer at a time preceding the arrival of granule cells (Fig. 4). These cells originate from the primary germinal matrix and they are proliferating glial cells (Fujita *et al.*, 1966). However, according to these authors, but not to any others (Swarz and Del Cerro, 1975) the external granular layer also gives rise to some glial cells, especially towards the end of the period of active cell proliferation.

III. Influence of Metabolic Factors on Cell Proliferation

Although the blueprint of the proliferation and differentiation of cells is genetically determined, these processes are also influenced by factors in the external and internal environments. Over the last few years we have studied the effects of hormones and nutrition on postnatal cell proliferation in the rat brain. The general approach in these studies was a combined application of morphological and biochemical techniques to the questions in hand. Autoradiographic techniques for tracing [³H]thymidine labelled cells have greatly advanced our knowledge on histogenesis in the brain. However, there are quantitative questions which can better be answered by using biochemical techniques, which also have great potential when problems are raised concerning molecular biological mechanisms underlying cell proliferation under normal and abnormal conditions. Much of the currently available information in this area has been obtained from studies on non-neuronal tissues, but important new results are now forthcoming especially on model systems such as nervous tissues, including various tumor lines in culture (for reviews, see McMorris, 1969; Sato, 1973; Prasad and Kumar, 1974; Nelson, 1975).

A. *Thyroid Deficiency*

The effect of neonatal hypothyroidism on cell acquisition is different in the various parts of the brain (Balázs *et al.*, 1968; Patel *et al.*, 1976). Cell acquisition is normal in the forebrain, its rate is reversibly retarded in the cerebellum, whereas cell numbers are persistently depressed in the olfactory bulbs (Fig. 5). It is known that in contrast to the forebrain (with the exception of the hippocampus), neurogenesis is a significant process in the cerebellum and the olfactory bulbs during the postnatal period. Thus, the results are consistent with the view that thyroid hormone is required for the formation and/or maintenance of nerve cells in the developing central nervous system.

In thyroid deficiency, the ultimate restoration of cell numbers to the normal level in the cerebellum results from the prolonged persistence of the germinal zone. This is shown by both histological studies (Legrand, 1967; Hamburgh, 1968; Nicholson and Altman, 1972; Lewis et al., 1976) and by estimating the rate of DNA synthesis which, towards the end of the period of active cell proliferation at 21 days of age, is approximately treble the control values (Patel et al., 1976) (see Fig. 5).

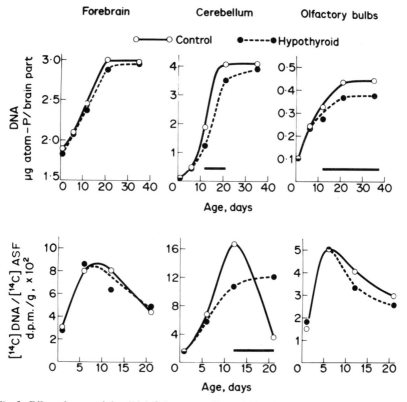

Fig. 5. Effect of neonatal thyroid deficiency on cell acquisition (top) and DNA synthesis rate in terms of [¹⁴C]DNA formation corrected for acid soluble ¹⁴C (bottom). Four control and hypothyroid rats at the ages indicated were given a subcutaneous injection of [2-¹⁴C]thymidine (15 μCi/100g body wt), and they were killed 30 min later. The results were analysed by analysis of variance, and the horizontal bars show the period when the differences between the experimental and control animals were significant (p < 0·01). (From Patel et al., 1976.)

We have found that two major factors are involved in the transient retardation of cell acquisition rate during the second week of life in the thyroid-deficient cerebellum (Lewis *et al.*, 1976). During that time, the number of cells in the external granular layer is only about 65% that of the control (see also Nicholson and Altman, 1972). Furthermore, cell loss is markedly increased in the internal granular layer: at day 12, the pyknotic index is 10–20 times greater than for controls. Since at the same time the pyknotic index is normal in both the external granular and the molecular layers, it would appear that thyroid deficiency does not affect the replicating and migrating cells, but interferes with the survival of a fraction of differentiating granule cells. The nature of the adverse conditions has been found in the influence of thyroid deficiency on the structural development of the cerebellar cortex. Significantly, the dendritic arborization of the Purkinje cells is severely retarded (Legrand, 1967): this results in a reduction in the availability of synaptic sites for the axons of the granule cells. We have proposed, therefore, that in accordance with the redundancy hypothesis of Hamburger and Levi-Montalcini (1949) death of a fraction of the granule cells is a consequence of a severe deficit in available postsynaptic sites for the termination of their axons. A similar mechanism has been suggested to operate in the developing cerebellum of the "staggerer" mutant mice (Sotelo and Changeux, 1974a). It is of interest that, in contrast to the effect of thyroid deficiency on the survival of cells, we have found no significant anomalies in the generation of cells in terms of cell cycle parameters (Lewis *et al.*, 1976).

It has to be emphasized that although cell numbers become ultimately normal the cellular composition in the cerebellar cortex is far from normal in thyroid deficiency. Significantly, there is a substantial deficit in basket cells and an increase in glial cells (Nicholson and Altman, 1972; Clos and Legrand, 1973). These changes in conjunction with the marked alterations in the development of synaptic organization (Hajós *et al.*, 1973) may be instrumental in the impaired motor coordination of the cretinous animals.

At this point it seems appropriate to discuss the significance of cell death in the nervous system. This phenomenon is implicated not only in the shaping of parts of the nervous system—"morphogenetic cell death" in the terminology of Glücksmann (1951)—but also in later stages of ontogenesis. Here it is seen as a result of cells failing to meet specific functional requirements. Such "histogenetic degeneration" may occur well into the postnatal period when it may be increased to biologically significant extent under abnormal circumstances. The example above demonstrates the importance of the achievement of synaptic contact for the maintenance of differentiating nerve cells. However, the structural and the molecular changes involved in cell death are quite obscure. Cell death does occur in the normal, postnatally developing cerebellum, and is seen both in the external granular layer and in the granule cell layer (Lewis, 1975; Lewis et al., 1976). It is also found in the forebrain subependymal layer. Degenerating cells have been shown to be postmitotic; macromolecule synthesis however is probably deranged before cells which are destined to die enter their last S phase (Pollak and Fallon, 1974). It has been calculated (Lewis, 1975) that only about 3% of newly formed neurones (cerebellum) or neuroglia (forebrain) are lost through this normal degenerative process. However, the extent of cell loss may be markedly increased under adverse metabolic conditions. The effect of thyroid deficiency has already been noted. In undernutrition, the loss of newly acquired cells may reach the 4–8% level in the second postnatal week (Lewis, 1975, see also Balázs, 1976), which may have implications in the long term for brain structure and function.

B. *Effect of Excess of Thyroid Hormone During Infancy*

When neonatal animals are treated with relatively high doses of thyroid hormone the major effect is a premature termination of cell proliferation (Balázs et al., 1971; Nicholson and Altman, 1972). We have recently extended these studies and found that at six days after birth, the external granular layer is thicker in animals treated with thyroid hormone than in controls, with comparable packing density and foliar development. This implies that at an earlier stage, cell proliferation may have been enhanced. There is evidence in support of this; an acceleration of increase of both thymidine kinase activity and DNA content in the cerebellum of thyroxine-treated rats have been demonstrated in the first five days of life (Gourdon et al., 1973; Weichsel, 1974). However, soon the rate of acquisition of new cells appears to be reduced, and this, together with premature emigration of cells from the germinal zone, as suggested by Balázs et al. (1971) and Nicholson and Altman (1972) could partly explain the marked reduction in thickness of this zone, which is observed at 12 days after birth.

Thyroid hormones have profound effects on the developing nervous system in amphibian larvae (Kollros, 1968; Pesetsky, 1976):

these include advanced differentiation of certain groups of neurones (e.g. nerve cells in the lateral motor column) and perhaps also an accelerated degeneration of motor neurones that have failed to make peripheral connections, but there is little evidence that thyroxine affects the rate of proliferation of neurones (for references see Jacobson, 1970). However, although thyroid hormone is not required for the generation of the germinal-cell pool destined to populate the external granular layer, it is instrumental in the investment of the surface of the cerebellum with these replicating cells in the tadpole (Gona, 1973).

C. *Effect of Growth Hormone*

It has been reported that administration of impure growth hormone preparations to tadpoles leads to a marked increase (44–126%) in cell numbers in the cerebral hemispheres (Zamenhof, 1941). Hunt and Jacobson (1971) have also observed that a purified preparation of growth hormone, as well as prolactin stimulate cell acquisition in the tadpole brain. The effects are very complex: the rate of cell acquisition is accelerated by growth hormone during the period of treatment (which was in case of both hormones at an early larval stage), whereas it is retarded in later stages of development, so that by the end of metamorphosis the DNA content is only slightly above the normal level. On the other hand, prolactin leads to an extensive rise in cell acquisition rate mainly after the termination of the treatment effecting ultimately a 50–80% increase in brain DNA over control frogs. Additional studies with [^{3}H]thymidine have indicated that the effect of both hormones is, at least in part, due to increased cellular proliferation. However, especially in the brain of the prolactin-treated tadpoles the extensive cell loss, which occurs normally during metamorphosis, was also substantially reduced.

Zamenhof *et al.* (1966) have claimed that in developing mammals (during gestation) as well as in amphibia, growth hormone administration results in an increase in the number of cells, especially of neurones, in the brain. These observations have been supported by Sara and Lazarus (1975), who found a marked increase in the labelled DNA content of the brains of seven-day-old rats which had been given a single injection of [^{3}H]thymidine during the period of growth hormone treatment at the 20th day of gestation. It has not been ascertained, however, whether the latter findings reflect a genuine increase in cell proliferation, or result from changes in the availability

of [³H]thymidine to the embryo. Furthermore, the claims that
growth hormone promotes cell proliferation in the foetal brain have
not been confirmed by the histological studies of Clendinnen and
Eayrs (1961) and by biochemical investigations in our laboratory
(Cotterrell, 1971). Brain weight, as well as DNA, RNA and protein
content did not differ significantly from controls during the period
from birth to 35 days of age in the young of mother rats treated with
bovine growth hormone (3·2 mg per day) from 7th to 19th day of
pregnancy. Zamenhof et al. (1971) have recently reported results
similar to our negative findings, but they now claim that treatment
with growth hormone prevents the depression of cell acquisition
caused by nutritional deprivation in pregnant rats.

D. Undernutrition

Undernutrition frequently accompanies abnormal hormonal states
during development, and we have therefore investigated its effect on
cell proliferation in the brain (Patel et al., 1973; Lewis et al., 1975).
Our findings confirmed previous observations on the irreversible

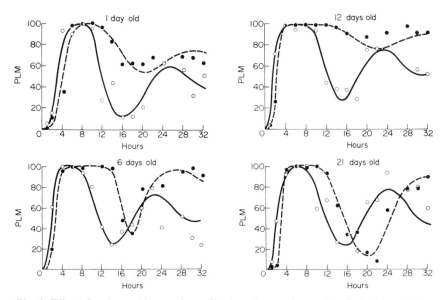

Fig. 6. Effect of undernutrition on the replication of external granule cells in the cerebellar
cortex. Computer generated curves are superimposed on the data of percentage labelled mitoses
(PLM) observed 1–32 h after injection of [³H]thymidine at the different ages indicated.
Control, O——O and undernourished, ●–––●, rats. Mean estimates of cell cycle parameters
are given in Table 1. (From Lewis et al., 1975.)

depression of cell acquisition caused by undernutrition during the suckling period (Winick, 1969; Dobbing and Smart, 1974). However, we also obtained a puzzling result, which ultimately was of great value in establishing that the mechanisms underlying disturbed cell proliferation in undernutrition are clearly distinct from those in abnormal hormonal states, such as thyroid deficiency. It was observed that in contrast to the moderate depression of cell numbers throughout the brain (approximately 15% deficit) undernutrition resulted in a severe reduction in the rate of DNA synthesis *in vivo*, which at its nadir was only about 20% (forebrain) to 30% (cerebellum) of the control values (Patel *et al.*, 1973). Further studies

Table 1

Effect of undernutrition (UN) on the length of cell cycle phases in the cerebellar external granular layer of developing rat brain

	Treatment	Age (d)			
		1–2	6–7	12–13	21–22
S phase	Control	9·3	9·9	10·7	10·0
	UN	14·7	13·8	19·6	12·8
G_2 phase	Control	3·1	1·8	1·6	2·2
	UN	4·2	2·7	2·4	3·0
G_1 phase	Control	8·5	5·3	5·6	5·3
	UN	2·8	1·1	0·5	6·2
Cell cycle time	Control	20·9	17·0	17·9	17·5
	UN	21·7	17·6	22·5	22·0

Mean values are given. The estimate of the length of the cell cycle phases (in h) were obtained by fitting computer generated curves to the data representing the percentage labelled mitoses at 1–32 h after injection of [^{3}H]thymidine (see Fig. 6).

showed that the discrepancy between the effect of undernutrition on the rate of cell acquisition and the rate of DNA synthesis could be largely accounted for by a disproportionately greater prolongation of the DNA synthesis (S) phase of the cell cycle than of the turnover time of the germinal cells (Lewis *et al.*, 1975). Cell cycle times were also only slightly affected (Fig. 6 and Table 1). This relatively small effect of the treatment on cell cycle time, in spite of the prolongation of the DNA synthesis phase, was a consequence of a severe curtailment of the length of the G_1 phase of the cell cycle.

1. Estimation of cell cycle parameters

In these studies, we took advantage of the circumscribed localization of the secondary germinal sites, the subependymal layer in the forebrain and the external granular layer in the cerebellum, to obtain reliable estimates of the cell cycle parameters of the germinal cells by determining the time-course of the appearance and disappearance of the wave of labelled mitoses in these sites after a single injection of [^{3}H]thymidine (with the construction of a percentage labelled mitosis, PLM, curve see e.g. Cleaver, 1967). The results expected for an ideal case, i.e. when the labelled precursor is present for a very short time and the replicating cells constitute a homogeneous population, is depicted in Fig. 7. The successive waves of labelled mitoses correspond to consecutive divisions of the fraction of the cell population that was in S phase during the availability of [^{3}H]thymidine. No labelled mitoses can be found during the period of G_2 (t_2): at first the cells exposed to the precursor near to the end of the S phase show labelled mitoses. Then the fraction of mitotic figures labelled increases rapidly to 100% in a period equal to the duration of mitosis (t_m). The labelled fraction remains at 100% for the period equal to the length of the S phase minus t_m, and subsequently falls to zero as the cells, which had just started to synthesize DNA at the time of exposure to [^{3}H]thymidine, finished division. The second wave of labelled mitotic figures appears after a period equal to G_1 and G_2. It is indicated in Fig. 7 that the construction of the PLM curve, for which computer programmes are available (e.g. Steel and Hanes, 1971), provides estimates for the cell cycle parameters. There are also other techniques, which have been applied to the CNS as well, for the determination of cell cycle parameters (e.g. continuous labelling method, Fujita et al., 1966; for review, see Cleaver, 1967). The results indicate that the cell cycle time of the germinal cells gradually becomes more prolonged during development: it is about 11 h in the neural tube (mouse foetus at 11 days; Kauffman, 1968; Atlas and Bond, 1965), and 12 h in the rhombic lip (rat foetus at 14 days; Ellenberger et al., 1969). However, the cell cycle time is nearly double this value in the secondary germinal sites in the postnatal brain (Table 1). It is of interest that the cell cycle times are similar in the subependymal layer in the forebrain and the external granular layer in the cerebellum, and they do not seem to change significantly during the whole postnatal period of active cell proliferation (Fujita et al., 1966; Lewis et al., 1975). It has been claimed, however, that glioblast proliferation is slow in

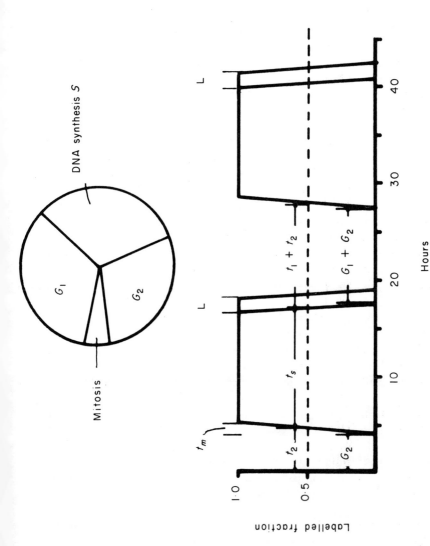

Fig. 7. *Above*: the four phases of the cell cycle cells progress clockwise around the cycle. *Below*: fraction of mitoses labelled after a pulse of [^{3}H]thymidine. The drawing represents an ideal cell population which is homogenous in terms of replication kinetics. L: duration of precursor availability; t_m, t_1, t_2 and t_s stand respectively for the length of mitosis and the duration of the different phases, G_1, G_2 and S, of the cell cycle. (Illustration from Cleaver, 1967— by permission of the publisher.)

comparison with the mean values obtained in the secondary germinal sites. For example, in the neonatal mouse cell cycle times for glial cells of 55–120 h in the cerebellar cortex and of 65 h in the subependymal layer have been reported by Fujita et al. (1966) and Sidman (1970). This low rate is not consistent either with more recent estimates of the generation time of subependymal germinal cells, which are believed to differentiate mainly into glial cells (Lewis et al., 1975), or with observations on the recruitment of cells in the cerebellum. In the rat cerebellum only a small fraction of the final cell number is present at birth (3%). Since the neurone to glia ratio is approximately 1:1 both during development and in the adult (Lewis et al., 1976) the postnatal generation of glial cells and neurones seems to progress in a parallel fashion. As noted earlier Fujita et al. (1966) have suggested that glial cells are formed from the external granular layer only towards the end of the proliferation period, whereas according to other authors (Swarz and Del Cerro, 1975) only neurones are generated from this layer. Thus at least in the first two weeks gliogenesis must have occurred predominantly in other sites (such as the internal granular layer and white matter). The similar increase in the number of glial cells and neurones would suggest that the turnover time of these two cell types is unlikely to differ by a factor of 3–7, the discrepancy in cell cycle times, especially as the pyknotic indices appear to be even lower in the internal granular layer than in the external granular layer (Lewis et al., 1976).

While autoradiographic estimates of turnover time of astrocytes in the granular layer are not easy to obtain, it is nevertheless feasible to measure the cell cycle parameters by constructing PLM curves, since mitotic figures resembling those seen in astrocytes elsewhere in the brain (Cavanagh, 1970) can be found commonly in the granule cell layer at day 6 and occasionally at day 12 (see Fig. 4). In six-day-old rats, the PLM curve gives figures of: cell cycle time 19 h, DNA synthesis phase 8·5 h, t_{G_2} ($+0·5\ t_m$) 2·5 h; t_{G_1} ($+0·5\ t_m$) 8 h. These parameters are indeed comparable to those obtained from glial cells in the subependymal layer and are consistent with the findings on recruitment of cells into cerebellar cortex.

In mammalian cells the prolongation of the cell cycle time during development is mainly due to the lengthening of the G_1 phase. Thus, the multiplying cells in the brain of undernourished rats seem in this respect to have reverted to an embryonic pattern of replication. This effect may have very important functional consequences, for it has been shown recently that certain processes occurring during a limited period in the G_1 phase are critical in terms of the full expression of the normal differentiated functions of some cells (Vonderhaar and Topper, 1974).

2. Thymidine metabolism in the brain—possible errors in estimation of cell cycle parameters

Before further considering the effects of undernutrition on cell proliferation in the brain, an important methodical question must be clarified. An implicit assumption in estimating cell cycle parameters by the PLM method is that the tissue is exposed to a pulse of the radioactive precursor. This is evidently never achieved *in vivo*, and the protracted availability of the labelled precursor results in distortions in the PLM curve. This may cause errors in the estimates of cell cycle parameters, especially when different experimental conditions are compared. If the duration of the labelling period is not negligible then the length of the waves of labelled mitoses will be extended, resulting in an overestimate of the length of the S phase and underestimate of that of the G_1 and G_2 phases by amounts equal to the duration of the labelling period. However, relevant information can be obtained from kinetic observations on [^{14}C]thymidine metabolism with respect to the validity of comparison of experimental conditions. Although cell proliferation has been extensively studied by using autoradiographic techniques, the cerebral metabolism of thymidine, especially in relation to different brain regions and various experimental conditions, has attracted hitherto relatively little attention (Mori *et al.*, 1970; Yamagami *et al.*, 1973; Muzzo and Brasel, 1973; for review see Millard, 1974). Our studies in which the fate of [2-^{14}C]thymidine was followed in the brain clearly showed that the labelling period was not negligible (Patel *et al.*, 1976; Fig. 8). The concentration of [^{14}C]thymidine decayed with a fast ($t_{1/2}$ about 20 min) and a slow component ($t_{1/2}$ about 100). The radioactivity content of DNA increased more or less linearly for 0·5–1 h and became constant by 1–2 h, depending on region. Thus, although [^{14}C]thymidine was present for a relatively long time, [^{14}C]DNA formation was only detectable during the period of the fast decay of [^{14}C]thymidine. The results also indicated quantitative differences in thymidine metabolism in different brain regions. The rate of conversion of [^{14}C]thymidine into [^{14}C]thymidine nucleotides, and of these in turn to [^{14}C]DNA, is faster in the cerebellum than in the forebrain, where cell proliferation occurs on a smaller scale. Consequently, in the forebrain nearly linear DNA synthesis rate is maintained for a longer time than in the cerebellum (1 h v. 0·5 h), and

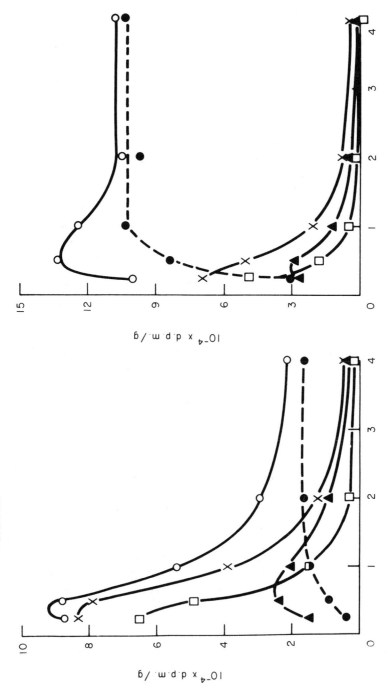

Fig. 8. Time-course of incorporation of [2-¹⁴C]thymidine into main constituents of forebrain and cerebellum of 14-day-old rats which received a subcutaneous injection of [2-¹⁴C]thymidine (15 µCi/100 g body wt) and were killed by immersion into −150° Freon at the times indicated. The results are the mean of two to three animals at each timepoint. Whole tissue, O——O; DNA, ●——●; acid soluble, ×——×; thymidine nucleotides (the sum of the ¹⁴C content of thymidine mono-, di-, and triphosphates), ▲——▲; and thymidine, □——□. (From Patel et al., 1976—by permission of Brain Research.)

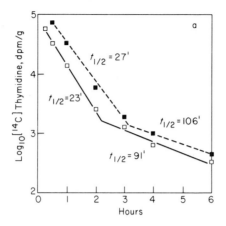

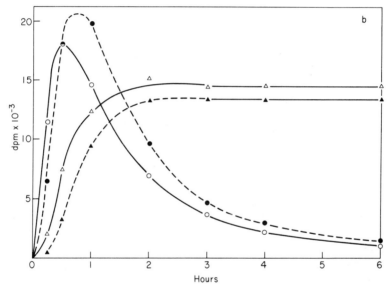

Fig. 9. Thymidine metabolism in the forebrain of 12-day-old undernourished rats. Two control and experimental animals were killed by immersion into −150° Freon at the times indicated after a subcutaneous injection of [2-^{14}C]thymidine (15μCi/100 g body wt), and the constituents were isolated as described by Patel *et al.*, (1976). The standard errors of the logarithmically transformed data for [^{14}C]thymidine (a), [^{14}C]thymidine nucleotides and [^{14}C]DNA (b) were 0·053, 0·025 and 0·027 respectively. The semilogarithmic plot of [^{14}C]thymidine decay is shown in (a): the half-lives ($t_{1/2}$) of the fast and slow decay components were calculated from the slopes of the regression lines. The radioactivity contents are expressed in terms of g fresh wt for thymidine and the sum of thymidine nucleotides, whereas [^{14}C]DNA refers to the whole forebrain. Control: [^{14}C]thymidine, □——□; [^{14}C]thymidine nucleotides, ○——○; [^{14}C]DNA, △——△. Undernourished rats: [^{14}C]thymidine ■– – –■; [^{14}C]thymidine nucleotides, ●– – –●; [^{14}C]DNA, ▲– – –▲. Unpublished observations from our laboratory.)

since less ^{14}C is conserved in DNA a significant efflux of unconverted [^{14}C]thymidine is evident.

We studied the kinetics of [^{14}C]thymidine metabolism in the brain of 12-day-old undernourished rats, when the prolongation of the S phase of the cell cycle was most pronounced (Fig. 9). The concentration of [^{14}C]thymidine was elevated in the undernourished brain, probably as a result of lower utilization of thymidine in the body as a whole, but it decreased rapidly with a decay constant similar to control. In comparison with the untreated animals the rate of conversion of [^{14}C]thymidine into [^{14}C]thymidine nucleotides was slightly slower, since the peak of [^{14}C]thymidine concentration was reached about 15 min later, but the ^{14}C content of these compounds was even higher in the undernourished brain after 30 min. The initial rate of brain [^{14}C]DNA formation was severely depressed. However, because of the longer availability of the precursor, [^{14}C]DNA formation proceeded with a rapid rate for 15–30 min longer in the undernourished brain, and thus the difference, in comparison with controls, was diminishing from 0·5 h onwards and the labelling of DNA reached a plateau slightly later at approximately two hours after the injection of [^{14}C]thymidine. Considering together the time-courses of the concentration of [^{14}C]thymidine, [^{14}C]thymidine nucleotides and [^{14}C]DNA, it seems that undernutrition caused a displacement on the time axis by 10–30 min. Since the cell cycle time and the length of the DNA synthesis phase are about 1200 min and 600 min respectively, it is unlikely that the slight prolongation of the availability of the precursor to the brain in undernutrition could introduce substantial errors, in comparison with controls, in the estimation of cell cycle parameters by the autoradiographic technique.

Besides the cell cycle parameters, important characteristics of growth in the germinal zones are provided by estimates of the turnover time for the dividing cells (100 × S-phase length/labelling index) and by those of the growth fraction (cell cycle time/turnover time). The results indicated that undernutrition consistently prolonged the turnover times in the external granular layer, but not in the subependymal layer (Lewis et al., 1975). However, the growth fractions were similar to control in both layers. It is evident from the considerations above that both the cell cycle parameters used in these calculations and the labelling indices would be subject to error if, in comparison with control, the DNA precursor availability were altered in the undernourished brain. As already discussed, the influence of this factor on the computed S-phase length is slight, and it would appear from Fig. 9 that the effect on the labelling indices, which were estimated one hour after the injection of labelled thymidine, must also be small. The decrease in labelled thymidine nucleotide concentrations in the first 15 min may have been balanced by their increase after 30 min. Furthermore, the alterations in the concentration of labelled DNA precursors during the one hour period would result in a rise or decrease in the radioactivity content of DNA produced per cell, rather than a change in the number of labelled cells. The latter would only apply to that relatively small fraction of cells which were synthesizing DNA for too short a time to accumulate enough radioactivity to be counted under the experimental conditions in controls (i.e. cells which either entered into S phase too late or were too near to the termination of DNA synthesis), and this would be unlikely to introduce substantial error.

3. Possible mechanisms involved in the effect of undernutrition on cell proliferation

The kinetic analyses gave, therefore, strong support to the observation that S phase is selectively prolonged in the replicating cells in the brain of undernourished animals. It has been observed previously that food deprivation results in slowing of DNA synthesis in organs other than brain (Howard, 1965; Mendes and Waterlow, 1958; Wiebecke et al., 1969). It would appear that in developing organs the reduction in the acquisition of cells is usually more severe than that observed in the brain, implying that in these organs, in contrast to brain, undernutrition effected a marked prolongation not only of the S phase, but also the cell cycle time.

A selective prolongation of the S phase, although without a concomitant curtailment of the length of G_1, has been observed in hepatoma cells (Reuber H35 cells) cultured in presence of dibutyryl cyclic AMP (DBcAMP) (Van Wijk et al., 1973). However, the mechanisms underlying the effect of cAMP seem to differ from those operating in undernutrition. DBcAMP results in a severe reduction of the conversion of thymidine to thymidine triphosphate in the hepatoma cells. In contrast, as described above, the conversion of [^{14}C]thymidine to [^{14}C]thymidine nucleotides is only slightly affected in the undernourished brain. Nevertheless, it should be noted that recent unpublished observations from our laboratory have indicated that the activity of thymidine kinase is significantly depressed in the brain of 12-day-old undernourished animals suggesting a repression of the proliferative machinery in the tissue (for other results on thymidine kinase activity in the undernourished brain see also Giuffrida *et al.*, 1975 and Weichsel and Dawson, 1976).

It is known that thymidine kinase is one of the enzymes whose activity closely reflects whether or not a cell is in the replicating state (for review Cleaver, 1967). Baril *et al.* (1974) have shown that a set of these enzymes associated with DNA synthesis (thymidine kinase, thymidilate synthetase, ribonucleotide reductase, and DNA polymerase II) also share subcellular localization on submicrosomal membranes. However, it has not yet been established how far these conclusions apply also to the replicating cells in brain, although studies on some of the enzymes have indicated that these activities are also sensitive markers of the proliferative potential in the CNS.

Recent observations of Short *et al.* (1974) may provide an important lead towards the understanding of the mechanisms underlying the overall effect of undernutrition on cell proliferation. These authors have found that blood-borne factors play a crucial role in inducing cell proliferation in a basically resting population of cells, such as prevail in the adult liver. It is possible to elicit marked cell replication in the liver by giving high protein containing food to animals which were kept for three days previously on a protein-free diet. The critical factors have been ultimately reduced to thyroid hormone and three amino acids in the diet, isoleucine, threonine and tryptophan.

IV. Drugs and Cell Proliferation in the Brain

A. *Effect of Reserpine*

It has been observed that reserpine in relatively small doses inhibits the growth of different tumors in experimental animals (Goldin *et al.*, 1957; West *et al.*, 1961), and depresses cell proliferation in the regenerating liver (Čihák and Vaptzarova, 1973). In recent studies (Patel *et al.*, 1977 and Lewis *et al.*, 1977,) we have followed up this observation by investigating the effect of reserpine, a powerful DNA depressant, on cell replication in the developing brain.

Initial experiments on 11-day-old rats showed that reserpine also caused a severe depression in the rate of *in vivo* brain DNA synthesis, which was used in these studies as a marker of cell proliferation. However, the side-effects of the drug made interpretation of the results difficult: the treated animals were hypothermic, and since they were sedated they did not suckle properly. Furthermore, reserpine in adult animals results in a significant elevation of the level of blood corticosteroids, which in high concentration are known to interfere with cell proliferation in certain tissues including the brain (for reviews see Balázs and Richter, 1973; Howard, 1974). In the next series of experiments it was possible to exclude that these side-effects had a significant role in the interference with cell proliferation in the brain of reserpine-treated rats. Marked depression in DNA synthesis was observed in reserpinized animals which were maintained at normal body temperature and were artificially fed during the experimental period (up to 36 h). The concentration of corticosterone in the blood was also determined: this was very low in the neonatal rat and was only slightly elevated by reserpine more or less to the normal adult level (11–14 μg/100 ml plasma). These observations are consistent with previous results and indicate a relative "silence" of adrenal cortical response to stimuli, which in the adult lead to a marked increase of corticosteroid secretion (for reference see Balázs and Richter, 1973). We have found earlier that, in order to produce a

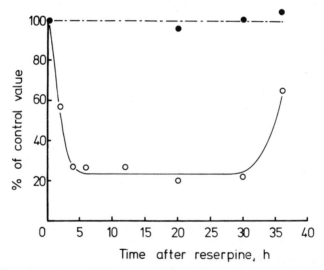

Fig. 10. Effect of reserpine on DNA synthesis in the forebrain. 11-day-old rats received either a single subcutaneous injection of reserpine (2·5 mg.kg.) or vehicle (controls). Both groups of animals were removed from the dams and kept at 31–32°: they were fed overy 3 h through a stomach tube with 0·5 ml cows' milk supplemented with 6% casein and 6% soya bean oil. At the indicated times after the administration of reserpine, the animals (2–6 for each point) received a subcutaneous injection of [³H]thymidine and were killed 30 min later. The amount of [³H]DNA per g wet wt was corrected on the basis of ³H₂O-free acid soluble radioactivity concentration, and the results in the reserpinized animals were expressed as a percentage of the Control values. (From Patel et al., 1977.)

significant retardation of cell acquisition in the brain, neonatal rats had to be treated with a minimal daily dose of 0·2 mg cortisol (approximately 2–3 mg/100 g) over a period of a few days (Cotterrell *et al.*, 1972). Thus, it is unlikely that the effect of reserpine on cell proliferation in the brain would be mediated through corticosteroids.

The depression of DNA synthesis rate was already detectable at two hours after the administration of reserpine and the rate was only 25% of control during the period 4–30 h (Fig. 10). Reserpine had no marked effect on the entry of labelled thymidine from blood to brain, but the drug caused some retardation in the rate of conversion of [^{3}H]thymidine into [^{3}H]thymidine nucleotides. Thymidine kinase activity was therefore determined, but it was found to be normal. If thymidine kinase were taken as a marker of the proliferative potential of the tissue (see e.g. Cleaver, 1967) the results indicate that reserpine did not interfere with the overall genetic expressions associated with replication. Rather, reserpine may have influenced regulatory processes such as the availability of ATP for the conversion of thymidine monophosphate to the proper DNA precursor thymidine triphosphate (Gwóźdź *et al.*, 1973; Dyduch, 1973; Maina, 1974). However, the results indicated that the interference with thymidine nucleotide formation was too small to account for the massive reduction in DNA synthesis rate. Possible mechanisms, in which reserpine plays an indirect role, are considered in the next section: these may have wider implications concerning the regulation of cell proliferation in the brain. Nevertheless, at the present time a direct action of the drug on the replicating cells cannot be excluded.

B. *Cyclic Nucleotides, Drugs Affecting Neurohumor Receptors and Cell Proliferation*

In attempting to elucidate the mechanism of reserpine action it is worth recalling that one of the main pharmacological effects of this drug is the depletion of the monoamine stores leading, in turn, to a feedback stimulation of those neuronal pathways which impinge upon the monoaminergic cells. It has recently been shown by Axelrod and his coworkers that increased impulse traffic through the presynaptic cholinergic fibres is instrumental in reserpinized animals in the induction of critical enzymes of catecholamine synthesis (tyrosine hydroxylase and dopamine β-hydroxylase) in postsynaptic cells in the sympathetic ganglia or the adrenal medulla (for review see

Axelrod, 1971/2). By using immunological techniques it has also been shown that the observed rise in transmitter enzyme activity is the result of increased *de novo* synthesis (Joh *et al.*, 1973; Hoeldtke *et al.*, 1974). Since the trans-synaptic induction can be blocked by actinomycin D, the results are consistent with the view that the transcription of the genetic material is affected. It is important in the present context that it has been demonstrated that trans-synaptic induction of tyrosine hydroxylase also occurs in the central nervous system (Thoenen, 1970; Zigmond *et al.*, 1974; Reis *et al.*, 1974; Black, 1975).

Cyclic nucleotides seem to be involved in the mechanisms underlying tyrosine hydroxylase induction (Mackay and Iversen, 1972; Guidotti *et al.*, 1975; however see Otten *et al.*, 1974). In "adrenergic" neuroblast clones and cultured superior cervical ganglia cAMP is able to induce this enzyme (Mackay and Iversen, 1972; Richelson, 1973), although in the adrenal medulla the reserpine-induced increase in tyrosine hydroxylase persists even after the rise in cAMP has been virtually abolished with a β-adrenergic blocker (Otten *et al.*, 1974). However, recent observations have indicated that alterations in the ratio of endogenous cAMP to cGMP mediated through the stimulation of specific hormone receptors are instrumental in leading to the changes in the expression of the tyrosine hydroxylase genome (Guidotti *et al.*, 1975). Other factors are also involved in the enzyme induction: for example, corticosteroids seem to have a "permissive" role in the superior cervical ganglion (Guidotti *et al.*, 1975) whereas, at high concentration, they can inhibit induction in cultured adrenal medulla (Goodman *et al.*, 1975). Here we should like to consider only the hormone receptor mediated changes in the concentration of cyclic nucleotides. It would appear that the increase in the cAMP/cGMP ratio must reach a certain magnitude (about fourfold), and persist for some time (about one hour) to induce tyrosine hydroxylase (Guidotti *et al.*, 1975). It is not yet known how these changes affect gene expression, but it has been postulated that cyclic-nucleotide-dependent protein kinases may influence the posphorylation of nuclear proteins (Greengard *et al.*, 1971), which seem to play an important role in the regulation of gene expression in eukaryotic cells (for reviews see e.g. Allfrey, 1974; Le Stourgeon *et al.*, 1974; Gilmour, 1974).

1. *Adrenergic and cholinergic mechanisms in the
control of proliferation of various cell types*

Cyclic nucleotides have been implicated not only in the regulation of
the expression of differentiated functions (Rutter *et al.*, 1973), but also
in the control of cell proliferation (Pastan *et al.*, 1975), which seems to
be influenced in various types of cells by neurohumors through
interaction with specific receptors. This has been shown to occur in
both stem cells (e.g. haemopoietic stem cells, Byron, 1974) and
actively cycling cells (e.g. a population of thymic lymphoblasts,
MacManus *et al.*, 1971), as well as resting cells stimulated to
proliferate (e.g. hepatocytes in regenerating liver, MacManus *et al.*,
1973; Thrower and Ord, 1974) (Table 2).

Mouse bone marrow contains uncommitted germinal cells (stem
cells) which after transplantation produce colonies in the spleen of
heavily irradiated mice; each colony arises from a single cell (Becker
et al., 1963). Under normal conditions the stem cells are in the resting
state and are insensitive to the cytocidal actions of high specific
activity [^{3}H]thymidine or inhibitors of DNA synthesis (e.g.
hydroxyurea) which, however, kill the cells if they have been
triggered by various agents from G_0 into the proliferating state.
Therefore, after treatment with mitogens, the number of colonies
formed in the host spleen is reduced in comparison with the G_0-bone-
marrow cells exposed only to the cytocidal agents, and substances
which are able to induce the transition into the replicating state can be
screened. Using this technique, Byron (1974) has shown that neuro-
hormones can initiate DNA synthesis in haemopoietic stem cells. The
mechanisms seem to involve hormone receptors and cyclic nucleotide-
mediated intracellular reactions. Cell proliferation is triggered by very
low concentrations (10^{-14}–10^{-13} M) of both β-adrenergic agents—
isoproterenol (isoprenaline) or more specifically by β_1-adrenergic
agents, such as salbutamol and cholinergic agents. The action of
isoproterenol is inhibited by the β-receptor blocker, propranolol, and
that of acetylcholine by the nicotinic cholinergic receptor blocker
tubocurarine. In target cells β-adrenergic and cholinergic agents often
lead to elevated concentrations of cAMP and cGMP respectively (for
reviews Robison *et al.*, 1971; Goldberg *et al.*, 1974). Byron (1974) has
further observed that the proliferation of haemopoietic stem cells can
be triggered both by low concentrations of exogenous cyclic nucleotides (dibutyryl derivatives of cAMP or cGMP, DBcAMP or
DBcGMP) and by an elevation of the endogenous level of cyclic
nucleotides by phosphodiesterase inhibitors. Moreover, the stimu-

Table 2

Neurohumor receptors and cell proliferation

	Adrenergic agents	Cholinergic agents
Haemopoietic stem cells	$\beta_1\uparrow$ (Effect blocked by P)[1]	$\uparrow$ (Effect blocked by nicotinic blockers)[1]
Intact liver	IPR$\uparrow$[2]	
Lens epithelium	$\beta\downarrow$ (Effect blocked by P)[3]	
Epidermis	$\beta\downarrow$[4,5] (Effect blocked by P)	
Salivary glands (adults)	IPR$\uparrow$ (Effect not influenced by P)[2,6]	
Salivary glands (infant)	IPR$\downarrow$[7]	
Peripheral blood lymphocytes	IPR$\downarrow$; (moderate effect at high conc.)[8]	
Peripheral blood lymphocytes (PHA stimulation)	IPR 0[8] $\alpha\uparrow$, $\beta\updownarrow$ (During induction period)[9] $\alpha\uparrow$, $\beta\uparrow$ (At the peak of transformation)[9]	$\uparrow$ (Effect blocked by muscarinic blockers)[14]
Peripheral blood lymphocytes (chronic lymphocytic leukaemia)	IPR$\downarrow$[8,10]	
Thymic lymphoblasts	Adrenaline$\uparrow$[11]	
Regenerating liver	α-blockers $\downarrow$[12,13]	

The effects refer to the action of agents acting on neurohumor receptors: cell proliferation is stimulated $\uparrow$, inhibited $\downarrow$ or unaltered 0 (slight effects are indicated with dashed arrows). IPR, isoproterenol; P, propranolol; PHA, phytohaemagglutinin. IPR is mainly a β-adrenergic agonist; however, it seems advisable to refer to IPR action rather than β-adrenergic stimulation in those cases in which the influence of β-blockers on IPR action was not tested.

References: 1 Byron (1974); 2 Barka (1965); 3 Sallmann and Grimes (1974); 4 Bullough (1965); 5 Voorhees et al. (1974); 6 Durham et al. (1974); 7 Schneyer (1973); 8 Abell et al. (1970); 9 Hadden et al. (1970); 10 Johnson and Abell (1970); 11 MacManus et al. (1971); 12 MacManus et al. (1973); 13 Thrower and Ord (1974); 14 Goldberg et al. (1974).

lation of phosphodiesterase activity with imidazole suppressed the action of both the cholinergic agents and of DBcGMP. Cycloheximide but not actinomycin D, inhibited DBcGMP-induced cell proliferation suggesting that *de novo* protein synthesis is required, although the information for DNA synthesis is already present in the stem cells.

MacManus *et al.* (1971) have observed that adrenaline stimulates the proliferation of a subpopulation of rat thymic lymphoblasts. Again cyclic nucleotide systems are implicated: the effect of suboptimal concentrations of adrenaline is potentiated by phosphodiesterase inhibitors, and it is inhibited by phosphodiesterase stimulators such as imidazole. Furthermore, adrenaline stimulates the activity of adenylate cyclase and results in a rise in the concentration of cAMP which, when added at low concentrations $(10^{-8}–10^{-6}$ M), enhances the proliferation of thymic lymphoblasts (MacManus and Whitfield, 1969).

Goldberg *et al.* (1974) have tested the effects of acetylcholine on the transformation of human peripheral blood lymphocytes. The rate of precursor incorporation into RNA, protein and DNA is stimulated by the hormone, but acetylcholine on its own is not mitogenic. However, cholinergic agents potentiate the phytohaemagglutinin (PHA)-induced stimulation of DNA synthesis. Hadden *et al.* (1970) have observed that under special circumstances—short exposure of lymphocytes prior to PHA to adrenergic agents in presence of 10^{-5} M cortisol—the mitogenic action of PHA is somewhat potentiated by drugs stimulating α-adrenergic receptors, whereas it is inhibited by β-adrenergic agents. However, at the peak of lymphocyte transformation, both α- and β-adrenergic agonists slightly stimulate the incorporation of labelled thymidine.

The action of cholinergic agents in the lymphocytes has been found to be associated with an elevation of cellular cGMP concentration: this is much greater after PHA, about tenfold, than in the presence of acetylcholine, two- to threefold. Exogenous cGMP on its own can also promote RNA synthesis rate in the lymphocytes. It would appear that the mechanism underlying the intracellular expression of cGMP action has an obligatory requirement for increased translocation or transport of Ca^{2+} in the cells (Goldberg *et al.*, 1974). The involvement of Ca^{2+} in mitogenic mechanisms triggered by adrenergic receptor stimulation believed to be mediated through cAMP in thymic lymphoblasts has also been proposed by MacManus *et al.* (1975).

In the adult rat, mitotic activity is very low in the liver. Isoproterenol has been reported to stimulate significantly the proliferation of hepatocytes in intact animals (Barka, 1965). It is well known that in the liver a dramatic increase in cell proliferation can be effected at 18–24 h after partial hepatectomy. α-Adrenergic blocking agents (phenoxybenzamine or phentolamine) cause a significant delay in the onset of the first wave of DNA synthesis (MacManus *et al.*, 1973; Thrower and Ord, 1974), whereas β-adrenergic blocking agents fail to influence cell proliferation.

The early information on the effect of hormones (adrenaline) on the mouse epidermis has led to the hypothesis of the regulation of cell proliferation by tissue specific endogenous mitotic inhibitors (Bullough, 1965; for a recent review see Lozzio *et al.*, 1975). These hypothetical intracellular regulators may well be part of the control system involving mechanisms initiated by the stimulation of neuro-humor receptors and mediated through reactions triggered by changes in cyclic nucleotide systems. Caution must nevertheless be exercised in the general acceptance of the involvement of neurohumor receptors and cyclic nucleotide systems in the regulation of cell proliferation, since many receptor stimulating and blocking agents are notorious for non-specific binding at a variety of macromolecular sites producing effects by non-specific interactions (Triggle, 1971), and cyclic nu-cleotides, especially in the relatively high concentrations frequently used, may have non-physiological action. A case in point is the induction of DNA synthesis in the adult parotid gland by isoprotere-nol, which is a powerful β-adrenergic agent and leads to an elevation of cellular cAMP levels. However, Durham *et al.* (1974) have shown that isoproterenol induction is not prevented by the β-adrenergic blocker, propranolol, although the rise in cAMP concentration is inhibited. These authors have also observed that, in contrast to most other tissues, the nuclear fraction in the parotid gland retains a great proportion, about one quarter, of the tissue isoproterenol. Further-more, the effect of a mitogen may also depend on the development stage, for example, the mitotic activity is great in the salivary glands of infant rats (mitotic index, M.I. about 3%), whereas it is low after weaning (M.I. 0·1–0·2%). In contrast to the adult, in the infant rat isoproterenol suppresses mitotic activity in the parotid gland (Schneyer, 1973).

In Tables 2 and 3 we have attempted to give a simplified tabulation of the observations on the involvement of neurohumor receptors and and cyclic nucleotides on cell proliferation in different tissues. At present, the results are still equivocal: it seems that the response, for example, to β-adrenergic receptor stimulation depends on the cell type, and that the original proposal that cAMP is an obligatory

Table 3

Cyclic nucleotides and cell proliferation

	cAMP	cGMP
Haemopoietic stem cells	↑[1]	↑[1]
Peripheral blood lymphocytes		
Porcine	↑[2]	
Horse	0[3]	
Human	↑[4]	
Human, PHA stimulated	↓[4], 0[5], ↑[19]	↑[6]
Human (leukaemic), PHA stimulated	↓[5]	
Splenic lymphocytes	0[7]	↑[7]
Concanavalin A stimulated	↓[7]	↑[7]
Thymic lymphoblasts	↑[8]	↑[8]
Epidermis	↓[9]	↑[9]
Lens epithelium	↓[10]	
Fibroblasts	↓[11]	↑[16], ↓[17][b]
Hepatocytes (in vitro)	↑[12]	↑[12]
Regenerating liver	↑[8, 13][a]	0[8]
Neuroblastoma	↓[14, 15]	↓[18]
Glial tumors	↓[14, 15]	

This table is an obviously oversimplified representation of the relationship between cyclic nucleotides and cell replication: it mainly includes data concerning the growth response to exogenous cycle nucleotides, but in a few instances the direction of the change in the concentration of endogenous cyclic nucleotides upon mitogenic stimulation is also indicated. Cell proliferation is stimulated ↑, inhibited ↓ or unaltered 0 (slight effects are indicated with dashed arrows).

a Although there are cyclic changes in the hepatic concentration of cAMP preceeding cell proliferation after hepatectomy it is not certain that the phenomena are causally related (Thrower and Ord, 1974).

b Growth stimulation by serum is associated with a decrease in cGMP levels.

References: 1 Byron (1974); 2 Cross and Ord (1971); 3 Averner et al. (1972); 4 Hirschhorn et al. (1970); 5 Johnson and Abell (1970); 6 Goldberg et al. (1974); 7 Weinstein et al. (1974); 8 MacManus et al. (1975); 9 Voorhees et al. (1974); 10 Sallmann and Grimes (1974); 11 Anderson and Pastan (1975); 12 Armato et al. (1974); 13 Thrower and Ord (1974); 14 Jaffe et al. (1972); 15 McIntyre et al. (1972); 16 Seifert and Rudland (1974); 17 Miller et al. (1975); 18 Prasad and Kumar (1974); 19 Gallo and Whang-Peng (1974).

negative effector in cell proliferation must be substantially qualified (for review see Pastan et al., 1975). The effect of elevated cAMP concentration on cell proliferation is not necessarily inhibitory, rather it depends upon the period in the cell cycle when the concentration has been modified, for example, an increase in cAMP may be needed in late G_1 to initiate S phase (Willingham *et al.*, 1972). Similarly, stimulation of DNA synthesis by cAMP in thymic lymphoblasts (MacManus and Whitfield, 1969) and peripheral blood lymphocytes (Cross and Ord, 1971) may result from affecting a previously activated subpopulation of these cells (Abell and Monahan, 1973). Furthermore, not all mitogenic actions are mediated through changes in cAMP levels (e.g. transformation of lymphocytes by PHA; Novogrodsky and Katchalski, 1970). The effect of cAMP may also depend on the concentration of Ca^{2+}, which according to some investigators plays a major role in the control of mitotic activity (Goldberg *et al.*, 1974; MacManus *et al.*, 1975). An important expansion of the original hypothesis is the dualistic model of the regulation in which cAMP and cGMP function together in a reciprocal fashion to control growth and other cellular functions (Yin-Yang hypothesis, Goldberg *et al.*, 1974). However, even this hypothesis seems to fall short of matching the complexity of the problem (e.g. Miller *et al.*, 1975), and recent advances in this field indicate that the regulation of cell proliferation cannot be ascribed exclusively to modifications in the concentration of a few effector molecules.

In spite of these limitations, the working hypothesis implicating in the control of cell proliferation mechanisms mediated through neurohumor receptors—including receptors for growth stimulating hormone-like polypeptides, which because of limitation in space could not be considered in the present discussion (however for current review see e.g. Holley, 1975)—offers important experimental avenues for future research. Guided by this hypothesis we have been recently testing the effect of various neurohumor receptor stimulating and blocking agents, in an attempt to further the understanding of the action of reserpine on DNA synthesis in the brain. Preliminary results (Patel, Béndek and Balázs, unpublished results) indicate that cell proliferation in the brain is sensitive to cholinergic agents and to exogenous cyclic nucleotides.

It is evident that in order to further the elucidation of the control mechanisms involved in cell proliferation in the brain it would be of great value to have access to isolated replicating cells whose properties could be studied under conditions much simpler than prevailing *in vivo* when the operation of secondary regulatory mechanisms may induce many variables. Recent efforts in our laboratory are concentrated in this direction. We have succeeded in the preparation of ultrastructurally well-preserved perikarya from dissociated cerebellar tissue of developing rats (Cohen *et al.*, 1974; Balázs *et al.*, 1975b; Wilkin *et al.*, 1976). Furthermore, it was possible to separate a fraction which is greatly enriched in proliferating cells (Cohen, Dutton, Currie, Hajós and Balázs, unpublished observations). Approximately 30% of the cells in this fraction are engaged, under *in vitro* conditions, in replicative DNA synthesis and they also incorporate amino acids into histones which are known to be produced predominantly during the *S* phase of the cell cycle. These observations open up exciting experimental possibilities concerning not only the role of hormone receptors in the proliferation of germinal cells from the brain, but also the factors underlying differentiation of these cells.

References

Abell, C. W. and Monahan, T. M. (1973). *J. Cell. Biol.* **59**, 549–558.
Abell, C. W., Kamp, C. W. and Johnson, L. D. (1970). *Cancer Res.* **30**, 717–723.
Addison, W. H. F. (1911). *J. Comp. Neurol.* **21**, 459–485.
Allfrey, V. G. (1974). In "Acidic Proteins of the Nucleus" (I. L. Cameron and J. R. Jeter, jun., eds). Academic Press, New York and London, pp. 1–27.
Altman, J. (1969). In "Handbook of Neurochemistry" (A. Lajtha, ed.), Vol. 2. Plenum Press, New York, pp. 137–182.
Altman, J. and Anderson, W. J. (1971). *Exp. Neurol.* **30**, 492–509.
Anderson, W. B. and Pastan, I. (1975). In Advan. Cyclic Nucleotide Res. (G. I. Drummond, P. Greengard and G. A. Robison, eds), Vol. 5. Raven Press, New York, pp. 681–698.
Angevine, J. B., jun. (1965). *Exp. Neurol. Suppl.* **2**, 1–70.
Angevine, J. B., jun. and Sidman, R. L. (1961). *Nature (London)* **192**, 766–768.
Armato, V., Andreis, P. G., Draghin, E. and Meneghelli, V. (1974). *In vitro* **9**, 357.
Armstrong, D. M. and Schild, R. F. (1970). *J. Comp. Neurol.* **139**, 449–456.
Atlas, M. and Bond, V. P. (1965). *J. Cell Biol.* **26**, 19–24.
Averner, M. J., Brock, M. L. and Jost, J.-P. (1972). *J. Biol. Chem.* **247**, 413–417.
Axelrod, J. (1971/2) *Harvey Lect.* **67**, 175–197.
Balázs, R. (1976). In "Perspectives in Neurobiology" (M. A. Corner and D. F. Swaab, eds). Elsevier Press, Amsterdam.
Balázs, R. and Richter, D. (1973). In "Biochemistry of the Developing Brain" (W. Himwich, ed.), Vol. 1. Dekker, New York, pp. 253–299.
Balázs, R., Kovács, S., Teichgräber, P., Cocks, W. A. and Eayrs, J. T. (1968). *J. Neurochem.* **15**, 1335–1349.
Balázs, R., Kovács, S., Cocks, W. A., Johnson, A. L. and Eayrs, J. T. (1971). *Brain Res.* **25**, 555–570.
Balázs, R., Hajós, F., Johnson, A. L., Tapia, R. and Wilkin, G. (1974). *Biochem. Soc. Trans.* **2**, 682–687.
Balázs, R., Lewis, P. D. and Patel, A. J. (1975a). In "Growth and Development of the Brain. Nutritional, Genetic and Environmental Factors" (M. A. B. Brazier, ed.). Raven Press, New York, pp. 83–115.
Balázs, R., Wilkin, G. P., Wilson, J. E., Cohen, J. and Dutton, G. R. (1975b). In "Metabolic Compartmentation and Neurotransmission. Relation to Brain Structure and Function" (S. Berl, D. D. Clarke and D. Schneider, eds). Plenum Press, New York, pp. 437–448.

Baril, E., Baril, B., Elford, H. and Luftig, R. B. (1974). *In* "Mechanism and Regulation of DNA Replication" (A. R. Kolber and M. Kohiyama, eds). Plenum Press, New York, pp. 275–291.

Barka, T. (1965). *Exp. Cell Res.* **37**, 662–679.

Becker, A. J., McCulloch, E. A. and Till, J. E. (1963). *Nature (London)* **197**, 452–454.

Berry, M. (1974). *In* "Aspects of Neurogenesis. Studies on the Development of Behavior and the Nervous System" (G. Gottlieb, ed.), Vol. 2. Academic Press, New York and London, pp. 7–67.

Berry, M. and Hollingworth, T. (1973). *Experientia* **29**, 204–207.

Berry, M. and Rogers, A. W. (1966). *In* "Evolution of the Forebrain" (R. Hassler and H. Stephan, eds). Thieme, Stuttgart, pp. 197–205.

Berry, M., Rogers, A. W. and Eayrs, J. T. (1964). *Nature (London)* **203**, 591–593.

Bignami, A. and Dahl, D. (1974). *J. Comp. Neurol.* **155**, 219–230.

Black, I. B. (1975). *Brain Res.* **95**, 170–176.

Boulder Committee (1970). *Anat. Record* **166**, 257–262.

Bullough, W. S. (1965). *Cancer Res.* **25**, 1683–1727.

Byron, J. W. (1974). *In* "Cell Cycle Controls" (G. M. Padilla, I. L. Cameron and A. Zimmerman, eds). Academic Press, New York and London, pp. 87–99.

Cavanagh, J. B. (1970). *J. Anat.* **106**, 471–487.

Cihák, A. and Vaptzarova, K. (1973). *Brit. J. Pharmacol.* **49**, 253–257.

Cleaver, J. E. (1967). "Thymidine Metabolism and Cell Kinetics". North-Holland, Amsterdam.

Clendinnen, B. G. and Eayrs, J. T. (1961). *J. Endocrinol.* **22**, 183–193.

Clos, J. and Legrand, J. (1973). *Brain Res.* **63**, 450–455.

Cohen, J., Dutton, G. R., Wilkin, G. P., Wilson, J. E. and Balázs, R. (1974). *J. Neurochem.* **23**, 899–901.

Cotterrell, M. (1971). M. Phil. Thesis. Council for National Academic Awards, London.

Cotterrell, M., Balázs, R. and Johnson, A. L. (1972). *J. Neurochem.* **19**, 2151–2167.

Cross, M. E. and Ord, M. G. (1971). *Biochem. J.* **124**, 241–248.

Dobbing, J. and Smart, J. (1974). *Brit. Med. Bull.* **30**, 164–168.

Durham, J. P., Baserga, R. and Butcher, F. R. (1974). *In* "Control of Proliferation in Animal Cells" (B. Clarkson and R. Baserga, eds). Cold Spring Harbour Laboratory, pp. 595–607.

Dyduch, A. (1973) *Acta Physiol.* **24**, 503–516.

Eccles, J. C., Ito, M. and Szentágothai, J. (1967). "The Cerebellum as a Neuronal Machine". Springer, Berlin.

Ellenberger, C., jun., Hanaway, J. and Netsky, M. G. (1969). *J. Comp. Neurol.* **137**, 71–88.

Ford, D. H. (1975). "Anatomy of the Central Nervous System in Review". Elsevier Press, Amsterdam.

Fujita, S. (1969). *In* "Neurobiology of Cerebellar Evolution and Development" (R. Llinas, ed.). AMA Educ. Res. Found. Chicago, pp. 743–747.

Fujita, S., Shimada, M. and Nakamura, T. (1966). *J. Comp. Neurol.* **128**, 191–208.

Gallo, R. C. and Whang-Peng, J. (1971). *J. Nat. Cancer Inst.* **47**, 91–94.

Gilmour, S. R. (1974). *In* "Acidic Proteins of the Nucleus" (I. L. Cameron and J. R. Jeter, jun., eds). Academic Press, New York and London, pp. 297–317.

Giuffrida, A. M., Cambria, A., Avitabile, M., Serra, I. and Vanella, A. (1975). 5th Int. Meet. Int. Soc. Neurochem., Barcelona, p. 425.

Glücksmann, A. (1951). *Biol. Rev.* **26**, 59–86.

Goldberg, N. D., Haddox, M. K., Dunham, E., Lopez, C. and Hadden, J. W. (1974). *In* "Control of Proliferation in Animal Cells" (B. Clarkson and R. Baserga, eds). Cold Spring Harbour Laboratory, pp. 609–625.

Goldin, A., Burton, R. M., Humphreys, S. R. and Venditti, J. M. (1957). *Science* **125**, 156–157.

Gona, A. G. (1973). *Exp. Neurol.* **38**, 494–501.

Goodman, R., Otten, V. and Thoenen, H. (1975). *J. Neurochem* **25**, 423–427.

Gourdon, J., Clos, J., Coste, C., Dainat, J. and Legrand, J. (1973). *J. Neurochem.* **21**, 861–871.

Greengard, P., Kuo, J. F. and Miyamoto, E. (1971). *Advan. Enzyme Regul.* **9**, 113–125.

Guidotti, A., Hanbauer, I. and Costa, E. (1975). *In* "Advan. Cyclic Nucleotide Res." (G. I. Drummond, P. Greengard and G. A. Robison, eds), Vol. 5. Raven Press, New York, pp. 619–639.

Gwóźdź, B., Dyduch, A. and Kozielski, J. (1973). *Pol. J. Pharmacol. Pharm.* **25**, 341–344.

Hadden, J. W., Hadden, E. M. and Middleton, E. (1970). *Cell. Immunol.* **1**, 583–595.

Hamburger, V. and Levi-Montalcini, R. (1949). *J. Exp. Zool.* **111**, 457–500.

Hamburgh, M. (1968). *Gen. Comp. Endocrinol.* **10**, 198–213.

Hicks, S. P. and D'Amato, C. J. (1968). *Anat. Record* **160**, 619–634.

Hirschhorn, R., Grossman, J. and Weissmann, G. (1970). *Proc. Soc. Exp. Biol. Med.* **133**, 1361–1365.

Hoeldtke, R., Lloyd, T. and Kaufman, S. (1974). *Biochem. Biophys. Res. Commun.* **57**, 1045–1053.

Hajós, F., Patel, A. J. and Balázs, R. (1973). *Brain Res.* **50**, 387–401.

Holley, R. W. (1975). *Nature (London)* **258**, 487–490.

Howard, E. (1965). *J. Neurochem.* **12**, 181–191.

Howard, E. (1974). *In* "Biochemistry of the Developing Brain" (W. Himwich, ed.), Vol. 2. Dekker, New York, pp. 1–68.

Hunt, R. K. and Jacobson, M. (1971). *Develop. Biol.* **26**, 100–124.

Jacobson, M. (1970). "Developmental Neurobiology". Holt, Rinehart and Winston, Inc., New York.

Jaffe, B. M., Philpott, G. W., Hamprecht, B. and Parker, C. W. (1972). *Advan. Biol. Sci.* **9**, 179–182.

Joh, T. H., Geghman, G. and Reis, D. (1973). *Proc. Nat. Acad. Sci. U.S.A.* **70**, 2767–2771.

Johnson, L. D. and Abell, C. W. (1970). *Cancer Res.* **30**, 2718–2723.

Karfunkel, P. (1974). *Int. Rev. Cytol.* **38**, 245–271.

Kauffman, S. L. (1968). *Exp. Cell Res.* **49**, 420–424.

Kollros, J. J. (1968). *In* "Ciba Foundation Symposium on Growth of the Nervous System" (G. E. W. Wolstenholme and M. O'Connor, eds). Churchill, London, pp. 179–192.

Legrand, J. (1967). *Arch. Anat. Microsc. Morphol. Exp.* **56**, 205–244.

Le Stourgeon, W. M., Totten, R. and Fores, A. (1974). *In* "Acidic Proteins of the Nucleus" (I. L. Cameron and J. R. Jeter, jun., eds). Academic Press, New York and London, pp. 159–190.

Lewis, P. D. (1975). *Neuropath. Appl. Neurobiol.* **1**, 21–29.

Lewis, P. D., Balázs, R., Patel, A. J. and Johnson, A. L. (1975). *Brain Res.* **83**, 235–247.

Lewis, P. D., Patel, A. J., Johnson, A. L. and Balázs, R. (1976). *Brain Res.* **104**, 49–62.

Lewis, P. D., Patel, A. J., Bénedek, G. and Balázs, R. (1976b). *Brain Res.* (in press).

Lozzio, B. B., Lozzio, C. B., Bamberger, E. G. and Lair, S. V. (1975). *Int. Rev. Cytol.* **42**, 1–47.

Mackay, A. V. P. and Iversen, L. L. (1972). *Brain Res.* **48**, 424–426.
MacManus, J. P. and Whitfield, J. F. (1969). *Exp. Cell. Res.* **58**, 188–191.
MacManus, J. P., Whitfield, J. F. and Youdale, T. (1971). *J. Cell Physiol.* **77**, 103–116.
MacManus, J. P., Braceland, B. M., Youdale, T. and Whitfield, J. F. (1973). *J. Cell Physiol.* **82**, 157–164.
MacManus, J. P., Whitfield, J. F., Boynton, A. L. and Rixon, R. H. (1975). *In* "Advan. Cyclic Nucleotide Res." (G. I. Drummond, P. Greengard and G. A. Robison, eds), Vol. 5. Raven Press, New York, pp. 719–734.
Maina, G. (1974). *Biochim. Biophys. Acta* **333**, 481–486.
McIntyre, E. H., Wintersgill, C. J., Perkins, J. P. and Vatter, A. E. (1972). *J. Cell Sci.* **11**, 639–667.
McMorris, F. A., Nelson, P. G. and Ruddee, F. H. (eds) (1973). "Contributions of Clonal Systems to Neurobiology", NRP Bull. Vol. 11(5). NRP, Boston.
Mendes, C. B. and Waterlow, J. C. (1958). *Brit. J. Nutr.* **12**, 74–88.
Miale, I. L. and Sidman, R. L. (1961). *Exp. Neurol.* **4**, 277–296.
Millard, S. A. (1974). *In* "Reviews in Neurosciences" (S. Ehrenpreis and I. J. Kopin, eds), Vol. 1. Raven Press, New York, pp. 115–136.
Miller, Z., Lovelace, E., Gallo, M. and Pastan, I. (1975). *Science* **190**, 1213–1215.
Mori, K., Yamagami, S. and Kawakita, Y. (1970). *J. Neurochem.* **17**, 835–843.
Muzzo, J. and Brasel, J. A. (1973). *Endocrinology* **92**, 155A.
Nelson, P. G. (1975). *Physiol. Rev.* **55**, 1–61.
Nicholson, J. L. and Altman, J. (1972). *Brain Res.* **44**, 13–23.
Novogrodsky, A. and Katchalski, E. (1970). *Biochim. Biophys. Acta* **215**, 291–296.
Otten, V., Mueller, R. A., Oesch, F. and Thoenen, H. (1974). *Proc. Nat. Acad. Sci. U.S.A.* **71**, 2217–2221.
Palay, S. L. and Chan-Palay, V. (1974). "Cerebellar Cortex, Cytology and Organization". Springer, Berlin.
Pastan, I. H., Johnson, G. S. and Anderson, W. B. (1975). *Ann. Rev. Biochem.* **44**, 491–522.
Patel, A. J., Balázs, R. and Johnson, A. L. (1973). *J. Neurochem.* **20**, 1151–1165.
Patel, A. J., Rabié, A., Lewis, P. D. and Balázs, R. (1976). *Brain Res.* **104**, 33–48.
Patel, A. J., Bénedek, G., Balázs, R. and Lewis, P. D. (1976b). *Brain Res.* (in press).
Pesetsky, I. (1976). *In* "Thyroxine and Brain Development" (G. D. Grave, ed.) (in press).
Phelps, C. H. and Pfeiffer, S. E. (1975). *In* "Cell Cycle and Cell Differentiation" (J. Reinert and Holtzer, H., eds). Springer, Berlin, pp. 63–83.
Pollak, R. D. and Fallon, J. F. (1974). *Exp. Cell Res.* **86**, 9–14.
Prasad, K. N. and Kumar, S. (1974). *In* "Control of Proliferation in Animal Cells" (B. Clarkson and R. Baserga, eds). Cold Spring Harbor Laboratory, pp. 581–594.
Raaf, J. and Kernohan, J. W. (1944). *Amer. J. Anat.* **75**, 151–172.
Rakic, P. (1971a). *Brain Res.* **33**, 471–476.
Rakic, P. (1971b). *J. Comp. Neurol.* **141**, 283–312.
Ramon y Cajal, P. (1890). *Int. Monatschr. Anat. Physiol (Leipzig)* **7**, 12–31.
Richelson, E. (1973). *Nature, New Biol.* **242**, 175–177.
Reis, D. J., Joh, T. H., Ross, R. A. and Pickel, V. M. (1974). *Brain Res.* **81**, 380–386.
Robison, G. A., Butcher, R. W. and Sutherland, E. W. (1971). "Cyclic AMP". Academic Press, New York and London.
Rutter, W. J., Pictet, R. L. and Morris, P. W. (1973). *Annu. Rev. Biochem.* **42**, 601–646.

Sallmann, von. L. and Grimes, P. (1974). *Invest. Ophthalmol.* **13**, 210–218.
Sara, V. R. and Lazarus, L. (1975). *Develop. Psychobiol.* **8**, 489–502.
Sato, G. (ed.) (1973). "Tissue Culture of the Nervous System". Plenum Press, New York.
Sauer, F. C. (1935). *J. Comp. Neurol.* **62**, 377–405.
Sauer, F. C. (1936). *J. Morphol.* **60**, 1–11.
Schneyer, C. A. (1973). *Proc. Soc. Exp. Biol. Med.* **143**, 899–904.
Seifert, W. E. and Rudland, P. S. (1974). *Nature (London)* **248**, 138–140.
Short, J., Armstrong, N. B., Kolitsky, M. A., Mitchell, R. A., Zemel, R. and Lieberman, I. (1974). *In* "Control of Proliferation in Animal Cells" (B. Clarkson and R. Baserga, eds). Cold Spring Harbor Laboratory, pp. 37–48.
Sidman, R. L. (1970). *In* "Contemporary Research Methods in Neuroanatomy" (W. J. H. Nauta and S. O. E. Eddesson eds). Springer, Berlin, pp. 252–274.
Smolyaninov, V. V. (1971). *In* "Models of the Structural–Functional Organization of Certain Biological Systems" (I. M. Gelfand, V. S. Gurfinkel, S. V. Fomin and M. L. Tsetlin, eds). MIT Press, Cambridge, Massachusetts and London, pp. 250–423.
Sotelo, C. and Changeux, J.-P. (1974a). *Brain Res.* **67**, 519–526.
Sotelo, C. and Changeux, J.-P. (1974b). *Brain Res.* **77**, 484–491.
Spemann, H. (1938). "Embryonic Development and Induction". Yale Univ. Press, New Haven, Conn.
Steel, G. G. and Hanes, S. (1971). *Cell Tissue Kinet.* **4**, 93–105.
Swarz, J. R. and Del Cerro, M. (1975). "Neuroscience Abstracts, 5th Ann. Meet. Soc. Neurosci". Soc. Neurosci., Bethesda, p. 760.
Taber-Pierce, E. (1967). *J. Comp. Neurol.* **131**, 27–54.
Theonen, H. (1970). *Nature (London)* **228**, 861–862.
Thrower, S. and Ord, M. G. (1974). *Biochem. J.* **144**, 361–369.
Triggle, D. J. (1971). "Neurotransmitter-Receptor Interactions". Academic Press, New York and London.
Van Wijk, R., Wicks, W. D., Bevers, M. M. and Van Rijn, J. (1973). *Cancer Res.* **33**, 1331–1338.
Vonderhaar, B. K. and Topper, Y. J. (1974). *J. Cell Biol.* **63**, 707–712.
Voorhees, J. J., Colburn, N. H., Stawiski, M., Duell, E. A., Haddox, M. and Goldberg, N. D. (1974). *In* "Control of Proliferation of Animal Cells" (B. Clarkson and R. Baserga, eds). Cold Spring Harbor Laboratory, pp. 635–648.
Weichsel, M. E., jun. (1974). *Brain Res.* **78**, 455–465.
Weichsel, M. E., jun. and Dawson, L. (1976). *J. Neurochem.* **26**, 675–681.
Weinstein, Y., Chambers, D. A., Bourne, H. R. and Melmon, K. L. (1974). *Nature (London)* **251**, 352–353.
West, W. L., Baird, G. M., Steward, J. D. and Pradhan, S. N. (1961). *J. Pharmacol. Exp. Ther.* **131**, 171–178.
Weston, J. A. (1971). *In* "Cellular Aspects of Neural Growth and Differentiation" (D. C. Pease, ed.), UCLA in Medical Sciences, No. 14, pp. 1–19.
Wiebecke, B., Heybowitz, R., Löhrs, U. and Eder, M. (1969). *Virchows Arch. Abt. B. Zellpath.* **4**, 164–175.
Wilkin, G. P., Balázs, R., Wilson, J., Cohen, J. and Dutton, G. R. (1976). *Brain Res.* **115**, 181–199.
Willingham, M. C., Johnson, G. S. and Pastan, I. (1972). *Biochem. Biophys. Res. Com.* **48**, 743–748.
Winick, M. (1969). *J. Pediat.* **74**, 667–679.

Woodard, J. S. (1960). *J. Comp. Neurol.* **115**, 65–73.

Yamagami, S., Kiriike, N. and Nawakita, Y. (1973). 4th Int. Meet. Int. Soc. Neurochem., Tokyo, p. 430.

Zamenhof, S. (1941). *Growth* **5**, 123–139.

Zamenhof, S., Mosley, J. and Schuller, E. (1966). *Science* **152**, 1396–1397.

Zamenhof, S., Marthens, van E. and Grauel, L. (1971). *Science* **174**, 954–955.

Zigmond, R. E., Schon, F. and Iversen, L. L. (1974). *Brain Res.* **70**, 547–552.

Chapter 4

Cyclic Nucleotides and Neuronal Function: Cyclic-GMP-Dependent Photoreceptor Degeneration in Inherited Retinal Diseases

RICHARD N. LOLLEY AND DEBORA B. FARBER

Developmental Neurology Laboratory, Veterans Administration Hospital, Sepulveda, California 91343, and Department of Anatomy, University of California School of Medicine at Los Angeles, California 90024, U.S.A.

I. Introduction

Our interest in cyclic nucleotide metabolism of neuronal tissue has grown over the years as it has become evident that adenosine 3′,5′-monophosphate (cyclic AMP) and guanosine 3′,5′-monophosphate (cyclic GMP) are potential regulators of neuronal function. The body of information accumulated on this subject is extensive and varied, but one important generalization to consider from the very beginning is that cyclic AMP and cyclic GMP regulate different and probably opposing systems within a neurone.

To those of us who are interested in diseases of the nervous system, it follows that a regulator of neuronal function is a potential candidate for promoting neuronal dysfunction. Several diseases in which cyclic nucleotide abnormalities occur have already been described and it is possible that others will follow. In our particular case, we have information that links an abnormality in cyclic nucleotide metabolism with the inherited disorders of the retina which cause photoreceptor cell degeneration and blindness.

The retina is a region of the central nervous system that is highly specialized for the reception of light and the transmission of encoded visual information to the brain. Its metabolism of cyclic nucleotides is similar in some respects to that of other regions of the central nervous system and, for that reason, we will provide background information that applies to the metabolism of cyclic AMP and cyclic GMP in the brain. In other respects, the metabolism of cyclic nucleotides in the retina is unusual, and it is in the specialization of cyclic GMP metabolism in photoreceptor cells that we find a dysfunction which leads to photoreceptor cell degeneration.

II. Cyclic Nucleotides in the Central Nervous System (CNS)

For the sake of clarity, we will discuss separately the metabolism of cyclic AMP and cyclic GMP. Such a separation is not intended to suggest that the cyclic nucleotides always act independently for it is known that there are cases in which their combined action is necessary for effective control of physiological events. Such interactions and the Ying-Yang hypothesis will be mentioned at the close of this section.

A. *Cyclic AMP*

1. *Metabolism*

The concentration of cyclic AMP in the brain, spinal cord or retina is controlled largely by the relative activities of adenylate cyclase and cyclic nucleotide phosphodiesterase, the enzymes responsible, respectively, for the formation of cyclic AMP from ATP and for its degradation to 5′-AMP. Of all the mammalian tissues studied, brain has been shown to contain the highest levels of both adenylate cyclase and cyclic nucleotide phosphodiesterase activities (Sutherland *et al.*, 1962; Butcher and Sutherland, 1962; Breckenridge and Johnston,

1969; Williams et al., 1969). Both enzymes are concentrated in grey matter (Weiss and Costa, 1968) and, particularly, in subcellular fractions rich in synaptic elements (DeRobertis et al., 1967). It has been observed that most regions of the brain possess a capacity to degrade cyclic AMP which is greater than that for its synthesis. Exceptions are found in cerebellum, corpora quadrigemina and pineal gland (Weiss and Costa, 1968). The steady-state level of cyclic AMP that results from the balanced activity of adenylate cyclase and phosphodiesterase also varies between regions of the brain. The factors that control it appear to be complex since there are agents which modify the activity both of adenylate cyclase and phosphodiesterase or which sequester cyclic AMP from its degrading enzyme. The following discussion will touch upon some of these factors in an effort to present the dynamics of cyclic AMP metabolism in the central nervous system (CNS).

The rate at which cyclic AMP is synthesized in the CNS is dependent upon the degree to which adenylate cyclase is activated by divalent cations (Bradham, 1972), neurotransmitter agents or drugs. For example, the formation of cyclic AMP in brain slices has been shown to be stimulated by putative neurotransmitters such as epinephrine, norepinephrine, histamine, serotonin and adenosine (Kakiuchi and Rall, 1968a, 1968b; Sattin and Rall, 1970; Huang et al., 1971; Forn and Krishna, 1971; Schultz and Daly, 1973). Cyclic AMP synthesis is increased also by prostaglandin E_1 or electrical stimulation (Kakiuchi et al., 1969; Shimizu et al., 1970; Berti et al., 1973). Depolarizing agents such as ouabain, veratridine, glutamate or high concentrations of potassium ions also increase cyclic AMP synthesis by indirectly causing the release of adenosine (Shimizu and Daly, 1972; Huang et al., 1972). The ability of these agents to stimulate adenylate cyclase activity in neural tissue is dependent upon the morphological integrity of the tissue because, when homogenates of brain are tested, little if any stimulation of cyclic AMP formation is produced by the biogenic amines, adenosine or prostaglandin E_1 (Sattin and Rall, 1970; McCune et al., 1971; Drummond et al., 1971). The extent to which these agents stimulate adenylate cyclase activity in homogenates depends upon the method used for tissue disruption and upon the procedures which are employed for testing the activity of adenylate cyclase. Recently, tissue homogenization and cell fraction-ation techniques have been described which produce a cell-free particulate preparation from brain that retains a hormone-responsive adenylate cyclase (Chasin et al., 1974).

Another putative neurotransmitter that has been studied extensively for its ability to stimulate adenylate cyclase activity is dopamine. Brown and Makman (1972) have shown that dopamine stimulates adenylate cyclase activity in retinal homogenates of various mammalian species and that, in the intact retina, dopamine stimulation results in an increased formation of cyclic AMP (Mishra et al., 1974; Makman et al., 1975). Similarly, Kebabian et al. (1972) have demonstrated a dopamine-sensitive adenylate cyclase in homogenates of caudate nucleus of rat brain, and Clement-Cormier et al. (1974) have reported analogous results in homogenates of olfactory tubercle and nucleus accumbens of mammalian brain. Recently, the action of dopaminergic agonists on adenylate cyclase has been studied in detail using homogenates of rat striatum (Iversen et al., 1975; Miller and Iversen, 1974). A dopamine-sensitive adenylate cyclase has been described also in homogenates of bovine superior cervical ganglia (Kebabian and Greengard, 1971) and of thoracic ganglia from insects (Nathanson and Greengard, 1973). In the latter, the adenylate cyclase is also sensitive to octopamine and serotonin (Nathanson and Greengard, 1973, 1974).

Several models have been proposed for the adenylate cyclase system in an attempt to explain the regulation of adenylate cyclase activity by specific hormones. Robison et al. (1967) have suggested that the enzyme is an integral part of the plasma membrane, with a regulatory subunit facing the external milieu of the cell and a catalytic subunit exposed on the inner surface. Hormone interaction with the receptor unit causes an alteration in the receptor which in turn alters the catalytic subunit in a way that leads to increased enzyme activity. They suggested that both α- and β-adrenergic receptors are regulatory subunits of adenylate cyclase.

A model proposed by Hechter and Halkerson (1964) differs from that of Robison et al. (1967) only in that it considers intermediate moieties functioning between the hormone receptor and the catalytic unit. In another model, adenylate cyclase is a regulatory enzyme formed by a hormone discriminator (receptor), a transducer, and an amplifier (catalytic subunit) (Birnbaumer et al., 1970; Rodbell, 1971). The discriminator would be an allosteric site for hormone interaction on a regulatory subunit. The transducer component is visualized as the alterations in enzyme conformation which result in changes in activity of the catalytic subunit. Perkins (1973) suggested still another model in which the adenylate cyclase system would be composed of distinct receptor and catalytic moieties which would be physically separated but capable of interaction as a result of their location in a dynamic lipid matrix (the plasma membrane).

Each of these models accept that the activity of adenylate cyclase in brain is regulated via receptors linked to the membrane-bound enzyme. Furthermore, drugs can compete with hormones for the receptor sites. It follows from these observations that pharmacologically-active agents, which are agonists or antagonists at such receptors, owe their activity to their ability to alter the level of cyclic AMP. In addition to α- or β-adrenergic blocking agents, like phentolamine (α) or propanolol (β), several other drugs have been reported to compete for the receptor sites and prevent the accumulation of cyclic AMP in brain tissue. Phenothiazines and phenothiazine metabolites, for example, inhibit central adrenergic receptors as well as norepinephrine-induced (Kakiuchi and Rall, 1968a; Gordon, 1967; Free *et al.*, 1974; Palmer *et al.*, 1971; Palmer and Manian, 1974a, 1974b; Uzunov and Weiss, 1971) and dopamine-induced (Makman *et al.*, 1975) stimulation of adenylate cyclase. Antihistamines, like chlorphreniramine and pyrilamine, block histamine-stimulated increases of cyclic AMP (Chasin *et al.*, 1971). Theophylline not only acts on cyclic AMP levels by inhibiting phosphodiesterase but also by competitively blocking the adenosine-stimulated accumulation of cyclic AMP (Sattin and Rall, 1970; Sattin *et al.*, 1975).

Another agent that increases the activity of adenylate cyclase in brain homogenates is sodium fluoride (Perkins and Moore, 1971). Even though the mechanism of this stimulation remains unclear, it seems to be different from the activation by hormones. Fluoride, unlike hormones, does not stimulate adenylate cyclase activity of intact cells, having an effect only on broken cell preparations. Furthermore, inhibition of hormone-dependent enzyme activation does not prevent stimulation by fluoride. Additionally, the activity of adenylate cyclase increases when brain homogenates are treated with detergents and it cannot be further stimulated by fluoride. On the other hand, the activity of fluoride-stimulated adenylate cyclase can be increased further by detergents, indicating that sodium fluoride does not cause full expression of enzyme activity. These data are interpreted to indicate that sodium fluoride alters the state of the adenylate cyclase enzyme complex within the membrane structure. Perkins and Moore (1971) suggest that in the membrane the adenylate cyclase enzyme exists in an inhibited state. Hormones, interacting with the regulatory subunit, reduce the normal inhibition imposed on the catalytic subunit. Agents such as sodium fluoride or conditions such as freezing-and-thawing, which disrupt the structure of the membrane, cause a dissociation of the adenylate cyclase complex and, correspondingly, reduce the inhibition imposed on the catalytic subunit. Therefore, adenylate cyclase can be activated either through the physiological activity of hormones *in situ* or through non-specific perturbations of the membrane *in vitro*.

This brief introduction to the adenylate cyclase enzyme which synthesizes cyclic AMP is intended to convey the picture that adenylate cyclase is a part of a large membrane complex. This complex has the capacity to bind specific agents, and the chemical binding initiates a series of molecular changes that result in the activation of adenylate cyclase. The system is dynamic and subject to rapid and reversible change.

Studies of the developing CNS show that the activity of adenylate cyclase increases during postnatal life and that the capacity for hormone stimulation of adenylate cyclase is demonstrable after a basal level of adenylate cyclase activity is established (Schmidt *et al.*, 1970). In brain slices (Schmidt *et al.*, 1970), retina (Makman *et al.*, 1975) and pineal gland (Weiss, 1971) of rat and in retina of mice (Lolley *et al.*, 1974), the capacity for hormone stimulation is demonstrable by the second week of postnatal life. Thereafter, until there are changes with aging (Walker and Walker, 1973), hormone sensitivity of the adenylate cyclase system appears to remain relatively constant.

The hydrolytic cleavage of cyclic AMP to 5'-AMP, catalysed by cyclic nucleotide phosphodiesterase, is the only well-established mechanism by which the biologic actions of cyclic AMP are terminated. Several lines of evidence suggest that there are multiple forms of cyclic nucleotide phosphodiesterase in brain tissue. Brooker *et al.* (1968) and Thompson and Appleman (1971a, 1971b) provided kinetic data which showed that homogenates of brain exhibit at least two K_m values for cyclic AMP. Additional evidence that multiple forms of phosphodiesterase do exist in brain tissue was found in the separation of these enzymes using gel filtration (Thompson and Appleman, 1971b; Kakiuchi *et al.*, 1972), starch gel electrophoresis (Mann and Christiansen, 1971) and polyacrylamide gel electrophoresis (Uzunov and Weiss, 1972; Campbell and Oliver, 1972).

Different areas of brain have their own unique pattern and ratios of the multiple forms of phosphodiesterase. Rat cerebellum has six (Uzunov and Weiss, 1972), rat cerebrum, four (Uzunov *et al.*, 1974), and rat caudate nucleus only two (Fertel and Weiss, 1974) major forms of phosphodiesterase activity. These isoenzymes have distinguishing properties, for example, different stabilities, substrate specificities, kinetics and sensitivities to an endogenous activator and to several inhibitors.

The existence of a heat-stable non-dialysable protein activator of phosphodiesterase isolated from bovine brain, originally described by Cheung (1971), has been confirmed by several other investigators (Kakiuchi et al., 1972; Uzunov and Weiss, 1972; Weiss et al., 1974). The activator specifically enhances the activity of only one of the major forms of phosphodiesterase in brain (Uzunov and Weiss, 1972; Kakiuchi et al., 1973; Lin et al., 1974). The activity of this enzyme is also controlled by Ca^{2+}. Lin et al. (1974) suggest that the active form of the protein activator of phosphodiesterase is a Ca^{2+}-activator complex. Since the level of activator in brain tissue is usually in excess of the enzyme (Smoake et al., 1974), phosphodiesterase activity in vivo may be modulated by Ca^{2+}:

$$Ca^{2+} + \text{activator} \rightleftharpoons Ca^{2+} \cdot \text{activator}$$

$$(\text{Enzyme})_{\text{inactive}} + (Ca^{2+} \cdot \text{activator}) \rightleftharpoons [\text{Enzyme} \cdot (Ca^{2+} \cdot \text{activator})]_{\text{active.}}$$

The following observations are relevant to the stoichiometry of the reaction. The enzyme-activator complex has an apparent molecular weight of 200 000 when it is isolated by gel filtration (Teshima and Kakiuchi, 1974). In the presence of EGTA, it dissociates into two components having apparent molecular weights of 150 000 (inactive enzyme) and 28 000 (protein activator). These data suggest that more than one activator molecule may bind to one molecule of phosphodiesterase. In support of this conclusion, it was observed that the Hill interaction coefficient of the effect of the activator on the enzyme was approximately two. While most of the isoenzymes of phosphodiesterase from neural tissue can hydrolyse both cyclic AMP and cyclic GMP in vitro, the form of phosphodiesterase which requires the protein activator appears to prefer cyclic GMP as its substrate (Teshima and Kakiuchi, 1974).

Biochemical and cytochemical investigations of brain phosphodiesterases suggest that they are either soluble enzymes or loosely associated with membranes. After homogenization of brain tissue and centrifugation, phosphodiesterase activity is found in the 100 000-g soluble supernatant (Strada et al., 1974). Localization of phosphodiesterase in brain, observed by EM cytochemistry, shows activity restricted primarily to the postsynaptic region of nerve endings, with most of it immediately adjacent to the synaptic membrane (Florendo et al., 1971; Adinolfi and Schmidt, 1974).

In terms of cyclic nucleotide metabolism in the CNS, it is relevant to consider the ways by which the activity of cyclic nucleotide phosphodiesterase can be modified. Schultz (1975) has reported the regulation of phosphodiesterase by calcium in cerebral cortical slices of guinea-pig. He suggests that an increase in intracellular cyclic

AMP levels following hormonal stimulation results in an elevation of available intracellular Ca^{2+}. The free calcium then enhances phosphodiesterase activity and promotes the hydrolysis of cyclic AMP. Such a mechanism would constitute a kind of self-regulatory system in which cyclic AMP stimulates its own breakdown.

Many compounds of diverse chemical structure have been found which differentially inhibit the phosphodiesterase enzymes (Beer *et al.*, 1972; Chasin *et al.*, 1972; Pichard *et al.*, 1972; Schultz, 1974a, 1974b; Berndt and Schwabe, 1973; Uzunov and Weiss, 1971; Vernikos-Danellis and Harris, 1968), e.g. theophylline, isobutyl-methylxanthine, papaverine, neuroleptic and tricyclic antidepressive agents, phenothiazines, reserpine and benzodiazepines. In addition, SQ 20009, 1-ethyl-4-(isopropylidenehydrazino)-1H-pyrazolo-1 (3,4-b) pyridine-5-carboxylic acid, ethyl ester, hydrochloride), and compounds belonging to a family of 4-(3,4,-dialkoxybenzyl)-2-imidazolidinenes, like Ro 20-1724 and Ro 20-2926, have been shown to be very powerful phosphodiesterase inhibitors. All of these inhibitors not only produce different degrees of inhibition of the various forms of phosphodiesterase but seem to achieve the inhibition by the following mechanisms (Weiss, 1975a): 1. competitively blocking access of the substrate to the active site of the enzyme (e.g., theophylline and low concentrations of papaverine); 2. acting as non-competitive antagonists of the substrate (high concentrations of papaverine and inhibitors which are structurally unrelated to the substrate fall into this group) and 3. interfering with the activation of phosphodiesterase (phenothiazines, trifluoperazine and compounds which specifically bind calcium ions might be in this category).

During postnatal development of brain, the activity of cyclic nucleotide phosphodiesterase increases significantly (Strada *et al.*, 1974). The postnatal increase may result from a selective increase in one or more of the enzyme forms or from an increase in the concentration of the Ca^{2+}-activator complex. Strada *et al.* (1974) reported differences between patterns and ratios of phosphodiesterase activities in the 100 000-g soluble supernatants from brains of newborn and adult rats. They also showed postnatal changes in the activity of the phosphodiesterase activator: it increases with age in cerebellum and decreases in cerebrum and brain stem.

This synopsis of cyclic nucleotide phosphodiesterase in the CNS is intended to inform the reader of the multiple forms of the enzyme and of their individuality with respect to kinetics, activator requirements and drug susceptibility. Their postsynaptic localization and potential for controlling cyclic nucleotide levels in this dynamic region are features which emphasize the importance of phosphodiesterase activity in the biochemistry and function of the synapse.

2. Role and mechanism of action

The content of cyclic AMP in rat brain exhibits considerable regional variation, with the highest levels observed in cerebellum (Cramer *et al.*, 1971; Schmidt *et al.*, 1971). A comment here about the methods used to fix the tissues is in order, since the levels of cyclic AMP increase severalfold within a minute after decapitation of animals (Breckenridge, 1964; Ditzion *et al.*, 1970). Microwave irradiation seems to be the most appropriate way to stop adenylate cyclase and phosphodiesterase activities (Schmidt *et al.*, 1971). Freezing the animals in isopentane, cooled with liquid nitrogen, has drawbacks, e.g. it is extremely difficult to dissect a frozen brain accurately and inactivation of the deeper structures of the brain is not instantaneous. Since it has been reported that even at 0° phosphodiesterase retains considerable activity (O'Dea *et al.*, 1971), the levels of cyclic AMP could be artificially low in deeper brain areas.

The level of cyclic AMP in brain increases with age (Schmidt *et al.*, 1970), following a developmental pattern similar to that observed for the activities of adenylate cyclase (Schmidt *et al.*, 1970) and cyclic nucleotide phosphodiesterase (Weiss, 1971). The greatest increase occurs in the postnatal period when the brain is undergoing biochemical and morphological maturation (Davison and Dobbing, 1968).

Evidence accumulated within the past few years indicates an involvement of cyclic AMP in the functioning of the nervous system, particularly in the mediation of the action of some neurotransmitters at certain types of synapses. Several reviews on the subject have appeared in recent volumes edited by Greengard and Costa (1970), by Robison *et al.* (1974), by Greengard *et al.* (1972) and by Drummond *et al.* (1975).

A model illustrating a possible role and mechanism of action of cyclic AMP in synaptic transmission has been proposed by Greengard (1975) (Fig. 1). According to Greengard, neurotransmitter released from a presynaptic nerve terminal activates an adenylate cyclase in the postsynaptic membrane and, thereby, causes accumulation of cyclic AMP in the postsynaptic neurone. The physiological effects of cyclic AMP are believed to be mediated

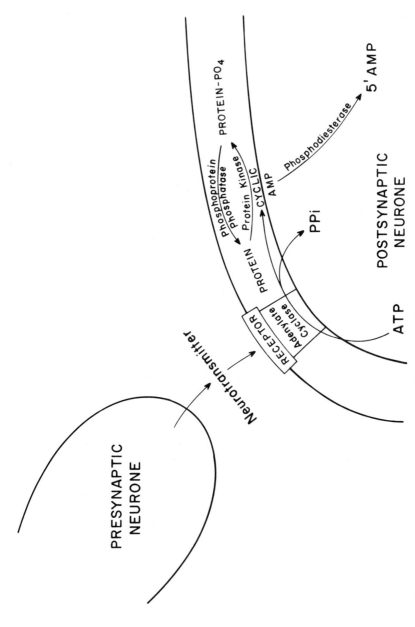

Fig. 1. Model of the proposed mechanism by which cyclic AMP may mediate synaptic transmission at certain types of synapses. Courtesy of Paul Greengard (1975) and Raven Press.

through the action of protein kinases (Kuo and Greengard, 1969). These enzymes which catalyse phosphorylation of proteins are composed of at least two subunits that interact with each other and with cyclic AMP.

$$RC + \text{cyclic AMP} \rightleftharpoons R \cdot \text{cyclic AMP} + C$$

In this equation, RC represents an inactive protein kinase, R · cyclic AMP, the regulatory subunit to which cyclic AMP is bound, and C, the free active catalytic subunit. The model indicates that the newly formed cyclic AMP activates a protein kinase which in turn transfers a phosphate group from ATP to a specific protein constituent of the plasma membrane. The phosphorylation of the plasma membrane of the postsynaptic neurone causes an alteration in the movement of ions across the membrane, resulting in a change in membrane potential of the cells. This is a transient potential, and the restoration of the postsynaptic membrane to its pre-excitation state is accomplished by the combined action of two enzymes, i.e. a phosphodiesterase which destroys the cyclic AMP formed in the postsynaptic neurone, and a phosphoprotein phosphatase which dephosphorylates the specific membrane protein.

Considerable evidence supports this model. For instance, sub-cellular fractions rich in synaptic membranes contain high levels of cyclic-AMP-dependent protein kinase (Maeno *et al.*, 1971), substrate protein for cyclic-AMP-dependent protein kinase (Johnson *et al.*, 1971), and phosphoprotein phosphatase (Maeno and Greengard, 1972). Adenylate cyclase, phosphodiesterase and cyclic AMP itself have also been shown to be enriched in the same fractions (DeRobertis *et al.*, 1967; Weiss and Costa, 1968; Lust and Goldberg, 1970). Therefore, the emerging picture is one of a highly compartmentalized system, in which enzymes for the synthesis and degradation of cyclic AMP are found in close proximity to the ones responsible for its biological activity.

Moreover, several investigators have reported that the major cyclic-AMP-generating sites in brain are postsynaptic since the accumulations of cyclic AMP elicited by norepinephrine or other agents are unaffected when the noradrenergic presynaptic terminals are destroyed with 6-hydroxy-dopamine (Dismukes and Daly, 1975; Huang *et al.*, 1973; Kalisker *et al.*, 1973; Palmer, 1972; Weiss and Strada, 1972) or when norepinephrine levels are depleted with reserpine (Dismukes and Daly, 1975; Palmer *et al.*, 1973). In addition, Kebabian *et al.* (1975a) demonstrated by the use of an immunofluorescent assay that dopamine increases cyclic AMP in the bovine superior cervical ganglion and that this increase is localized in the postganglionic neurones.

While most of the observations using preparations of brain tissue *in vitro* or *in situ* are consistent with the above model, studies with cultured cells, derived from neuronal tissue, offer a somewhat different view of cyclic nucleotide metabolism as it relates to function. For example, the effects of catecholamines, adenosine and prostaglandins have been determined in monolayer cultures of foetal rat brain (Gilman and Schrier, 1972), in reaggregated brain cells from embryonic mouse brain (Seeds and Gilman, 1971), and in cell lines derived from neuroblastomas and gliomas, primarily astrocytomas (Perkins, 1973; Gilman, 1972; Schultz and Hamprecht, 1973; Blume *et al.*, 1973). In brain cell aggregates, where the proportions of neurones and glia are comparable to brain tissue *in situ*, the responses to catecholamines are similar to those observed in brain slices. But in monolayer cultures, which contain a preponderance of glial cells, the intracellular concentration of cyclic AMP is greatly increased after treatment with catecholamines, adenosine and prostaglandin E_1. Although results obtained with neuroma cells cannot be extrapolated to what happens in normal brain tissue, since many times the tumor cell lines show altered enzyme levels or hormone responsiveness, it is interesting that clones of glial cells increased their content of cyclic AMP when stimulated by catecholamines; biogenic amines did not have any effect on neuroblastoma cells. In view of these observations, Gilman (1972) has hypothesized that accumulations of cyclic AMP elicited in brain by catecholamines may occur primarily in glial cells, and that glia would be effector cells of neurones. Perhaps cyclic AMP plays a role in the regulation of the metabolism or function both of neuronal and glial cells.

Siggins *et al.* (1971a) investigated the physiological role of cyclic AMP in central nervous system *in vivo*. They studied the effects of iontophoretically-applied cyclic AMP or of agents known to stimulate its formation or block its degradation on the electrical activity of individual neurones. Such studies demonstrated that norepinephrine released from presynaptic terminals inhibited spontaneous discharge of cerebellar Purkinje cells (Siggins *et al.*, 1971b; Hoffer *et al.*, 1972) and hippocampal pyramidal cells (Segal and Bloom, 1974a, 1974b; Oliver and Segal, 1974), while dopamine has a similar effect on neurones in the caudate nucleus (Siggins *et al.*, 1974). Furthermore, iontophoretically-applied cyclic AMP and its analogues (Siggins and Hendriksen, 1975) can mimic the inhibitory effects of norepinephrine and dopamine. The duration and magnitude of those responses are increased by the administration of phosphodiesterase inhibitors (Siggins *et al.*, 1971a, 1971b; Hoffer *et al.*, 1972; Segal and Bloom, 1974a), but are not antagonized by the actions of prostaglandins (Hoffer *et al.*, 1969; Siggins *et al.*, 1971a, 1971b; Segal and Bloom, 1974a) nor neuroleptic drugs which antagonize the responses to norepinephrine or dopamine (Freedman and Siggins, 1974; Siggins *et al.*, 1974). However, since the response to iontophoretically-applied norepinephrine or cyclic AMP can be seen in animals pretreated with 6-hydroxy-dopamine to remove the endogenous catecholamine nerve terminals, all of these results indicate a direct postsynaptic activation of adenylate cyclase as one step in the molecular mechanisms causing the inhibition by norepinephrine (Siggins *et al.*, 1971a). In addition, immunocytochemical studies (Wedner *et al.*, 1972) show that topical application of norepinephrine increases the proportion of cerebellar Purkinje cells with detectable intracellular cyclic AMP. This supports the proposal of Siggins *et al.* (1971a) that cyclic AMP can mediate the intracellular actions of catecholamines at some central synapses *in vivo*.

B. *Cyclic GMP*

1. *Metabolism*

It is only in the last few years that cyclic GMP has gained a place of importance in cyclic nucleotide research comparable to that of cyclic AMP. By now, numerous studies have demonstrated that cyclic GMP is involved in the biochemistry of many mammalian tissues (Goldberg *et al.*, 1973b) and that it may have an important role in central nervous system function (Ferrendelli, 1975).

Guanylate cyclase, the enzyme that catalyses the formation of cyclic GMP from GTP, is quite active in brain. However, highest levels of guanylate cyclase activity in the CNS have been demonstrated in the retina, particularly in rod outer segments of photoreceptor cells (Goridis *et al.*, 1973).

In contrast to adenylate cyclase, which is associated predominantly with membranes, guanylate cyclase seems to be concentrated in soluble fractions of brain (Goridis and Morgan, 1973). However, evidence obtained from the treatment of homogenates of retina (Bensinger *et al.*, 1973) and of other tissues (White, 1975) with detergents such as Triton X-100 indicates that some guanylate cyclase may be bound also to membranes and that its activity becomes fully expressed only upon solubilization.

When homogenates of brain are separated by differential centrifugation, the distribution of guanylate cyclase resembles that of soluble enzymes which are considered neuronal markers (Goridis and Morgan, 1973) such as glutamate decarboxylase (Fonnum, 1965) and tyrosine hydroxylase (Kuczenski and Mandell, 1972), and it is different from that of soluble non-specific cytoplasmic markers such as lactate dehydrogenase. Additionally, studies of chick embryo brain cells in culture show that guanylate cyclase activity is always higher in those cultures which contain a significant ratio of neurones to glia. In cultures where only glial or meningeal cells are present, guanylate cyclase activity is below the limit of detection (Goridis et al., 1974a). These results suggest that guanylate cyclase activity might be mainly, if not exclusively, concentrated in neurones.

The first substance found to produce an increase in cyclic GMP content of neural tissue was acetylcholine. This effect has not been fully clarified but it may be associated with activation of guanylate cyclase rather than inhibition of phosphodiesterase. It should be noted, though, that a hormone- or neurotransmitter-sensitive guanylate cyclase has not been demonstrated as yet in any neuronal or non-neuronal tissue (Beam and Greengard, 1975). Kuo et al. (1972) showed that, in slices of cerebral and cerebellar tissues, cyclic GMP levels were elevated 70–300% after 30 and 60 sec of exposure to acetylcholine. Ferrendelli et al. (1970) tested the possibility of a relationship between acetylcholine action and cyclic GMP accumulation by monitoring the changes in brain tissue cyclic nucleotide levels following the administration of oxotremorine, a drug whose effects in the CNS are believed to derive from a release of acetylcholine. Oxotremorine increases cyclic GMP content in mice cerebral cortex and cerebellum. These elevations of cyclic GMP can be antagonized by atropine (Ferrendelli et al., 1970; Lee et al., 1972) which suggests that the effect of acetylcholine or other muscarinic cholinergic agonists (Kuo et al., 1972; Lee et al., 1972) may be related to the activation of muscarinic receptors. Evidence also suggests that an elevation of acetylcholine levels, in situ, increases cyclic GMP content. Administration of maaloxone, a centrally-active cholinesterase inhibitor, promotes accumulation of acetylcholine in the CNS and, correspondingly, causes an increase in cyclic GMP levels in the cerebellum (Goldberg et al., 1973a). These observations imply than an elevation of cyclic GMP is linked to the activation of muscarinic receptors with guanylate cyclase acting presumably as the intermediate enzyme. The association or interaction between the muscarinic receptor and the guanylate cyclase remains to be identified.

The finding that d-amphetamine, chlorpromazine and reserpine, drugs which influence CNS monoaminergic neurotransmission processes, alter the levels of cyclic GMP in mouse cerebellum *in vivo* suggests that cyclic GMP may also be involved in the actions of neurotransmitters other than acetylcholine (Ferrendelli *et al.*, 1972). d-Amphetamine produces a twofold increase in cyclic GMP levels, whereas chlorpromazine and reserpine reduced cyclic GMP levels 62 and 73%, respectively. It has been reported that there may be species-related variation in the response of brain slices to norepinephrine. For example, Ferrendelli *et al.* (1975) demonstrated recently that as little as 1 μM norepinephrine is capable of increasing the level of cyclic GMP in incubated slices of mouse cerebellum. Kuo *et al.* (1972), on the other hand, have shown with rabbit cerebellum that cyclic GMP levels are diminished after exposure to norepinephrine. These groups have also shown using brain slices that histamine increases cyclic GMP levels of cerebral cortex, while serotonin and dopamine have no effect on cyclic GMP levels of cerebellum except at high concentrations (1 mM) where they cause depression of the cyclic GMP content.

Among the agents that produce an increase in cyclic GMP levels in brain slices are the putative amino acid neurotransmitters–(glutamate, γ-aminobutyric acid (GABA) and glycine (Ferrendelli *et al.*, 1974)— and the compounds that cause membrane depolarization–veratridine, ouabain and high levels of K^+ (Ferrendelli *et al.*, 1973). Hydroxylamine, a compound that increases the concentration of GABA in brain, also increases markedly cyclic GMP levels in slices of cerebral cortex (Kimura *et al.*, 1975). It is probably an important observation that most of the agents already mentioned, which cause an accumulation of cyclic GMP in brain, produce this effect through a Ca^{2+}-dependent mechanism (Ferrendelli, 1975; Ferrendelli *et al.*, 1973, 1974, 1975). The elevation of cyclic GMP levels by sodium azide appears to be an exceptional case since sodium azide activates guanylate cyclase in the absence of added calcium in slices from the cerebral cortex and cerebellum (Kimura *et al.*, 1975). Demonstration of a Ca^{2+}-independent mechanism for the accumulation of cyclic GMP has been related to the presence of two forms of guanylate cyclase (Kimura and Murad, 1974, 1975). It is argued that guanylate cyclase may show different requirements for Ca^{2+} when it is membrane associated or when it is soluble.

Mao *et al.* (1974a) have shown that cyclic GMP concentrations increase in various brain regions of rats exposed to cold (4°) *in situ*. In cerebellum, where the increase reaches its maximum within 5 min of cold exposure, this change does not appear to require the participation of adrenergic, cholinergic or serotonergic synaptic mechanisms. However, the extent of cyclic GMP increase elicited by cold is modulated when the cerebellar concentrations of GABA are increased or decreased by drugs. Thus, when GABA levels are depressed below normal by injection of convulsive or subconvulsive doses of isonicotinic acid hydrazide, or when GABA receptors are blocked by administration of picrotoxin, the basal cyclic GMP concentrations in cerebellum are elevated (Mao et al., 1974b). Moreover, the mechanism that promotes the increase of cerebellar cyclic GMP concentration during cold exposure seems inoperative when GABA levels are reduced. Conversely, when GABA levels are elevated by treatment with aminooxyacetic acid, hydroxylamine or hydrazine, the mechanism that elevates cyclic GMP in cerebellum of rats exposed to cold is inhibited. In addition, there is evidence for an involvement of GABA in the mediation of the cerebellar cyclic GMP decrease caused by the anticonvulsant action of diazepam and some other benzodiazepines (Mao et al., 1975a; Costa et al., 1975b). Diazepam is at least 50 times more active than phenobarbital in lowering the cerebellar content of cyclic GMP (Costa et al., 1975a).

Studies on the cyclic GMP system in a strain of mutant mice, with a number of cerebellar Purkinje cells reduced to 10% of normal, suggest that the regulation of a substantial portion of the cyclic GMP content of cerebellum depends on the presence of Purkinje cells (Mao et al., 1975b). On the basis of these results, it was postulated that the pool of cyclic GMP in the Purkinje cells is regulated by the excitatory input reaching these cells via the climbing or parallel fibres, or both.

Studies with 3-acetylpyridine, a drug that destroys the climbing fibres (Guidotti et al., 1975a), or with harmaline, an alkaloid that selectively activates the climbing fibres (Mao et al., 1974b, 1975c), suggest that activation of the olivo-cerebellar tract is important in the regulation of cerebellar cyclic GMP content. In this regard, the increase produced by harmaline in the cyclic GMP level of rat cerebellum can be antagonized by diazepam but not by anticholinergic drugs. In addition, doses of diazepam, greater than the minimal required to reduce the increase of cyclic GMP elicited by harmaline, decrease the cyclic GMP content of cerebellum (Mao et al., 1974b). Amino acids other than GABA may also be associated with alterations in cyclic GMP levels since taurine also antagonizes the harmaline-induced tremor and the increase of cerebellar cyclic GMP (Guidotti et al., 1976). These data suggest that both GABA and taurine may act in the modulation of the functional state of the olivo-cerebellar pathway.

The hydrolytic cleavage of cyclic GMP to 5′-GMP, catalysed by phosphodiesterase, is the only well-established mechanism by which the biological actions of cyclic GMP can be terminated. *In vitro*, this reaction is subject to modulation and control by endogenous agents and drugs that have been described in a previous section dealing with the hydrolysis of cyclic AMP by phosphodiesterase. For example, in terms of cyclic GMP metabolism, the phosphodiesterase which shows specificity for cyclic GMP in brain is characterized by its association with a Ca^{2+}-dependent protein activator (Teshima and Kakiuchi, 1974). In general, it may be possible that the neuronal cells selectively control the tissue steady-state levels of the two cyclic nucleotides by means of independent regulatory mechanisms.

2. Role and mechanism of action

There is considerable regional variation in cyclic GMP content within the brain, with cerebellum being the region where it is especially concentrated (Kuo *et al.*, 1972; Goldberg *et al.*, 1970; Steiner *et al.*, 1970; Ferrendelli *et al.*, 1970, 1972; Mao *et al.*, 1974a; Steiner *et al.*, 1972; Murad *et al.*, 1971). In terms of the CNS, however, the retina has been shown to possess the highest level of cyclic GMP (Farber and Lolley, 1974; Goridis *et al.*, 1974b).

Weight *et al.* (1974) have shown that cyclic GMP is associated with synaptic transmission in neural tissue. Brief stimulation of cholinergic preganglionic nerve fibres increases the levels of cyclic GMP in bullfrog sympathetic ganglion. When the release of synaptic transmitter is prevented by a high-magnesium, low-calcium Ringer solution, stimulation of the preganglionic fibres does not increase cyclic GMP in the ganglion. Atropine also blocks the cyclic GMP increase. These results indicate that the increase in cyclic GMP is associated with synaptic transmission rather than with impulse conduction along the preganglionic nerve fibres, and that it involves the activation of muscarinic postsynaptic receptors. In support of this conclusion, either acetylcholine or bethanechol, a muscarinic agonist, can increase the content of cyclic GMP in slices of bovine sympathetic ganglia, and this response is antagonized by atropine (Kebabian *et al.*, 1975b). The nicotinic agonist, N,N'-dimethylphenylpiperazinium, does not alter the level of cyclic GMP, and hexamethonium, the nicotinic antagonist, does not block the increase caused by the cholinergic agents (Kebabian *et al.*, 1975b). Moreover, by using a histochemical procedure for localizing cyclic GMP (Fallon *et al.*, 1974), evidence has been obtained that the acetylcholine-induced accumulation of cyclic GMP occurs in the postganglionic neurones (Kebabian *et al.*, 1975a).

The physiological effects of cyclic GMP seem to be dependent upon the action of protein kinases. These enzymes have been found in mammalian brain, uterus and bladder (Greengard and Kuo, 1970), as well as in a variety of invertebrate tissues (Greengard and Kuo, 1970; Kuo and Greengard, 1970; Kuo *et al.*, 1971). The mechanism of activation of cyclic-GMP-dependent protein kinases appears to be analogous to that by which cyclic AMP brings about the activation of cyclic-AMP-dependent protein kinases (see Fig. 1).

C. *Yin-Yang Hypothesis*

In the preceding discussion, we have considered cyclic AMP and cyclic GMP as if they were acting independently. However, it is important to realize that there are at least two basic types of cyclic nucleotide mechanisms which operate in most cells. These have been classified as unidirectional or bidirectional systems (Goldberg *et al.*, 1974). In unidirectional systems, control is exercised by a simple on–off principle. When the stimulus is present, the cells are switched on; when the stimulus is removed, they become quiescent. This type of control is usually found in cells which are regulated by a single stimulant. If there are added stimulants, these act in parallel with the primary stimulant and, if cyclic AMP and cyclic GMP are involved, they are thought to function in concert. This appears to be the case for the photoreceptor cells of the retina (Berridge, 1975) and, in a subsequent section, it will be emphasized that the metabolism of cyclic GMP is selectively influenced by the presence or absence of a light stimulant.

In bidirectional systems, cellular control is more dynamic since stimulation and recovery are mediated by separate stimulants. The final response is often determined by a balance between the two opposing stimulants. The appearance of one stimulant causes an increase in cell activity, whereas the second either mediates the recovery from or opposes the action of the first stimulant. Goldberg *et al.* (1975) described the intracellular basis of these control mechanisms in terms of interactions between cyclic AMP and cyclic GMP. Their Ying-Yang hypothesis is clearly summarized in the following quotation:

> We believe that this concept of biologic regulation through opposing actions of two cyclic nucleotides is well described by the ancient oriental concept embodied in the terms *yin yang*. Yin yang symbolizes a dualism between opposing natural forces but also takes into account that under

certain circumstances the forces may enter into a mutual interaction that results in a synthesis. In its simplest form the hypothesis defines cyclic GMP and cyclic AMP as biologic effectors involved in regulating cellular functions that are controlled bidirectionally (Goldberg *et al.*, 1975).

Neurones are subject to bidirectional influences of excitation and inhibition and several lines of evidence suggest that the relative concentrations of cyclic AMP and cyclic GMP may be important in the modulation of neuronal function. One example, which appears to support the Ying-Yang hypothesis in neural tissue, illustrates the importance of changes in the ratio of cyclic AMP to cyclic GMP when considering enzyme induction in the adrenal medulla.

Guidotti *et al.* (1975b) studied the induction of tyrosine hydroxylase under a variety of drug- or stress-induced conditions. Exposure of rats to 4° or the injection of reserpine produce opposing changes in cyclic AMP and cyclic GMP concentrations of the adrenal medulla. By 30 min after applying the stimulus, the cyclic AMP concentration has increased about five- to eightfold and that of cyclic GMP decreased about 50%. The cyclic AMP to cyclic GMP ratio of chromaffin cells increases from a basal value of approximately ten to values in the range of 150–180 within 30 min. Since the cyclic GMP content remains very low for more than one hour, the cyclic AMP/cyclic GMP increase at one hour is still approximately five times the basal value. Guidotti *et al.* (1975b) presented evidence which suggests that increases in the ratio of cyclic AMP to cyclic GMP to over 40 and maintenance of this ratio for at least one hour are associated with induction of tyrosine hydroxylase synthesis in the adrenal medulla. They stress the complexity of stimuli that can change the concentration ratio of the cyclic nucleotides and the possible involvement of neurotransmission and glucocorticoids in the process of regulating the concentration of the individual cyclic nucleotides.

Similar studies using sympathetic ganglia (Costa *et al.*, 1974) suggest that cyclic nucleotides may act in a comparable manner within other regions of the nervous system. The implication here is that cyclic AMP and cyclic GMP act as intracellular promoters of programmed cell function and that nucleotide concentrations inside ganglion cells may be regulated by transmitters released at synapses. The result of such changes, particularly those which produce alterations in cyclic AMP to cyclic GMP ratios of long duration, would alter the metabolic capabilities of postsynaptic neurones. In the example of tyrosine hydroxylase, metabolism of catecholamines would be modified due to induction of the enzyme which is rate-limiting to catecholamine synthesis.

III. Cyclic Nucleotides and Photoreceptor Degeneration in the Retina of C3H Mice

The adult retina is a layered structure with a limited number of cellular classes (Fig. 2). It develops embryonically from the primitive forebrain and becomes specialized for the reception and integration of visual stimuli. Light of the visible spectrum (400–650 nm) is absorbed by the visual pigment of the photoreceptor cell, and this event is converted by as yet unknown mechanisms into polarization changes across its

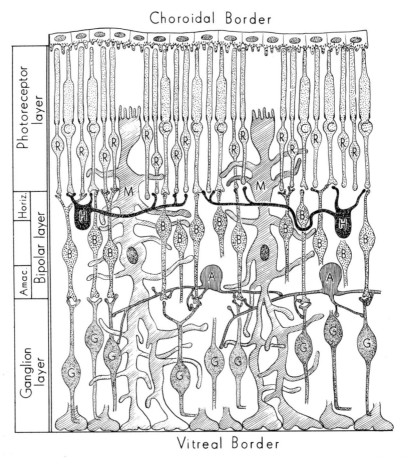

Fig. 2. The major constituents of the vertebrate retina and their synaptic relationships. The cells of the neural retina are designated as R: rods, C: cones, H: horizontal cells, B: bipolar cells, A: amacrine cells, G: ganglion cells and M: Müller cells. The outer layer of pigment epithelium cells is unlabelled. (From Lolley, 1969.)

plasma membrane. The response to light is reflected as a hyper-polarization of the membrane in photoreceptor cells of vertebrates (Werblin, 1974) or as a depolarization in invertebrates (Hagins, 1965; Knight et al., 1970). Photoreceptor cells make characteristic ribbon-synapses as well as conventional synapses with bipolar and horizontal cells (Dubin, 1974) and these synapses pass the electrophysiological response in turn to neighbouring cells of the photoreceptor layer and to those of the ganglion cell layer. The degree of interaction between neighbouring cells determines the degree of information processing in the retina and this appears to be species-dependent (Dubin, 1974; Dowling, 1968). From a flash of light, most of the cells of the retina show a polarization change, and only two cell classes, i.e. amacrine and ganglion cells, generate action potentials (Werblin and Dowling, 1969; Kaneko and Hashimoto, 1969). The integrated response of retinal cells to a flash of light can be measured as the electroretinogram (ERG).

Before discussing the inner layers of the retina, where processing of visual information occurs, let us consider some specialized features of photoreceptor cells. A photoreceptor cell functions as a unit but, for the sake of discussion, it can be subdivided into discrete, morphologi-cal compartments which appear to serve rather specific functions. According to such a subdivision, a photoreceptor cell is composed of an outer segment containing light-absorbing visual pigment, an inner segment rich in mitochondria, a nucleus located in the cell soma, and a synaptic ending joined to the soma by a short axon (Young, 1969a). The fine structural organization of the synapse suggests that the photoreceptor cell releases a chemical transmitter, but the nature of this transmitter is still unknown. Recent studies suggest further that the transmitter is released continuously in the dark and that release is diminished in the presence of light (Ripps et al., 1976; Baylor and Fuortes, 1970).

There are two general classes of photoreceptor cells, i.e. rods and cones, with subclasses having been identified in some species (Stell, 1972). In the retina of rodents, the vast majority of photoreceptor cells are rods. Photoreceptor cells are often classified according to the appearance of their outer segments. However, it has been shown that there are a number of morphological, chemical and biological features which distinguish a rod from a cone photoreceptor (Werblin, 1974; Dubin, 1974; Young, 1969a, 1969b; Young and Bok, 1969; Hogan et al., 1974).

The outer segments of rod photoreceptor cells have been studied extensively to gain insight into the mechanisms by which they absorb light, amplify this signal and generate a polarization change across their plasma membranes, i.e. carry out the visual process. In brief, these studies suggest that, in the dark, the visual pigment rhodopsin exists as a conjugate of the protein opsin with the chromophore 11-*cis* retinal, that light is absorbed by rhodopsin, and that the absorption of light by rhodopsin results in the isomerization of 11-*cis* retinal to the all-*trans* configuration. Rod outer segments are composed of tightly-packed membranous discs which are encased by but not attached to the plasmalemma of the cell. Most of the visual pigment is concentrated in the disc membranes with, possibly, some in the plasmalemma (Jan and Revel, 1974; Dewey *et al.*, 1969). The steps which follow rhodopsin bleaching (isomerization of 11-*cis* to all-*trans* retinal) and which lead to amplification of the initial light signal and to polarization of the cell plasmalemma are still unresolved. From physiological data, however, it is proposed that Ca^{2+} and, possibly, cyclic GMP may participate in these functions.

A model of a rod outer segment attempting to explain its function has been devised by Hagins and Yoshikami (1974). This model suggests that Ca^{2+} is the intracellular transmitter of the light signal. It proposes that Ca^{2+}, released from the disc membranes of the rod outer segment upon the absorption of light by rhodopsin (Mason *et al.*, 1974; Hendricks *et al.*, 1974), may interact with the plasmalemma, blocking the ion channels and reducing the net flow of Na^+ across the membrane. This results in hyperpolarization of the plasmalemma. Cyclic GMP may also be an intermediate in the visual process. Bitensky *et al.* (1973) suggest that cyclic nucleotides act by stimulating the phosphorylation of sodium channels in the plasmalemma sensitizing them to Ca^{2+}. Therefore, it seems that Ca^{2+} may act as an intracellular transmitter in the visual process but the role of cyclic GMP is still undefined.

Evidence is accumulating, however, which shows that the content and metabolism of cyclic GMP in the photoreceptor cells is influenced by light. The level of cyclic GMP in rod outer segments is about 100 times that of cyclic AMP (Krishna *et al.*, 1975) and it varies with the conditions of illumination. When dark-adapted retina or rod outer segments are exposed to light, there is a rapid reduction in cyclic GMP content (Fletcher and Chader, 1976) which is sustained while the light stimulus is maintained (Goridis *et al.*, 1974b). The mechanisms which cause this reduction in cyclic GMP content have been only partially resolved. Early studies suggested that light might inhibit the activity of guanylate cyclase (Pannbacker, 1973a; Bensinger *et al.*, 1973) but recent evidence appears to favour activation of phosphodiesterase by light (Bitensky *et al.*, 1975).

Phosphodiesterase activity of rod outer segments has been localized by EM histochemistry (Robb, 1974) and has been shown to be activated by light, in the presence of ATP (Goridis and Virmaux, 1974; Chader *et al.*, 1974b; Miki *et al.*, 1973), with an action spectrum like that of rhodopsin (Keirns *et al.*, 1975). The phosphodiesterase of rod outer segments has a relatively high apparent K_m for cyclic GMP, in the range of 10^{-4} M, which is not changed by light. It can be eluted from the rod outer segment membranes with buffers of low-ionic strength (Bitensky *et al.*, 1975) but, when separated from the discs, it loses the ability for light-activation. However, the soluble phosphodiesterase can be activated by protamine. While the enzyme is associated with rod outer segment membranes, certain polyanions such as heparin or silicates can substitute both for light and ATP in the activation process. These observations suggest that the phosphodiesterase of rod outer segments is linked through some mechanism, possibly requiring ATP, to the visual pigment, rhodopsin. Upon absorption of light by rhodopsin, phosphodiesterase is activated and the level of cyclic GMP is rapidly reduced.

The importance of the light-induced reduction in cyclic GMP levels to the visual process or light adaptation (Lipton, 1975) is still unknown. It may involve a protein kinase system and phosphorylation of membrane proteins or rhodopsin (Weller *et al.*, 1975) thus affecting membrane permeability in a manner which is analogous to that described earlier (see Fig. 1). There are data which show that protein kinases are present in isolated rod outer segments (Pannbacker, 1973b). Some controversy still exists, however, over whether the kinases are capable of stimulation by cyclic nucleotides (Pannbacker, 1973b; Chader *et al.*, 1975, 1976). This field of study looks promising, and possibly it may contribute significantly to our understanding of the visual process.

It is upon this background that we present our observations which relate to cyclic GMP metabolism in the normal mouse retina and in that of the C3H mouse, which is afflicted with an inherited disorder causing photoreceptor cell degeneration.

In the mouse retina, at birth, photoreceptor cells are immature but, in the subsequent two weeks, differentiate and become fully responsive to light (Fig. 3) (Noell, 1965). By the fourth postnatal day, signs of differentiation at both poles of the cell are evidenced by the development of an inner segment as well as ribbon synapses with horizontal cells (Blanks *et al.*, 1974a). A modified cilium, which will form the connection between the outer and inner segment, protrudes into the space between the inner segment and pigment epithelium by day 6 and

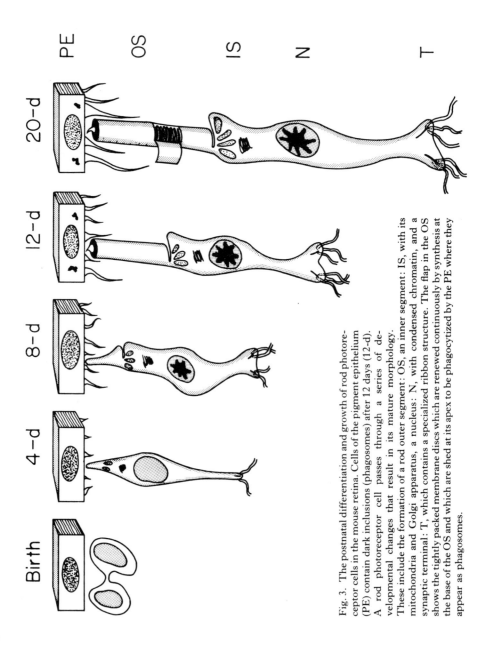

Fig. 3. The postnatal differentiation and growth of rod photoreceptor cells in the mouse retina. Cells of the pigment epithelium (PE) contain dark inclusions (phagosomes) after 12 days (12-d). A rod photoreceptor cell passes through a series of developmental changes that result in its mature morphology. These include the formation of a rod outer segment: OS, an inner segment: IS, with its mitochondria and Golgi apparatus, a nucleus: N, with condensed chromatin, and a synaptic terminal: T, which contains a specialized ribbon structure. The flap in the OS shows the tightly packed membrane discs which are renewed continuously by synthesis at the base of the OS and which are shed at its apex to be phagocytized by the PE where they appear as phagosomes.

outer segment discs begin to form by day 8 (Sonohara and Shiose, 1968; Olney, 1968). From day 8 to 20, the outer segments grow in length. Thereafter, their length remains stable, due to the balance between disc renewal and shedding which occurs throughout the life of the mouse (Young and Droz, 1968; Young and Bok, 1969; LaVail, 1973). Rod outer segment renewal will be discussed more fully in a subsequent section. By 14 days, the photoreceptor cell forms synaptic contacts with horizontal and bipolar cells (Blanks *et al.*, 1974a) and the ERG exhibits a pattern which is typical of the normal adult mouse retina (Noell, 1965).

Several investigations of cyclic nucleotide metabolism in the vertebrate retina have shown that photoreceptor cells are characterized by a high level of cyclic GMP metabolism (Goridis *et al.*, 1973; Chader

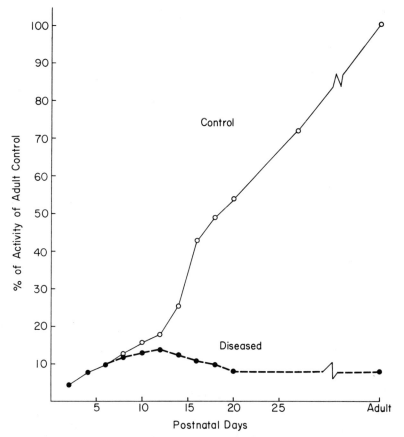

Fig. 4. Development of guanylate cyclase activity in retinas of control and diseased (C3H) mice as a function of postnatal age. The activity measured at 0·7 mM GTP is expressed in relation to that of adult control retina (0·24 nmol cyclic GMP formed/retina.min^{-1}).

et al., 1974a), while the metabolism of cyclic AMP is very low (Lolley *et al.*, 1974). In our studies of rodent retina, we found that cyclic AMP metabolism is restricted almost exclusively to the inner retinal layers.

The capacity for cyclic GMP metabolism in the mouse retina increases during the period of photoreceptor cell differentiation as indicated by the postnatal increase in the activity of guanylate cyclase (Fig. 4) and of cyclic GMP phosphodiesterase (PDE) (Fig. 5) (Farber and Lolley, 1976). Kinetic analyses of these enzymes in homogenates of whole retina or of microdissected retinal layers show that a different class of guanylate cyclase and cyclic-GMP-PDE is associated with the photoreceptor cells than with the other cells of the neural retina (Farber and Lolley, 1976). The guanylate cyclase of the photoreceptor cells shows a greater affinity for GTP, and the cyclic-GMP-PDE of the photoreceptor cells shows less affinity for cyclic GMP than the respective enzymes of the inner retinal layers.

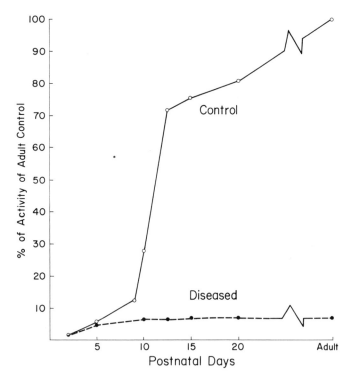

Fig. 5. Development of cyclic GMP phosphodiesterase activity in retinas of control and diseased (C3H) mice as a function of postnatal age. The activity measured at 0·4 mM cyclic GMP is expressed in relation to that of adult control retina (8·5 nmol cyclic GMP hydrolysed/retina.min^{-1}). (From Lolley and Farber, 1976b.)

The balance of synthesis and degradation of cyclic GMP as well as its possible compartmentation in the photoreceptor outer segments is reflected in the steady-state level of cyclic GMP (Fig. 6) (Farber and Lolley, 1974). The content of cyclic GMP in the adult retina is three- to fourfold greater than that of the adult cerebellum (Ferrendelli *et al.*, 1970; Murad *et al.*, 1971; Mao *et al.*, 1974a) and is localized predominantly in the photoreceptor cells. Accordingly, the content of cyclic GMP in the developing mouse retina increases during the period in which photoreceptor cells differentiate and rod outer segments grow in length and develop a physiological response to light.

In the inherited retinal degeneration of C3H/HeJ mice, a mutation has occurred which is carried as an autosomal recessive characteristic (Sidman and Green, 1965; LaVail and Sidman, 1974). The only morphological abnormality which has been ascribed to this mutation is the selective degeneration of retinal photoreceptor cells. The photoreceptor cells appear to form normally in the pre- and early postnatal

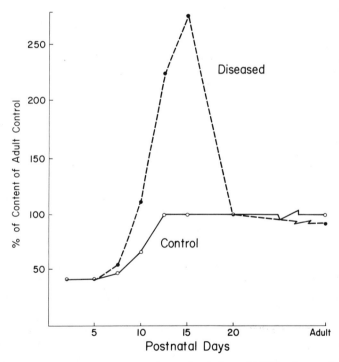

Fig. 6. Content of cyclic GMP in retinas of control and diseased (C3H) mice as a function of postnatal age. The content is expressed in relation to that of the adult control retina (72·1 pmol cyclic GMP/retina). (From Lolley and Farber, 1976b.)

period and to achieve some degree of differentiation as indicated by the development of rudimentary rod outer segments and a synaptic ribbon apparatus (Fig. 7) (Blanks *et al.*, 1974b). They are responsive to high-intensity illumination and they exhibit an attenuated ERG (Noell, 1965). The first signs of ultrastructural damage to the photoreceptor cells has been observed on the eighth postnatal day; a swelling of mitochondria of the inner segments (Sonohara and Shiose, 1968). Cellular death is apparent by the tenth day (Lolley, 1973) and, by day 20, virtually all of the photoreceptor cells have degenerated (Noell, 1965; Caley *et al.*, 1972; LaVail and Mullen, 1974). The rate of photoreceptor cell death is not affected by the level of illumination in which the mice are reared. Loss of photoreceptor cells is reflected in the loss of protein from the retina (Farber and Lolley, 1973). The few cells that still remain after 20 days of age appear to be of the cone class of photoreceptors. It has been proposed that death of the photoreceptor cells results from their "faulty" differentiation (Noell, 1965; Lolley, 1973; Wegmann *et al.*, 1971).

A biochemical abnormality in cyclic GMP metabolism occurs about two days before the C3H photoreceptor cells begin to degenerate. The photoreceptor cells are able to synthesize cyclic GMP via the guanylate cyclase reaction (see Fig. 4) from the onset of differentiation but they are always deficient in the capacity to hydrolyse cyclic GMP via the cyclic-GMP-PDE reaction (see Fig. 5) (Farber and Lolley, 1976). Kinetic studies show that the activity of cyclic-GMP-PDE, which is localized in the photoreceptor cells of normal retina, is missing from the C3H retina throughout the period of photoreceptor cell differentiation and degeneration. This imbalance in cyclic GMP metabolism results in the accumulation of cyclic GMP in the C3H photoreceptor cells (Farber and Lolley, 1974) during the period of postnatal life in which they degenerate (Fig. 6). We have proposed that high levels of cyclic GMP, acting through an accentuation of the metabolic or functional role of the cyclic nucleotide, may cause the degeneration of C3H photoreceptor cells.

In collaboration with Hollyfield *et al.* (1975), we have tested this hypothesis using eye rudiments of *Xenopus laevis* embryos in hanging-drop culture. Photoreceptor cells of these rudiments differentiate and grow normally but, when the phosphodiesterase inhibitor, isobutyl-methylxanthine (IBMX), is added to the culture medium, the photoreceptor cells undergo selective and dose-dependent degeneration (Lolley *et al.*, 1976). IBMX effectively inhibits PDE in this preparation, since cyclic GMP accumulates in the rudiments with increasing concentrations of the drug. This study shows that a drug-

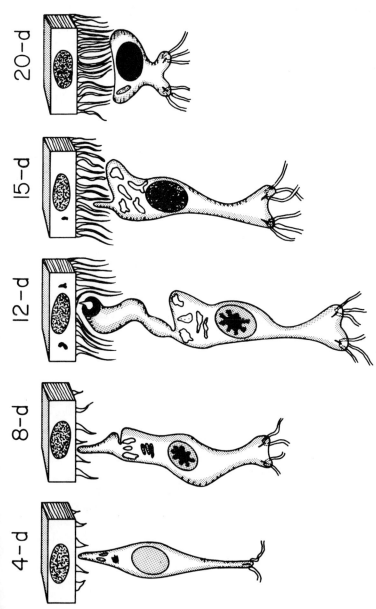

Fig. 7. The postnatal differentiation and subsequent degeneration of rod photoreceptor cells in the retina of C3H/HeJ mice. The photoreceptor cells appear morphologically normal in terms of synaptic terminal and outer segment development until 8 days (8-d). The first signs of pathology can be observed as swelling of the mitochondria of the inner segment. Rod outer segments shed and phagosomes are observed by 10–12 days (12-d) in the pigment epithelium. Subsequently, photoreceptor cells degenerate rapidly. The few photoreceptor nuclei and synaptic terminals which persist at 20 days (20-d) continue to degenerate, and the mature retina of C3H mice is composed solely of its inner layers.

induced disruption of cyclic GMP metabolism can cause photoreceptor cell degeneration, and it reinforces our proposal that an abnormality in cyclic GMP metabolism is causally involved in the degeneration of photoreceptor cells in the C3H retina.

IV. Cyclic Nucleotide Metabolism and Photoreceptor Degeneration in the Retina of RCS Rats

Morphological development of the photoreceptor cells of the rat retina is similar to that depicted for the photoreceptor cells of the mouse retina (Fig. 3) but it occurs a few days later in postnatal life (Bok, 1968).

In normal retina, membrane components of the discs of a rod outer segment are synthesized in the inner segment of the photoreceptor cell, transported to the outer segment, and assembled into disc membranes at the base of the outer segment (Young, 1969b). Once assembled, the discs are displaced proximally by the addition of new discs and, after about 9–10 days, the discs reach the tip of the outer segment where they are shed. The sheddings are then engulfed and phagocytized by cells of the pigment epithelium (Young and Bok, 1969). This process has been shown to occur in the retina of several species and seems to represent the normal mechanism of rod outer segment renewal (Young, 1967, 1969b; Young and Bok, 1969).

Royal College of Surgeons (RCS) rats possess an autosomal recessive mutation which selectively affects the photoreceptor cells of the retina (Dowling and Sidman, 1962). As illustrated in Fig. 8, the photoreceptor cells form, differentiate and develop their responsiveness to light before they degenerate.

In the RCS retina, the processes involved in rod outer segment renewal are out of balance due to the inability of the pigment epithelium to engulf and phagocytize the shed outer segment membranes (Bok and Hall, 1971). Autoradiographic studies show that synthesis, assemblage and displacement of rod outer segment discs are apparently normal in photoreceptor cells of RCS retinas throughout the early phases of the disease (Bok and Hall, 1971; Herron et al.,1971). As a consequence of the photoreceptor cell's steady production of rod outer segment material and the pigment epithelium's incompetence for phagocytizing shed membranes, debris accumulates in the space between the tip of the rod outer segments and the pigment epithelium. This debris constitutes the morphological characteristic of the RCS disorder (Dowling and Sidman, 1962; Bok and Hall, 1971).

There is still some controversy over whether the rod outer segments

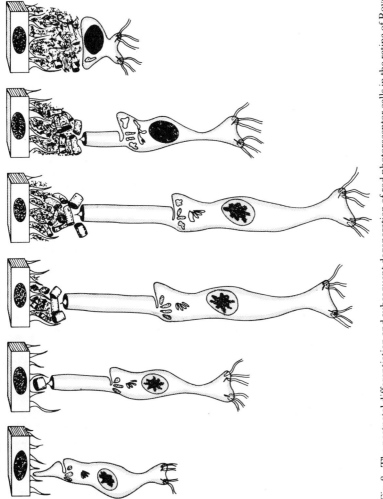

Fig. 8. The postnatal differentiation and subsequent degeneration of rod photoreceptor cells in the retina of Royal College of Surgeons (RCS) rats. The disorder is characterized morphologically by the accumulation of debris between the tips of the rod outer segments and the pigment epithelium. Debris forms from an inability of the pigment epithelium to engulf and phagocytize the shed rod outer segment membranes. Debris accumulation begins at about 12–14 days (12-d) and terminates after 30 days (30-d). Photoreceptor cell degeneration begins at about 20 days (20-d) and is nearly complete by 50–60 days (52-d). The adult retina of RCS rats is composed solely of its inner layers.

of RCS retina are abnormal in their composition, e.g. lacking appropriate surface molecules for recognition by pigment epithelium (Custer and Bok, 1975), or whether the pigment epithelium of the RCS retina is abnormal in its function, e.g. lacking recognition sites which initiate the process of endocytosis of rod outer segment membranes. The use of chimeric rats of normal and RCS parentage seems to favour the proposal that the pigment epithelium is abnormal in its function (LaVail, 1975). If this is the case, why do RCS photoreceptor cells degenerate?

Earlier, it was thought that accumulating debris could create a barrier to the flow of nutrients into the photoreceptor cells from the pigment epithelium and choroid vasculature and that the photoreceptor cells would die from deprivation of essential metabolites. In this regard, the photoreceptor layer is avascular and obtains the major share of its metabolites from the choroid circulation with a lesser contribution from the retinal vasculature (Lolley and Schmidt, 1974). Herron et al. (1971), in their study of rod outer segment renewal, suggest that passage of amino acids from blood to photoreceptor cells is apparently normal in RCS retina during the period of debris accumulation. This observation indicates that a barrier is not created to the exchange of amino acids between the retina and choroid by the RCS debris, and it implies that the passive-barrier hypothesis is inadequate to explain why photoreceptor cells degenerate in the rat disorder.

An alternative hypothesis which suggests that the accumulating RCS debris affects specific aspects of photoreceptor cell metabolism or function seems more in keeping with recent biochemical findings. The data indicate that the metabolism of cyclic GMP in the RCS photoreceptor cells is modified at the time in development when debris accumulates. The full impact of this induced abnormality in cyclic GMP metabolism is unclear but the inference is made that disruption in cyclic GMP metabolism is hazardous to the continued viability of photoreceptor cells. In this regard, the RCS rat disorder has a common feature with that of the inherited retinal degeneration of C3H mice; namely, they both possess abnormalities in cyclic GMP metabolism which are evident a few days before the photoreceptor cells degenerate.

Debris starts accumulating in the RCS retina at about 12–14 days of postnatal life (Dowling and Sidman, 1962; Bok and Hall, 1971). By 20–24 days, the photoreceptor cells begin to degenerate and the majority of them have disappeared by day 50. The degeneration of the photoreceptor cell population is reflected in a loss of protein from the RCS retina (Lolley and Farber, 1975).

The RCS rat disorder appears to be more complex than that of the C3H mouse since, in the rat, debris is formed through a dysfunction in the process of photoreceptor renewal. The debris, or one of its components, then acts upon the photoreceptor cells to limit their capacity to metabolize cyclic GMP. Without means of removing the debris, the photoreceptor cells are confronted with the possibility of functioning under this condition of suppressed cyclic GMP metabolism or degenerating. The morphological data show that they succumb and that the course of the disease is accelerated by light (LaVail and Battelle, 1975).

The following biochemical evidence is presented in support of the proposal that the capacity of RCS photoreceptor cells to metabolize

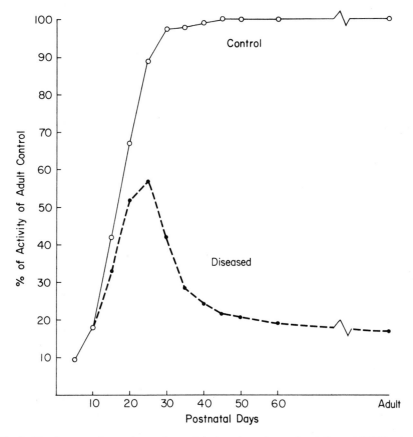

Fig. 9. Development of guanylate cyclase activity in retinas of control and diseased (RCS) rats as a function of postnatal age. The activity measured at 0·7 mM GTP is expressed in relation to that of adult control retina (0·58 nmol cyclic GMP formed/retina.min^{-1}).

cyclic GMP is limited upon the formation of debris at 12–14 postnatal days. The activity of guanylate cyclase (Fig. 9) is comparable to that of control retina for the first ten days and falls below that of the control by day 15. Later in life, when the photoreceptor cells are degenerating, it declines to a value which is observed in retina of adult RCS rats. The developmental pattern for cyclic-GMP-PDE (Fig. 10) is similar to that of guanylate cyclase, but cyclic-GMP-PDE activity is somewhat more stable between 10 and 40 days of postnatal life (Lolley and Farber, 1975). The steady-state balance between the synthesis and hydrolysis of cyclic GMP has been assessed by measuring the cyclic GMP content of these retinas (Fig. 11) (Lolley and Farber, 1976a).

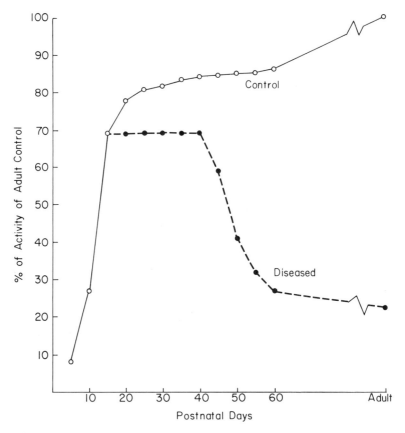

Fig. 10. Development of cyclic GMP phosphodiesterase activity in retinas of control and diseased (RCS) rats as a function of postnatal age. The activity measured at 0·4 mM cyclic GMP is expressed in relation to that of adult control retina (17 nmol cyclic GMP hydrolyzed/retina.min^{-1}).

The pattern of change in cyclic GMP content during development is very similar to that observed for the activity of cyclic-GMP-PDE.

That debris has the capacity to modify the activity and kinetic characteristics of the enzymes of cyclic GMP metabolism has been tested using cyclic-GMP-PDE. Figure 12(a and c) shows the K_m values which are observed in microdissected samples of photoreceptor and inner layers of control and RCS retina. Two points should be noted. First, the K_m values for cyclic-GMP-PDE of the inner layers are identical in control and RCS retinas, but the K_m value for cyclic-GMP-PDE of the RCS photoreceptor layer (1×10^{-4} M) is slightly lower than that of the control (5×10^{-4} M). Secondly, kinetic analysis of homogenates which contain all layers of the retina (Fig. 12b and d)

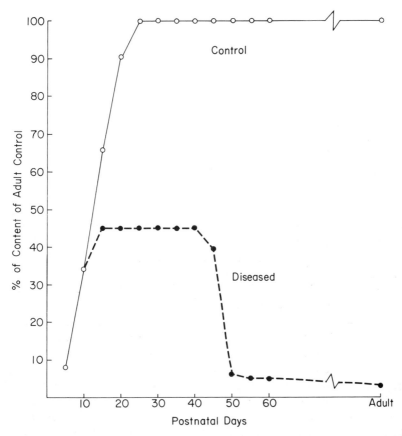

Fig. 11. Content of cyclic GMP in retinas of control and diseased (RCS) rats as a function of postnatal age. The content is expressed in relation to that of the adult control retina (32 pmol cyclic GMP/retina).

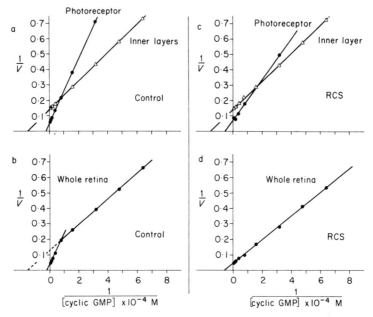

Fig. 12. Lineweaver-Burke plots of cyclic-GMP-PDE activity in: a. freeze-dried photoreceptor layer (○) and bipolar-plus-ganglion-cell layers (△) of control retinas; b. freeze-dried control retinas containing all layers; c. freeze-dried photoreceptor layer (○) and combined inner layers (△) of RCS retinas; and d. freeze-dried RCS retinas containing all layers. The enzyme activity, V, is expressed as nmol cyclic GMP hydrolysed/mg protein.min^{-1}. (From Lolley and Farber, 1975.)

shows two apparent K_m values for cyclic-GMP-PDE of control retina but only a single apparent K_m for that of RCS retina. The K_m value for the cyclic-GMP-PDE of RCS retina is identical to that of the RCS photoreceptor layer. From this we inferred that some component of the RCS photoreceptor layer is capable of modifying the kinetic characteristics of cyclic-GMP-PDE of the RCS inner layers.

A series of mixing experiments confirmed that RCS retina can modify the kinetic characteristics of cyclic-GMP-PDE of control retina (Lolley and Farber, 1976a). Subjecting the RCS retina to heat or dialysis showed that the active component of the RCS retina which enacted this modification was heat-denaturable and non-dialysable. It could be removed from the RCS retina by washing, implying that it was loosely associated. It is known that debris adheres in part to the RCS retina during dissection (Dowling and Sidman, 1962), and the biochemical data suggest that the RCS debris might be the source of the modulator.

Debris was isolated and tested for its ability to modify the kinetics of cyclic-GMP-PDE from control retina. Debris from the eye cup of 16 day and older RCS rats caused the kinetic modification (Lolley and Farber, 1976a). Debris does not alter the apparent kinetic characteristics of the PDE enzyme when cyclic AMP is used as substrate (Lolley and Farber, 1975). These observations suggest that a component of the RCS debris is capable of interacting with and modifying the kinetic characteristics of cyclic-GMP-PDE selectively.

Much is still to be learned about the RCS debris and the mechanism by which it interacts with the metabolism or function of the photoreceptor cells. The current state of our knowledge is presented here to emphasize that the RCS rat disorder appears to arise from a dysfunction in the renewal process of the photoreceptor outer segment. This dysfunction leads to the accumulation of debris which, in turn, acts back upon the neural retina to induce an abnormality in cyclic GMP metabolism in the RCS photoreceptor cells. It is our belief that the induced abnormality in cyclic GMP metabolism of the photoreceptor cells is associated with the biochemical events which lead to the degeneration of the RCS photoreceptor cells.

V. Cyclic AMP Metabolism in the Inner Layers of the Retina

The inner layers (bipolar-plus-ganglion) of the retina (Fig. 2), unlike the photoreceptor cells, possess a significant content of cyclic AMP and the enzymes for its metabolism (Lolley et al., 1974). Like grey matter of the CNS, the inner layers contain a variety of putative neurotransmitter agents (Graham, 1974). Dopamine is the predominant catecholamine in the retina and amacrine cells have been identified as the source of this neurotransmitter. In terms of cyclic AMP metabolism, it has been shown that the inner retinal layers possess an adenylate cyclase, stimulated by dopamine (Lolley et al., 1974) and by other pharmacological agents such as apomorphine and S 584 (the catabolic metabolite of the anti-Parkinson drug, piribecil) (Makman et al., 1975). The stimulation by dopamine is antagonized by relatively low concentrations of neuroleptic drugs. α-Adrenergic blocking agents antagonize this response at relatively high concentrations but β-adrenergic blocking agents are essentially without effect. Overall, the adenylate cyclase of the retina of several species is very similar to that found in brain caudate nucleus (Makman et al., 1975).

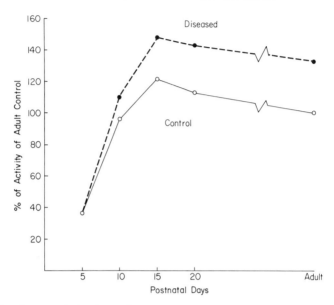

Fig. 13. Development of adenylate cyclase activity in retinas of control and diseased (C3H) mice as a function of postnatal age. The activity was measured at 1·2 mM ATP in the presence of 10 mM sodium fluoride, and it is expressed in relation to that of adult control retina (80 pmol cyclic AMP formed/retina.min^{-1}).

During postnatal maturation of the normal rodent retina, there is a steady increase in the activity of adenylate cyclase (Fig. 13) and of cyclic-AMP-PDE (Schmidt and Lolley, 1973), as well as of the content of cyclic AMP (Fig. 14) (Lolley et al., 1974). Postnatal changes in enzymes of cyclic AMP metabolism are less dramatic than those shown previously for cyclic GMP, possibly because the neurones of the inner layers, other than the bipolar cells, are more differentiated by birth than the photoreceptor cells (Hinds and Hinds, 1974; Sidman, 1961). However, there appears to be a trend of increasing sensitivity of adenylate cyclase to dopamine during early postnatal life. At birth, adenylate cyclase is refractive to dopamine. At five days, it is activated slightly and, at about day 15, the stimulation by dopamine is the greatest observed throughout the life of the animal. Makman et al. (1975) have interpreted the decrease in dopamine stimulation, which occurs after 15 days, to indicate a desensitization of retinal neurones which occurs following their innervation, i.e. the reverse of de-nervation hypersensitivity.

As has been already described (see Fig. 7), the retinas of C3H mice lose their photoreceptor cells through an inherited degeneration and

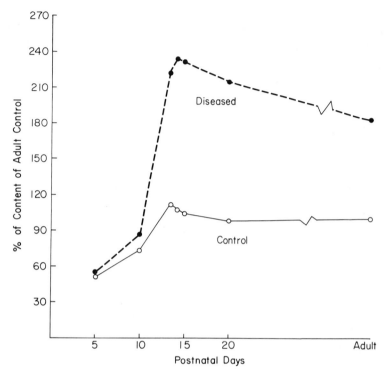

Fig. 14. Content of cyclic AMP in retinas of control and diseased (C3H) mice as a function of postnatal age. The content is expressed in relation to that of the adult control retina (8 pmol cyclic AMP/retina).

the inner layers remain as survivors of the disorder (Noell, 1965). Photoreceptor degeneration begins at about the tenth postnatal day, and it is essentially complete by day 20. During this time period, a normal mouse opens its eyes and its retinal photoreceptor cells form synapses with horizontal and bipolar cells (Blanks *et al.*, 1974a). Simultaneously, the mouse retina begins to exhibit an ERG pattern with adult characteristics (Noell, 1965). The C3H mouse opens its eyes at the appropriate time. It also shows some degree of sensitivity to light even though the synapse which characterizes the photoreceptor/bipolar cell contact does not fully develop (Blanks *et al.*, 1974b). It is still unclear what impact this synaptic abnormality might have upon bipolar cell development since the bipolar cells are as yet incompletely differentiated.

In terms of cyclic AMP metabolism in the surviving inner layers of the C3H retina, the loss of photoreceptor cells is an important event in their biochemical lives. Starting at about ten days, the activity of adenylate cyclase (Fig. 13) and, more strikingly, the content of cyclic AMP (Fig. 14) become greatly elevated (Lolley et al., 1974). They reach their maximum levels about the 15th postnatal day. Thereafter, both the activity of adenylate cyclase and the content of cyclic AMP decline somewhat with age but, even in the adult retina, their levels are above those of the normal retina. Kinetic data indicate that, throughout the life of the C3H mouse, the characteristics of the retinal adenylate cyclase are unchanged, particularly as they relate to the relative sensitivity of adenylate cyclase to dopamine stimulation. Unlike adenylate cyclase, the activity of cyclic-AMP-PDE does not appear to increase during this period.

The role or the physiological consequence of the high levels of cyclic AMP in the inner layers of the C3H retina is not understood but it is probably related to the denervation or lack of innervation of bipolar or horizontal cells by the photoreceptor cells. Photoreceptor cell death appears to place the surviving cells of the inner retinal layers upon a pathway of biochemical differentiation which is quantitatively different from that of the inner layers of control retina. Irrespective of the morphological or biochemical events which trigger this response, the alteration in cyclic AMP metabolism becomes a characteristic of the surviving cells of the adult C3H retina. Therefore, the disruption of the afferent input to a neurone, which occurs during its differentiation or upon initiation of function, may produce biochemical changes in that neurone which are manifest throughout its life.

As described in the previous section, the photoreceptor cells of the RCS retina are relatively mature, morphologically, when the first signs of the disease appear (Fig. 8), and they are functionally mature before they degenerate (Dowling and Sidman, 1962). In terms of cyclic AMP metabolism, the death of the photoreceptor cells has no influence on the content of cyclic AMP in the RCS retina (Fig. 15). This observation points out once again that cyclic AMP is localized almost exclusively in the inner layers of the retina, and it shows that the metabolism of cyclic AMP in the inner layers of the RCS retina responds differently to photoreceptor death than in the case of the C3H retina. We interpret these observations in the C3H mouse and RCS rat retina to indicate that there is a "critical period" in the biochemical maturation of neurones during which they are susceptible to variations in levels of afferent stimulation. This concept is commonplace in the field of neuroendocrinology and well documented in physiological studies of the developing visual system (Hubel, 1967). However, it has received little attention in biochemical investigations of the developing central nervous system. In our case, it was a neurochemical correlation which was unexpected and it was welcomed as a bonus to our work on inherited retinal degenerations.

VI. Cyclic Nucleotides and Neurological Disorders

The death of photoreceptor cells in the retina causes blindness but, in other regions of the CNS, the selective death of neurones may cause a variety of behavioural or perceptual abnormalities. For example, the Purkinje or granule cells of the cerebellum degenerate during postnatal development in several inbred strains of mice and their death alters the physiological signal being transmitted from the cerebellum. This

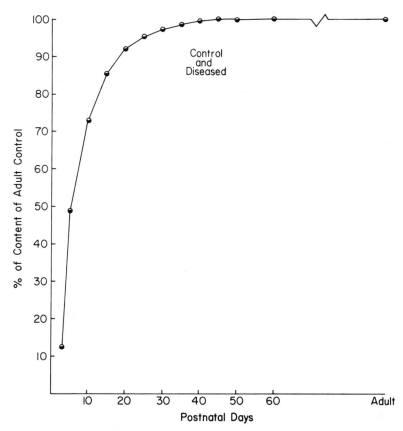

Fig. 15. Content of cyclic AMP in retinas of control and diseased (RCS) rats as a function of postnatal age. The content is expressed in relation to that of the adult control retina (6·7 pmol cyclic AMP/retina).

results in disorders which are characterized by a dysynchrony in motor function, and the strains of mice are often named for their unusual manner of locomotion, e.g. staggerer, nervous, reeler, weaver (Sidman, 1974).

Another type of abnormality involves adaptive changes in second order neurones, which could occur upon degeneration or impairment in the function of their primary afferent pathway. For example, in the absence of afferent stimuli, some classes of neurones in the CNS fail, during development, to migrate to their final position (Levi-Montalcini, 1964) and some may actually degenerate (Cowan, 1970). The dependence of a neurone upon appropriate afferent stimuli may be recognized even by more subtle criteria such as an impaired induction of synthetic enzyme activity (Black *et al.*, 1971) or an enhanced level of enzyme activity. An example of the latter form of adaptation is found in the changes in cyclic AMP metabolism which are observed within the inner layers of the C3H mouse retina as an apparent consequence of photoreceptor cell death. This effect occurs within a critical period of development and the death of the photoreceptor cells is imprinted in a lasting manner in the metabolism of the surviving cells so that it becomes a characteristic of these cells in adulthood.

As the earlier sections of this chapter have indicated, the most effective site at which an abnormality in cyclic nucleotide metabolism might be expressed in a neurone is at the synaptic junction. The apparent involvement of cyclic nucleotides in the generation and possible control of synaptic potentials places them at the critical site where information is transferred within the CNS. The synapse is also the site of action of a wide variety of drugs which effect both cyclic nucleotide metabolism and neuronal function. Even the hallucinogens, LSD and tetrahydrocannabinol, may exert their action through the cyclic nucleotide system (Dolby and Kleinsmith, 1974; von Hungen *et al.*, 1975; Da Prada *et al.*, 1975; Spano *et al.*, 1975).

Several lines of evidence indicate that cyclic AMP and cyclic GMP are associated with different classes of synapses. The respective synapses can act antagonistically in terms of their physiological response and they may be selectively modified by drugs. Under normal conditions, there is an integrated blend of postsynaptic potentials which are in part mediated by cyclic nucleotides. The summed depolarizations and hyperpolarizations which are generated at the active synapses determine whether the postsynaptic neurone will generate a propagated action potential. In an abnormal condition, which could be produced by drugs or which could arise from disruption in the metabolism of cyclic AMP or cyclic GMP, the function of the postsynaptic neurone would be distorted in proportion to its specific innervation and to its responsiveness to cyclic nucleotides. The net result of such an abnormality would be an altered input to a second order neurone and, ultimately, an alteration to information processing in the CNS. While the above case is hypothetical, it is likely that such alterations do exist in the living brain.

It has been reported that abnormalities in cyclic nucleotide metabolism can cause disease states in tissues throughout the body. Symposia have been devoted to this subject and the resulting books (Greengard and Robison, 1974; Weiss, 1975b) are useful guides to the interested reader. A few examples are cited to show the diversity of such diseases. In the eye, abnormalities in the metabolism of cyclic AMP have been implicated in the formation of cataracts and in the increased interocular pressure associated with glaucoma (Neufeld, 1976). Voorhees et al. (1974) have shown an imbalance in the ratio of cyclic AMP and cyclic GMP in the human proliferative skin disease, psoriasis. The cyclic nucleotides have been implicated also in smooth muscle disturbances such as hypertension and asthma (Bär, 1974). They have been suggested also as pathological agents in immunologic abnormalities (Parker et al., 1974), and there is strong evidence that cyclic nucleotides play a role in some types of cancer (Ryan and Heirdick, 1974).

We have provided a general outline of our present knowledge and a description of our current insight into inherited retinal degenerative diseases of rodent retina. Much is still to be learned, and it is our belief that the study of selected disease states of the CNS may both give insight into the normal role of cyclic nucleotides in the metabolism or function of neural tissue and provide an understanding of disease states from which their treatment may be formulated.

Acknowledgements

We wish to acknowledge the helpful criticisms of Drs Stanley G. Korenman and Robert A. Marcus and the thoughtful assistance of Ms Louise V. Eaton in the preparation of this chapter. Special thanks go to Mrs Elisabeth Racz, Mr George Sullivan and Mr Bruce Brown, for their technical assistance in the laboratory, and to the Veterans Administration, the National Eye Institute and the National Science Foundation, for supporting our research programme.

References

Adinolfi, A. M. and Schmidt, S. Y. (1974). *Brain Res.* **76**, 21–31.
Bär, H.–P. (1974). *In* "Advan. Cyclic Nucleotide Res." (P. Greengard and G. A. Robison, eds), Vol. 4. Raven Press, New York, pp. 195–238.
Baylor, D. A. and Fuortes, M. G. F. (1970). *J. Physiol. (London)* **207**, 77–92.
Beam, K. G. and Greengard, P. (1975). *Cold Spring Harbor Symp. Quant. Biol.* **40**, 157–168.
Beer, B., Chasin, M., Clody, D. E., Vogel, J. R. and Horovitz, Z. P. (1972). *Science* **176**, 428–430.
Bensinger, R. E., Fletcher, R. T. and Chader, G. J. (1973). *Science* **183**, 86–87.
Berndt, S. and Schwabe, U. (1973). *Brain Res.* **63**, 303–312.
Berridge, M. J. (1975). *In* "Advan. Cyclic Nucleotide Res." (P. Greengard and G. A. Robison, eds), Vol. 6. Raven Press, New York, pp. 1–98.
Berti, F., Trabucchi, M., Bernareggi, V. and Fumagalli, R. (1973). *In* "International Conference on Prostaglandins, Vienna, Advan. Biosci." (S. Bergström and S. Bernhard, eds), Vol. 9. Pergamon, Oxford, pp. 475–480.
Birnbaumer, L., Pohl, S. L., Krans, M. L. and Rodbell, M. (1970). *Advan. Biochem. Psychopharmacol.* **3**, 185–208.
Bitensky, M. W., Miki, N., Marcus, F. R. and Keirns, J. J. (1973). *Life Sci.* **13**, 1451–1472.
Bitensky, M. W., Miki, N., Keirns, J. J., Keirns, M., Baraban, J. M., Freeman, J., Wheeler, M. A., Lacy, J. and Marcus, F. R. (1975). *In* "Advan. Cyclic Nucleotide Res." (G. I. Drummond, P. Greengard and G. A. Robison, eds), Vol. 5. Raven Press, New York, pp. 213–240.
Black, I. B., Hendry, I. and Iversen, L. L. (1971). *Brain Res.* **34**, 229–246.
Blanks, J. C., Adinolfi, A. M. and Lolley, R. N. (1974a). *J. Comp. Neurol.* **156**, 81–93.
Blanks, J. C., Adinolfi, A. M. and Lolley, R. N. (1974b). *J. Comp. Neurol.* **156**, 95–106.
Blume, A. J., Dalton, C. and Sheppard, H. (1973). *Proc. Nat. Acad. Sci. U.S.A.* **70**, 3099–3102.
Bok, P. D. (1968). Ph.D. Thesis, University of California, Los Angeles.
Bok, D. and Hall, M. O. (1971). *J. Cell Biol.* **49**, 664–682.
Bradham, L. S. (1972). *Biochim. Biophys. Acta* **276**, 434–443.
Breckenridge, B. McL. (1964). *Proc. Nat. Acad. Sci. U.S.A.* **52**, 1580–1586.
Breckenridge, B. McL. and Johnston, R. E. (1969). *J. Histochem. Cytochem.* **17**, 505–510.
Brooker, G., Thomas, L. J., jun. and Appleman, M. M. (1968). *Biochemistry* **7**, 4177–4181.
Brown, J. Heller and Makman, M. (1972). *Proc. Nat. Acad. Sci. U.S.A.* **69**, 539–543.
Butcher, R. W. and Sutherland, E. W. (1962). *J. Biol. Chem.* **237**, 1244–1250.
Caley, D. W., Johnson, C. J. and Liebelt, R. A. (1972). *Amer. J. Anat.* **133**, 179–212.
Campbell, M. T. and Oliver, I. T. (1972). *Eur. J. Biochem.* **28**, 30–37.
Chader, G., Fletcher, R., Johnson, M. and Bensinger, R. (1974a). *Exp. Eye Res.* **18**, 509–515.
Chader, G. J., Herz, L. R. and Fletcher, R. T. (1974b). *Biochim. Biophys. Acta* **347**, 491–493.
Chader, G. J., Fletcher, R. T. and Krishna, G. (1975). *Biochem. Biophys. Res. Commun.* **64**, 535–538.
Chader, G. J., Fletcher, R. T., O'Brien, P. and Krishna, G. (1976). *Biochemistry* **15**, 1615–1620.

Chasin, M., Rivkin, I., Mamrak, F., Samaniego, S. G. and Hess, S. M. (1971). *J. Biol. Chem.* **246**, 3037–3041.

Chasin, M., Harris, D. N., Phillips, M. B. and Hess, S. M. (1972). *Biochem. Pharmacol.* **21**, 2443–2450.

Chasin, M., Mamrak, F. and Samaniego, S. G. (1974). *J. Neurochem.* **22**, 1031–1038.

Cheung, W. Y. (1971). *J. Biol. Chem.* **246**, 2859–2869.

Clement-Cormier, Y. C., Kebabian, J. W., Petzold, G. L. and Greengard, P. (1974). *Proc. Nat. Acad. Sci. U.S.A.* **71**, 1113–1117.

Costa, E., Guidotti, A. and Hanbauer, I. (1974). *Life Sci.* **14**, 1169–1188.

Costa, E., Guidotti, A., Mao, C. C. and Suria, A. (1975a). *Life Sci.* **17**, 167–186.

Costa, E., Guidotti, A. and Mao, C. C. (1975b). *In* "Mechanism of Action of Benzodiazepines" (E. Costa and P. Greengard, eds). Raven Press, New York, pp. 113–130.

Cowan, W. M. (1970). *In* "Contemporary Research Methods in Neuroanatomy" (W. J. H. Nauta and S. O. Ebbesson, eds). Springer-Verlag, New York, pp. 217–251.

Cramer, H., Paul, M. I., Silbergeld, S. and Forn, J. (1971). *J. Neurochem.* **18**, 1605–1608.

Custer, N. V. and Bok, D. (1975). *Exp. Eye Res.* **21**, 153–166.

Da Prada, M., Saner, A., Burkard, W. P., Bartholine, G. and Pletscher, A. (1975). *Brain Res.* **94**, 67–73.

Davison, A. N. and Dobbing, J. (1968). *In* "Applied Neurochemistry" (A. N. Davison and J. Dobbing, eds). F. A. Davis Company, Philadelphia, pp. 253–286.

DeRobertis, E., Rodriquez de Lores Arnaiz, G. A., Alberici, M., Butcher, R. W. and Sutherland, E. W. (1967). *J. Biol. Chem.* **242**, 3487–3493.

Dewey, M. M., Davis, P. K., Blasie, J. K. and Barr, L. (1969). *J. Mol. Biol.* **39**, 395–405.

Dismukes, R. K. and Daly, J. W. (1975). *Exp. Neurol.* **49**, 150–160.

Ditzion, B. R., Paul, M. I. and Pauk, G. L. (1970). *Pharmacology* **3**, 25–31.

Dolby, T. W. and Kleinsmith, L. J. (1974). *Biochem. Pharmacol.* **23**, 1817–1825.

Dowling, J. E. (1968). *Proc. Roy. Soc. Biol.* (*London*) *Ser. B* **170**, 205–228.

Dowling, J. E. and Sidman, R. L. (1962). *J. Cell Biol.* **14**, 73–109.

Drummond, G. I., Severson, D. L. and Duncan, L. (1971). *J. Biol. Chem.* **246**, 4166–4173.

Drummond, G. I., Greengard, P. and Robison, G. A. (eds) (1975). "Advan. Cyclic Nucleotide Res.," Vol. 5. Raven Press, New York.

Dubin, M. Wm. (1974). *In* "The Eye" (H. Davson and L. T. Graham, jun., eds), Vol. 6. Academic Press, New York and London, pp. 227–256.

Fallon, E. F., Agrawal, R., Furth, E., Steiner, A. L. and Crowden, R. (1974). *Science* **184**, 1089–1091.

Farber, D. B. and Lolley, (1973). *J. Neurochem.* **21**, 817–828.

Farber, D. B. and Lolley, R. N. (1974). *Science* **186**, 449–451.

Farber, D. B. and Lolley, R. N. (1976). *J. Cyclic Nucleotide Res.* **2**, 139–148.

Ferrendelli, J. A. (1975). *In* "Cyclic Nucleotides in Disease" (B. Weiss, ed.). University Park Press, Baltimore, London and Tokyo, pp. 377–390.

Ferrendelli, J. A., Steiner, A. L., McDougal, D. B., jun. and Kipnis, D. M. (1970). *Biochem. Biophys. Res. Commun.* **41**, 1061–1067.

Ferrendelli, J. A., Kinscherf, D. A. and Kipnis, D. M. (1972). *Biochem. Biophys. Res. Commun.* **46**, 2114–2120.

Ferrendelli, J. A., Kinscherf, D. A. and Chang, M. M. (1973). *Mol. Pharmacol.* **9**, 445–454.

Ferrendelli, J. A., Chang, M. M. and Kinscherf, D. A. (1974). *J. Neurochem.* **22**, 535–540.

Ferrendelli, J. A., Kinscherf, D. A. and Chang, M. M. (1975). *Brain Res.* **84**, 63–73.

Fertel, R. and Weiss, B. (1974). *Anal. Biochem.* **59**, 386–398.

Fletcher, R.T. and Chader, G. J. (1976). *Biochem Biophys. Res. Commun.* **70**, 1297–1302.

Florendo, N. T., Barrnett, R. J. and Greengard, P. (1971). *Science* **173**, 745–748.

Fonnum, F. (1965). *Biochem. J.* **106**, 401–412.

Forn, J. and Krishna, G. (1971). *Pharmacology* **5**, 193–204.

Free, C. A., Paik, V. S. and Shada, J. D. (1974). *Advan. Biochem. Psychopharmacol.* **9**, 739–748.

Freedman, R. and Siggins, G. R. (1974). *Fed. Proc.* **33**, 245.

Gilman, A. G. (1972). *In* "Advances in Cyclic Nucleotide Research" (P. Greengard, R. Paoletti and G. A. Robison, eds), Vol. 1. Raven Press, New York, pp. 389–410.

Gilman, A. G. and Schrier, B. K. (1972). *Mol. Pharmacol.* **8**, 410–416.

Goldberg, N. D., Lust, W. D., O'Dea, R. F., Wei, S. and O'Toole, A. G. (1970). *Advan. Biochem. Psychopharmacol.* **3**, 67–87.

Goldberg, N. D., Haddox, M. K., Hartle, D. K. and Hadden, J. W. (1973a). *In* "Pharmacology and the Future of Man" Proc. 5th Int. Congress Pharmacology, San Francisco, 1972, Vol. 5. Karger, Basel, pp. 146–169.

Goldberg, N. D., O'Dea, R. F. and Haddox, M. K. (1973b). *In* "Advan. Cyclic Nucleotide Res." (P. Greengard and G. A. Robison, eds), Vol. 3. Raven Press, New York, pp. 155–223.

Goldberg, N. D., Haddox, M. K., Dunham, E., Lopez, C. and Hadden, J. W. (1974). *In* "Control of Proliferation in Animal Cells" (B. Clarkson and R. Baserga, eds). Cold Spring Harbor Laboratory, New York, pp. 609–625.

Goldberg, N. D., Haddox, M. K., Nicol, S. E., Glass, D. B., Sanford, C. H., Keuhl, F. A., jun. and Estensen, R. (1975). *In* "Advan. Cyclic Nucleotide Res." (G. I. Drummond, P. Greengard and G. A. Robison, eds), Vol. 5. Raven Press, New York, pp. 307–330.

Gordon, M. (1967). *In* "Psychopharmacological Agents" (M. Gordon, ed.), Vol. 11. Academic Press, New York and London, pp. 1–198.

Goridis, C. and Morgan, I. G. (1973). *FEBS Lett.* **34**, 71–73.

Goridis, C. and Virmaux, N. (1974). *Nature (London)* **248**, 57.

Goridis, C., Virmaux, N., Urban, P. F. and Mandel, P. (1973). *FEBS Lett.* **30**, 163–166.

Goridis, C., Massarelli, R., Sensenbrenner, M. and Mandel, P. (1974a). *J. Neurochem.* **23**, 135–138.

Goridis, C., Virmaux, N., Cailla, H. L. and Delaage, M. A. (1974b). *FEBS Lett.* **49**, 167–169.

Graham, L. T., jun. (1974). *In* "The Eye" (H. Davson and L. T. Graham, jun., eds), Vol. 6. Academic Press, New York and London, pp. 283–333.

Greengard, P. (1975). *In* "Advan. Cyclic Nucleotide Res." (G. I. Drummond, P. Greengard and G. A. Robison, eds), Vol. 5. Raven Press, New York, pp. 585–601.

Greengard, P. and Costa, E. (eds) (1970). "Role of Cyclic AMP in Cell Function." Raven Press, New York.

Greengard, P. and Kuo, J. F. (1970). *Advan. Biochem. Psychopharmacol.* **3**, 287–306.

Greengard, P. and Robison, G. A. (eds) (1974). "Advan. Cyclic Nucleotide Res." Vol. 4. Raven Press, New York.

Greengard, P., Paoletti, R. and Robison, G. A. (eds) (1972). "Advan. Cyclic Nucleotide Res." Vol. 1. Raven Press, New York.

Guidotti, A., Biggio, G. and Costa, E. (1975a). *Brain Res.* **96**, 201–205.

Guidotti, A., Hanbauer, I. and Costa, E. (1975b). *In* "Advan. Cyclic Nucleotide Res." (G. I. Drummond, P. Greengard and G. A. Robison, eds), Vol. 5. Raven Press, New York, pp. 619–639.

Guidotti, A., Biggio, G., Naik, N. and Mao, C. C. (1976). *In* "Taurine" (R. Huxtable and A. Barbeau, eds). Raven Press, New York, pp. 243–251.

Hagins, W. A. (1965). *Cold Spring Harbor Symp. Quant. Biol.* **30**, 403–417.

Hagins, W. A. and Yoshikami, S. (1974). *Exp. Eye Res.* **18**, 299–305.

Hechter, O. and Halkerston, I. D. K. (1964). *In* "The Hormones" (G. Pinkus, K. V. Thimann and E. B. Astwood, eds), Vol. 5. Academic Press, New York and London, pp. 697–825.

Hendricks, Th., Daemen, F. J. M. and Bonting, S. L. (1974). *Biochim. Biophys. Acta* **345**, 468–473.

Herron, W. L., jun., Riegel, B. W. and Rubin, M. L. (1971). *Invest. Ophthalmol.* **10**, 54–63.

Hinds, J. W. and Hinds, P. L. (1974). *Dev. Biol.* **37**, 381–416.

Hoffer, B. J., Siggins, G. R. and Bloom, F. E. (1969). *Science* **166**, 1418–1420.

Hoffer, B. J., Siggins, G. R., Oliver, A. P. and Bloom, F. E. (1972). *In* "Advan. Cyclic Nucleotide Res." (P. Greengard, R. Paoletti and G. A. Robison, eds), Vol. 1. Raven Press, New York, pp. 411–423.

Hogan, J. J., Wood, I. and Steinberg, R. H. (1974). *Nature (London)* **252**, 305–307.

Hollyfield, J. G., Mottow, L. S. and Ward, A. (1975). *Exp. Eye Res.* **20**, 383–391.

Huang, M., Shimizu, H. and Daly, J. (1971). *Mol. Pharmacol.* **7**, 155–162.

Huang, M., Shimizu, H. and Daly, J. (1972). *J. Med. Chem.* **15**, 462–466.

Huang, M., Ho, A. K. S. and Daly, J. W. (1973). *Mol. Pharmacol.* **9**, 711–717.

Hubel, D. H. (1967). *The Physiologist* **10**, 17–45.

Iversen, L. L., Horn, A. S. and Miller, R. J. (1975). *In* "Advan. Neurology" (D. Calne, T. N. Chase and A. Barbeau, eds), Vol. 9. Raven Press, New York, pp. 197–212.

Jan, L. Y. and Revel, J.-P. (1974). *J. Cell Biol.* **62**, 257–273.

Johnson, E. M., Maeno, H. and Greengard, P. (1971). *J. Biol. Chem.* **246**, 7731–7739.

Kakiuchi, S. and Rall, T. W. (1968a). *Mol. Pharmacol.* **4**, 367–378.

Kakiuchi, S. and Rall, T. W. (1968b). *Mol. Pharmacol.* **4**, 379–388.

Kakiuchi, S., Rall, T. W. and McIlwain, H. (1969). *J. Neurochem.* **16**, 485–491.

Kakiuchi, S., Yamazaki, R. and Teshima, Y. (1972). *In* "Advan. Cyclic Nucleotide Res." (P. Greengard, R. Paoletti and G. A. Robison, eds), Vol. 1. Raven Press, New York, pp. 455–477.

Kakiuchi, S., Yamazaki, R., Teshima, Y. and Menishi, K. (1973). *Proc. Nat. Acad. Sci. U.S.A.* **70**, 3526–3530.

Kalisker, A., Rutledge, C. O. and Perkins, J. P. (1973). *Mol. Pharmacol.* **9**, 619–626.

Kaneko, A. and Hashimoto, H. (1969). *Vision Res.* **9**, 37–55.

Kebabian, J. W. and Greengard, P. (1971). *Science* **174**, 1346–1349.

Kebabian, J. W., Petzold, G. L. and Greengard, P. (1972). *Proc. Nat. Acad. Sci. U.S.A.* **69**, 2145–2149.

Kebabian, J. W., Bloom, F. E., Steiner, A. L. and Greengard, P. (1975a). *Science* **190**, 157–159.

Kebabian, J. W., Steiner, A. L. and Greengard, P. (1975b). *J. Pharmacol. Exp. Ther.* **193**, 474–488.

Keirns, J. J., Miki, N., Bitensky, M. W. and Keirns, M. (1975). *Biophys. J.* **15**, 168a, Abstract #TH-PM-Di.

Kimura, H. and Murad, F. (1974). *J. Biol. Chem.* **249**, 6910–6916

Kimura, H. and Murad, F. (1975). *Advan. Cyclic Nucleotide Res.* **5**, 822.
Kimura, H., Mittal, C. K. and Murad, F. (1975). *Nature (London)* **257**, 700–702.
Knight, B. W., Toyoda, J.-I. and Dodge, F. A., jun. (1970). *J. Gen. Physiol.* **56**, 421–437.
Krishna, G., Krishnan, Fletcher, R. and Chader, G. (1976). *J. Neurochem.* **27**, 712–722.
Kuczenski, R. T. and Mandell, A. J. (1972). *J. Biol. Chem.* **247**, 3114–3119.
Kuo, J. F. and Greengard, P. (1969). *Proc. Nat. Acad. Sci. U.S.A.* **64**, 1349–1355.
Kuo, J. F. and Greengard, P. (1970). *J. Biol. Chem.* **245**, 2493–2498.
Kuo, J. F., Wyatt, G. R. and Greengard, P. (1971). *J. Biol. Chem.* **246**, 7159–7167.
Kuo, J. F., Lee, T. P., Reyes, P. L., Walton, K. G., Donnelly, T. E., jun. and Greengard, P. (1972). *J. Biol. Chem.* **247**, 16–22.
LaVail, M. M. (1973). *J. Cell Biol.* **58**, 650–661.
LaVail, M. M. (1975). Personal Communication.
LaVail, M. M. and Battelle, B. A. (1975). *Exp. Eye Res.* **21**, 167–192.
LaVail, M. M. and Mullen, R. J. (1974). ARVO 1974 Meeting, p. 61.
LaVail, M. M. and Sidman, R. L. (1974). *Arch. Ophthalmol.* **91**, 394–400.
Lee, T.-P., Kuo, J. F. and Greengard, P. (1972). *Proc. Nat. Acad. Sci. U.S.A.* **69**, 3287–3291.
Levi-Montalcini, R. (1964). *In* "The Nature of Biological Diversity" (J. M. Allen, ed.). McGraw-Hill, New York, pp. 261–295.
Lin, Y. M., Lin, Y. P. and Cheung, W. Y. (1974). *J. Biol. Chem.* **249**, 4943–4954.
Lipton, S. A. (1975). ARVO 1975 Meeting, p. 4.
Lolley, R. N. (1969). *In* "Handbook of Neurochemistry" (A. Lajtha, ed.), Vol. 2. Plenum Press, New York, pp. 473–504.
Lolley, R. N. (1973). *J. Neurochem.* **20**, 175–182.
Lolley, R. N. and Farber, D. B. (1975). *Exp. Eye Res.* **20**, 585–597.
Lolley, R. N. and Farber, D. B. (1976a). *Exp. Eye Res.* **22**, 477–486.
Lolley, R. N. and Farber, D. B. (1976b). *Annu. Ophthalmol.* **8**, 469–473.
Lolley, R. N. and Schmidt, S. Y. (1974). *In* "The Eye" (H. Davson and L. T. Graham, jun., eds), Vol. 6. Academic Press, New York and London, pp. 343–378.
Lolley, R. N., Schmidt, S. Y. and Farber, D. B. (1974). *J. Neurochem.* **22**, 701–707.
Lolley, R. N., Farber, D. B., Rayborn, M. and Hollyfield, J. G. (1976). *Science* (in press).
Lust, W. D. and Goldberg, N. D. (1970). *Pharmacologist* **12**, 290.
Maeno, H. and Greengard, P. (1972). *J. Biol. Chem.* **247**, 3269–3277.
Maeno, H., Johnson, E. M. and Greengard, P. (1971). *J. Biol. Chem.* **246**, 134–142.
Makman, M. H., Brown, J. Heller and Mishra, R. K. (1975). *In* "Advan. Cyclic Nucleotide Res." (G. I. Drummond, P. Greengard and G. A. Robison, eds), Vol. 5. Raven Press, New York, pp. 661–679.
Mann, E. and Christiansen, R. O. (1971). *Science* **173**, 540–541.
Mao, C. C., Guidotti, A. and Costa, E. (1974a). *Mol. Pharmacol.* **10**, 736–745.
Mao, C. C., Guidotti, A. and Costa, E. (1974b). *Brain Res.* **79**, 510–514.
Mao, C. C., Guidotti, A. and Costa, E. (1975a). *Naunyn-Schmiedebergs Arch. Pharmakol. Exp. Pathol.* **289**, 369–378.
Mao, C. C., Guidotti, A. and Sandis, S. (1975b). *Brain Res.* **90**, 335–339.
Mao, C. C., Guidotti, A. and Costa, E. (1975c). *Brain Res.* **83**, 516–519.
Mason, W. T., Fager, R. S. and Abrahamson, E. W. (1974). *Nature (London)* **247**, 562–563.

McCune, R. W., Gill, T. H., von Hungen, K. and Roberts, S. (1971). *Life Sci.* **10**, Part II, 443–450.

Miki, N., Keirns, J. J., Marcus, F. R., Freeman, J. and Bitensky, M. W. (1973). *Proc. Nat. Acad. Sci. U.S.A.* **70** (12), 3820–3824.

Miller, R. J. and Iversen, L. L. (1974). *Naunyn-Schm. Arch. Pharmakol. Exp. Pathol.* **282**, 213–216.

Mishra, R. K., Katzman, R. and Makman, M. H. (1974). *Fed. Proc.* **33**, 494.

Murad, F., Manganiello, V. and Vaughan, M. (1971). *Proc. Nat. Acad. Sci. U.S.A.* **68**, 736–739.

Nathanson, J. A. and Greengard, P. (1973). *Science* **180**, 308–310.

Nathanson, J. A. and Greengard, P. (1974). *Proc. Nat. Acad. Sci. U.S.A.* **71**, 797–801.

Neufeld, A. H. (1976). *In* "Clinical Aspects of Cyclic Nucleotides" (L. Volicer, ed.), Vol. 14. Spectrum Publications, N.Y. (in press).

Noell, W. K. (1965). *In* "Biochemistry of the Retina" (C. N. Graymore, ed.). Academic Press, New York and London, pp. 51–72.

O'Dea, R. F., Haddox, M. K. and Goldberg, N. D. (1971). *Fed. Proc.* **30**, 219.

Oliver, A. P. and Segal, M. (1974). *Abstracts Society for Neuroscience (St. Louis)* **4**, 361.

Olney, J. W. (1968). *Invest. Ophthalmol.* **7**, 250–268.

Palmer, G. C. (1972). *Neuropharmacology* **11**, 145–149.

Palmer, G. C. and Manian, A. A. (1974a). *Neuropharmacology* **13**, 651–664.

Palmer, G. C. and Manian, A. A. (1974b). *Neuropharmacology* **13**, 851–866.

Palmer, G. C., Robison, G. A. and Sulser, F. (1971). *Biochem. Pharmacol.* **20**, 236–239.

Palmer, G. C., Sulser, F. and Robison, G. A. (1973). *Neuropharmacology* **12**, 327–337.

Pannbacker, R. G. (1973a). *Science* **182**, 1138–1140.

Pannbacker, R. G. (1973b). *In* "Prostaglandins and Cyclic AMP: Biological Action and Clinical Applications" (R. H. Kahn and W. E. M. Lands, eds). Academic Press, New York and London, pp. 251–252.

Parker, C. W., Sullivan, T. J. and Wedner, H. J. (1974). *In* "Advan. Cyclic Nucleotide Res." (P. Greengard and G. A. Robison, eds), Vol. 4. Raven Press, New York, pp. 1–80.

Perkins, J. P. (1973). *In* "Advan. Cyclic Nucleotide Research" (P. Greengard and G. A. Robison, eds), Vol. 3. Raven Press, New York, pp. 1–64.

Perkins, J. P. and Moore, M. M. (1971). *J. Biol. Chem.* **246**, 62–68.

Pichard, Anne-Lise, Hanoune, J. and Kaplan, J. C. (1972). *Biochim. Biophys. Acta* **279**, 217–220.

Ripps, H., Schakib, M. and MacDonald, E. D. (1976). *J. Cell Biol.* **70**, 86–96.

Robb, R. M. (1974). *Invest. Ophthalmol.* **13**, 740–747.

Robison, G. A., Butcher, R. W. and Sutherland, E. W. (1967). *Ann. N.Y. Acad. Sci.* **139**, 703–723.

Robison, G. A., Nahas, G. G. and Triner, L. (eds) (1971). "Cyclic AMP and Cell Function," Vol. 185, *Ann. N.Y. Acad. Sci.*

Rodbell, M. (1971). *In* "Colloquium on the Role of Adenyl Cyclase and Cyclic 3′,5′-AMP in Biological Systems" (P. Condliffe and M. Rodbell, eds). Fogarty International Centre, Government Printing Office, pp. 88–95.

Ryan, W. L. and Heirdick, M. L. (1974). *In* "Advan. Cyclic Nucleotide Res." (P. Greengard and G. A. Robison, eds), Vol. 4. Raven Press, New York, pp. 81–116.

Sattin, A. and Rall, T. W. (1970). *Mol. Pharmacol.* **6**, 13–23.

Sattin, A., Rall, T. W. and Zanella, J. (1975). *J. Pharmacol. Exp. Ther.* **192**, 22–32.

Schmidt, M. J., Schmidt, D. E. and Robison, G. A. (1971). *Science* **173**, 1142–1143.
Schmidt, S. Y. and Lolley, R. N. (1973). *J. Cell Biol.* **57**, 117–123.
Schultz, J. (1974a). *Pharmacol. Res. Commun.* **6**, 335–341.
Schultz, J. (1974b). *Arch. Biochem. Biophys.* **163**, 15–20.
Schultz, J. (1975). *J. Neurochem.* **24**, 495–501.
Schultz, J. and Daly, J. W. (1973). *J. Neurochem.* **21**, 573–579.
Schultz, J. and Hamprecht, B. (1973). *Naunyn-Schmiedebergs Archiv. Pharmakol. Exp. Pathol.* **278**, 215–225.
Seeds, N. W. and Gilman, A. G. (1971). *Science* **174**, 292.
Segal, M. and Bloom, F. E. (1974a). *Brain Res.* **72**, 79–97.
Segal, M. and Bloom, F. E. (1974b). *Brain Res.* **72**, 99–114.
Shimizu, H. and Daly, J. (1972). *Europ. J. Pharmacol.* **17**, 240–252.
Shimizu, H., Creveling, L. R. and Daly, J. W. (1970). *Proc. Nat. Acad. Sci. U.S.A.* **65**, 1033–1040.
Sidman, R. L. (1961). *In* "Structure of the Eye" (G. K. Smelser, ed.). Academic Press, New York and London, pp. 487–506.
Sidman, R. L. (1974). *In* "The Neurosciences, Third Study Program" (F. O. Schmitt and F. G. Worden, eds). The MIT Press, Cambridge, (Massachusetts) and London, pp. 743–758.
Sidman, R. L. and Green, M. C. (1965). *J. Hered.* **56**, 23–29.
Siggins, G. R. and Hendriksen, S. J. (1975). *Science* **189**, 559–561.
Siggins, G. R., Hoffer, B. J. and Bloom, F. E. (1971a). *Brain Res.* **25**, 535–553.
Siggins, G. R., Oliver, A. P., Hoffer, B. J. and Bloom, F. E. (1971b). *Science* **171**, 192–194.
Siggins, G. R., Hoffer, B. J. and Ungerstedt, V. (1974). *Life Sci.* **15**, 779–792.
Smoake, J. A., Song, S. Y. and Cheung, W. Y. (1974). *Biochim. Biophys. Acta* **341**, 402–411.
Sonohara, O. and Shiose, Y. (1968). *Folia. Ophth. Jap.* **19**, 77–86.
Spano, P. F., Kumakura, K., Tonon, G. C., Govoni, S. and Trabucchi, M. (1975). *Brain Res.* **93**, 164–167.
Steiner, A. L., Parker, C. W. and Kipnis, D. M. (1970). *Advan. Biochem. Psychopharmacol.* **3**, 89–111.
Steiner, A. L., Ferrendelli, J. A. and Kipnis, D. M. (1972). *J. Biol. Chem.* **247**, 1121–1124.
Stell, W. K. (1972). *In* "Handbook of Sensory Physiology" (M. F.G. Fuortes, ed.), Vol. 7, Part 2. Springer-Verlag, New York, pp. 111–213.
Strada, S. J., Uzunov, P. and Weiss, B. (1974). *J. Neurochem.* **23**, 1097–1103.
Sutherland, E. W., Rall, T. W. and Menon, T. (1962). *J. Biol. Chem.* **237**, 1220–1227.
Teshima, Y. and Kakiuchi, S. (1974). *Biochem. Biophys. Res. Commun.* **56**, 489–495.
Thompson, W. J. and Appleman, M. M. (1971a). *Biochemistry* **10**, 311–316.
Thompson, W. J. and Appleman, M. M. (1971b). *J. Biol. Chem.* **246**, 3145–3150.
Uzunov, P. and Weiss, B. (1971). *Neuropharmacology* **10**, 697–708.
Uzunov, P. and Weiss, B. (1972). *Biochim. Biophys. Acta* **284**, 220–226.
Uzunov, P., Shim, H. M. and Weiss, B. (1974). *Neuropharmacology* **13**, 377–391.
Vernikos-Danellis, J. and Harris, C. G. (1968). *Proc. Soc. Exp. Biol. Med.* **128**, 1016–1021.
von Hungen, K., Roberts, S. and Hill, D. F. (1975). *Brain Res.* **94**, 57–66.
Voorhees, J. J., Duell, E. A., Stawiski, M. and Harrell, E. R. (1974). *In* "Advan. Cyclic Nucleotide Res." (P. Greengard and G. A. Robison, eds), Vol. 4. Raven Press, New York, pp. 117–162.

Walker, J. B. and Walker, J. P. (1973). *Brain Res.* **54**, 391–396.

Wedner, H. J., Hoffer, B. J., Battenberg, E. F., Steiner, A. L., Parker, C. W. and Bloom, F. E. (1972). *J. Histochem. Cytochem.* **20**, 293–295.

Wegmann, T. G., LaVail, M. M. and Sidman, R. L. (1971). *Nature (London)* **230**, 333–334.

Weight, F. F., Petzold, G. and Greengard, P. (1974). *Science* **186**, 942–944.

Weiss, B. (1971). *J. Neurochem.* **18**, 469–477.

Weiss, B. (1975a). *In* "Advan. Cyclic Nucleotide Res." (G. I. Drummond, P. Greengard and G. A. Robison, eds), Vol. 5. Raven Press, New York, pp. 195–211.

Weiss, B. (ed.) (1975b). "Cyclic Nucleotides in Disease." University Park Press, Baltimore, London and Tokyo.

Weiss, B. and Costa, E. (1968). *Biochem. Pharmacol.* **17**, 2107–2116.

Weiss, B. and Strada, S. J. (1972). *In* "Advan. Cyclic Nucleotide Res." (P. Greengard, R. Paoletti and G. A. Robison, eds), Vol. 1. Raven Press, New York, pp. 357–374.

Weiss, B., Fertel, R., Figlin, R. and Uzunov, P. (1974). *Mol. Pharmacol.* **10**, 615–626.

Weller, M., Goridis, C., Virmaux, N. and Mandel, P. (1975). *Exp. Eye Res.* **21**, 405–408.

Werblin, F. S. (1974). *In* "The Eye" (H. Davson and L. T. Graham, jun., eds), Vol. 6. Academic Press, New York and London, pp. 257–281.

Werblin, F. S. and Dowling, J. E. (1969). *J. Neurophysiol.* **32**, 339–355.

White, A. (1975). *In* "Advan. in Cyclic Nucleotide Res." (G. I. Drummond, P. Greengard and G. A. Robison, eds), Vol. 5. Raven Press, New York, pp. 353–373.

Williams, R. H., Little, S. A. and Ensinck, J. W. (1969). *Amer. J. Med. Sci.* **258**, 190–202.

Young, R. W. (1967). *J. Cell. Biol.* **33**, 61–72.

Young, R. W. (1969a). *In* "The Retina: Morphology, Function and Clinical Characteristics" (B. R. Straatsma, M. O. Hall, R. A. Allen and F. Crescitelli, eds). University of California Press, Los Angeles, pp. 177–210.

Young, R. W. (1969b). *Invest. Ophthalmol.* **8**, 222–231.

Young, R. W. and Bok, D. (1969). *J. Cell Biol.* **42**, 392–403.

Young, R. W. and Droz, B. (1968). *J. Cell Biol.* **39**, 169–184.

Chapter 5

Neurotransmitter-related Pathways: the Structure and Function of Central Monoamine Neurones

T. J. CROW

Division of Psychiatry, Clinical Research Centre,
Watford Road, Harrow, Middlesex, and
Division of Physiology and Pharmacology,
National Institute for Medical Research,
The Ridgeway, Mill Hill, London, England

I. Introduction

Neurochemistry must concern itself not only with those ways in which neurones are chemically distinct from other tissues, but also the ways in which neurones may be distinguished from each other. Considering an organ with the anatomical complexity of the brain we may be sure that structural differentiation is paralleled by a high degree of chemical specificity at the cellular level, and that this specificity is intimately related to the detailed interactions between cells which are the *raison d'être* of the nervous system.

The chemical theory of nervous transmission suggests a functionally important way in which neurones may be distinguished. Since the concept of intercellular communication by way of a release of a chemical substance was first suggested by T. R. Elliot seventy years ago, after a slow start there has been a steady increase of interest in the mechanism of chemical release by nerve activity. Loewi (1921) demonstrated that stimulation of the frog's vagus nerve could release a substance into the ventricular fluid which, when pipetted into another heart, mimicked the action of the vagus. Dale had extracted the substance, acetylcholine, from horse spleen in 1929, and Feldberg and Krayer demonstrated the release of an acetylcholine-like substance (detected by its action on eserinized leech muscle) from the heart of a dog during stimulation of its vagal nerve. In a series of experiments a group of workers including Dale, Feldberg, Brown, Gaddum and Vogt were able to obtain crucial evidence that the substance acetylcholine was released by pre- and post-ganglionic parasympathetic fibres, by pre-ganglionic sympathetic fibres, and by the nerves innervating striated muscles. The accumulation of this evidence, together with observations that the actions of acetylcholine could be blocked by the substances atropine and curare which were already known to antagonize the effects of nervous transmission at the post-ganglionic parasympathetic and neuromuscular junction sites, respectively, served to establish the concept of neurohumoral transmission as a highly plausible hypothesis. The extension of the concept to sympathetic post-ganglionic transmission, stimulated by Loewi's discovery of an "acceleranstoff" in the heart, was achieved by Cannon and his coworkers in experiments on the release of the substance "sympathin" on electrical stimulation of sympathetic nerves.

The general principles of chemical transmission therefore were laid out for the peripheral nervous system in the 1930s. In order for a substance to be accepted as a neurohumoral transmitter at a particular site it should fulfil certain criteria—that its presence and the presence of the enzymes necessary for its synthesis should be demonstrated in the tissue concerned, that its release should follow nerve activity, that there should be a mechanism (e.g. cholinesterase) for its rapid disposal following release, and that the effects of nerve activity should be blocked by other substances known to block the pharmacological effects of the putative neurohumor.

Attempts to investigate neurohumoral transmission in th
focussed on the two substances known to have a transmitter ro
periphery. Acetylcholine was early shown to be present in many parts
of the nervous system (see Feldberg, 1950). Vogt (1954) demonstrated
that noradrenaline is also present, particularly in the hypothalamus,
and that its distribution in the brain cannot be accounted for by the
content of noradrenaline in sympathetic nerves accompanying cerebral blood vessels. Of particular historical significance was the finding of
Amin *et al.* (1954) of the indoleamine 5-hydroxytryptamine in various
brain areas.

At present acetylcholine, noradrenaline, adrenaline, dopamine, 5-
hydroxytryptamine, γ-aminobutyric acid and glycine, have a claim to
be considered central neurotransmitters, while others such as glutamic
and aspartic acids, are of doubtful status. Very recently there has been
interest in the possibility that certain polypeptides may have a central
neurohumoral role, a possibility made plausible by the fact that such
compounds function as pituitary hormone releasing factors in the
median eminence of the hypothalamus.

The information available on the localization and function of the
above substances in the central nervous system (CNS) varies widely.
Within the last few years it has become clear that very substantial
advances in knowledge are possible when a histochemical technique is
available for a particular neurohumor or an associated enzyme. In
these circumstances it is possible to define the particular neurones
which may release the substance, to study the effects of stimulation and
ablation, and in some cases to conduct electrophysiological studies. It
is for these reasons that our knowledge of the catecholamines and 5-
hydroxytryptamine is in many ways further advanced than that of
other neurotransmitters.

Neuronal systems containing the monoamines, dopamine, noradrenaline and 5-hydroxytryptamine have certain features in common. All
are small fibred, with axons of a few microns in diameter. In each case
the transmitter can be depleted by the drug reserpine, and this
presumably indicates that similar granular storage mechanisms are
involved (see e.g. Carlsson, 1965). The neural systems arise from well-
localized cell-body groups mainly within the brain stem. The axons
branch profusely to give rise to terminal networks with a very
widespread distribution to many areas of the brain and spinal cord, and
each monoamine system has an uptake mechanism with similar
characteristics, but some specificity, for the amine involved. These
common characteristics suggest that with the monoamine-containing
neurones we are dealing with a particular subset of neurones with

related phylogenetic origins and functions. More is now known of the anatomy and possible functions of these neurones than of other transmitter-related pathways, and the evidence relating to the structure of monoamine neurones and their possible functions will be described below.

II. Monoamine Pathways: Histochemical Techniques

Catecholamines were first visualized histochemically by an aqueous formaldehyde condensation technique (Eränkö, 1955). The development of this technique utilizing gaseous formaldehyde, by Falck and Hillarp and their colleagues (Falck et al., 1962), allowed the formation of a highly fluorescent derivative, in the presence of protein and in dry conditions, and permitting the visualization of the small amounts of catecholamines within peripheral and central catecholaminergic neurones. The reaction involves an initial condensation to form non-fluorescent 6, 7-dihydroxy-1, 2, 3, 4-tetrahydroisoquinolines, and subsequent dehydrogenation catalysed by protein to fluorescent 6, 7-dihydroxy-3, 4-dihydroisoquinolines (Jonsson, 1971). The products are in pH-dependent equilibrium with their tautomeric quinone structures, which are responsible for the strong fluorescence. The two catecholamines dopamine and noradrenaline have similar emission spectra but can be distinguished either by various drug pretreatments (e.g. Dahlström and Fuxe, 1964) or by treatment with HCl (Björklund et al., 1968), which causes a decrease in the fluorescence due to noradrenaline on account of the lability of the hydroxyl group in position 4. Fluorescent derivatives are also produced by the indoleamines, including 5-hydroxytryptamine, and these have an emission maximum at 525 nm, and can be distinguished by their yellowish fluorescence. In this case the fluorophore is more transient and the difficulties of precise anatomical studies are greater.

III. Catecholamine-containing neurones

The first application of the Falck–Hillarp technique to the central nervous system was made by Dahlström and Fuxe (1964) and their colleagues. These workers established the distribution of catecholamine-containing cell-bodies in the brain stem and hypothalamus, and the existence of diffuse catecholamine-containing terminal networks in the spinal cord, various brain stem nuclei, and large areas of the prosencephalon including a dense innervation of certain hypothalamic nuclei, the entire corpus striatum and the superficial layers of the cerebral cortex. Although fibres were not well visualized due to the very low concentrations of catecholamines within the axons, it was possible to determine the major pathways by studies in which the effects of lesions placed stereotaxically were observed on both terminals and cell-body groups. These studies demonstrated that many ascending monoamine fibres pass through the medial forebrain

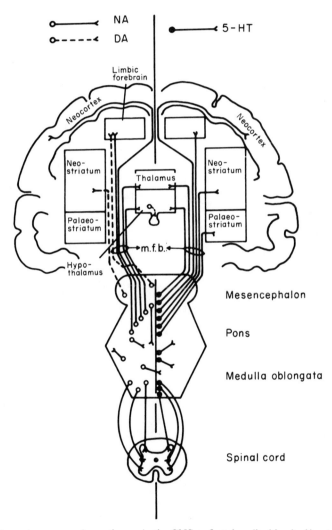

Fig. 1. The major monoamine pathways in the CNS as first described by Andén *et al.* (1966).

bundle in the lateral hypothalamic area on their way to be distributed to rostral structures. A useful summary of these findings is reproduced in Fig. 1, from Andén et al. (1966).

The fibre pathways were first mapped in detail by Ungerstedt (1971a).

A. The Dopamine Systems

These systems arise mainly from a large collection of cell bodies in the ventral mesencephalon (cell-body groups A_8 to A_{10} using the nomenclature originally introduced by Dahlström and Fuxe). These neurones form a continuous sheet of cell bodies extending across the mid-line over the interpeduncular nucleus out into the pars compacta of the substantia nigra on each side (the A_9 area). The mid-line portion is referred to as the A_{10} area and the caudal extension above and lateral to the pars compacta as the A_8 area. The cells of the A_9 area give rise to the dense network of terminals in the corpus striatum, forming the nigrostriatal pathway, and the cells of the A_{10} area give rise to terminals in the nucleus accumbens and olfactory tubercule, sometimes referred to as the "mesolimbic" dopamine area. More recently a dopaminergic innervation of the frontal cortex has been described using the glyoxylic acid fluorescence method (Lindvall and Björklund, 1974), and it appears that these terminals also originate from the cell bodies of the A_{10} area.

A small system of dopamine neurones arises from the arcuate nucleus of the hypothalamus with terminals distributed to the median eminence. This system almost certainly has a role in inhibiting prolactin release (Fuxe et al., 1969).

B. The Noradrenaline Systems

By contrast with the dopamine neurones the noradrenaline-containing cell-bodies of the brain stem send axons down into the spinal cord as well as rostrally into the forebrain. They are also distinguished by their very widespread terminal ramifications. Thus whereas the terminals of the dopamine systems innervate well-demarcated areas such as the striatum, the noradrenaline neurones have terminal distributions to wide areas of the cerebral cortex including the hippocampus, to the cerebellar cortex, to the olfactory bulbs, and to a number of hypothalamic and thalamic nuclei.

Dopamine

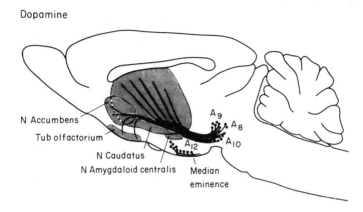

Fig. 2a. The ascending dopamine systems described by Ungerstedt (1971a). The cells of the A_9 area comprise the pars compacta of the substantia nigra and give rise to terminals in the corpus striatum. The terminals in the nucleus accumbens and tuberculum olfactorium arise mainly from the A_{10} area.

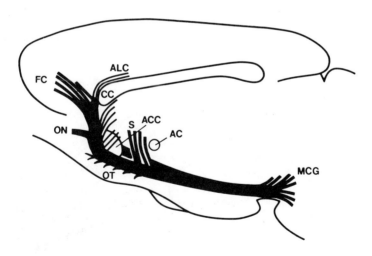

Fig. 2b. The more recently described extension of dopaminergic systems to innervate areas of the frontal cortex as revealed by the glyoxylic acid technique described by Lindvall and Björklund (1974). FC: frontal cortex, ALC: anterior limbic cortex, CC: corpus callosum, ACC: nucleus accumbens, S: septum, ON: olfactory nuclei, OT: olfactory tubercle, AC: anterior commissure, MCG: mesencephalic cell-groups.

Two major ascending noradrenaline pathways were first described by Ungerstedt (1971a). A dorsal bundle arising mainly from the locus coeruleus (the A_6 area), a small nucleus lying in the lateral part of the floor of the fourth ventricle in the mid-pons; and a ventral bundle arising mainly from the A_1, A_2 and A_3 cell-body groups in the caudal brain stem. The dorsal bundle gives rise to the innervation of the cerebellar and cerebral cortices and the hippocampus, and the ventral bundle innervates various hypothalamic nuclei. Although some details of the distribution of these systems are still obscure it appears that whereas the dorsal bundle originates mainly from cell-body groups placed dorsally in the brain stem (in particular the A_6 group, the locus coeruleus) and has a major terminal distribution to the dorsal parts of the nervous system including the cortices, the ventral bundle arises, to a large extent at least, from ventrally placed cell-body groups (mainly from cell-body groups A_1, A_2 and A_3 in the caudal medulla), and has its terminal distribution to ventral areas including the hypothalamus.

The outline of the ascending noradrenergic systems as described by Ungerstedt (Fig. 3) using the Falck–Hillarp formaldehyde technique has been amplified somewhat by studies with glyoxylic acid method, which provides more detail, particularly concerning the path followed by catecholamine-containing fibres (Lindvall and Björklund, 1974).

Lindvall and Björklund remark on the extent to which catecholamine-containing fibre systems, as revealed by the glyoxylic acid method follow non-adrenergic fibre tracts identified by classical

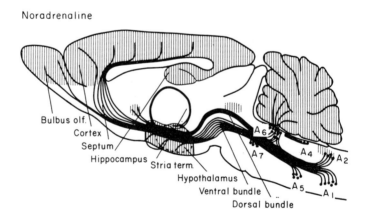

Fig. 3. The ascending noradrenaline-containing pathways as described by Ungerstedt (1971a).

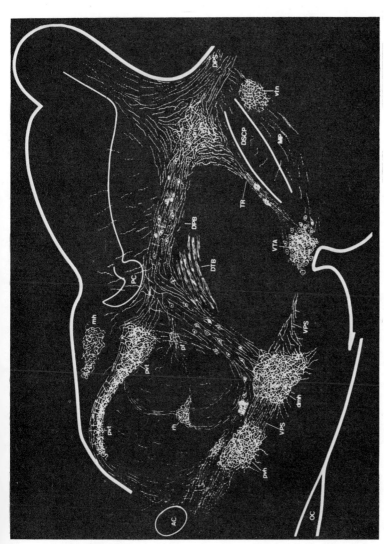

Fig. 4. The periventricular systems of noradrenaline neurones as described with the glyoxylic acid fluorescence technique by Lindvall and Björklund (1974). AC: anterior commissure, DPB: dorsal periventricular bundle, TR: tegmental radiations, DSCP: decussation of the superior cerebellar peduncle, DTB: dorsal tegmental bundle, MP: mammillary peduncle, OC: optic commissure, DPS: dorsal periventricular system, VPS: ventral periventricular system, VTA: ventral tegmental area; dmh: dorsomedial hypothalamic nucleus, drn: dorsal raphé nucleus, pf: parafascicular nucleus, pvh: paraventricular hypothalamic nucleus, pvt: periventricular thalamic nucleus, mh: medial habenular nucleus, rh: rhomboid nucleus, vtn: ventral tegmental nucleus.

neuroanatomical methods. They describe four major ascending conduction pathways:

1. the dopaminergic nigrostriatal pathway.
2. the medial forebrain bundle system, in the lateral hypothalamus, which receives fibres ascending from a variety of origins in the brain stem,
3. the central tegmental tract coursing up the brain stem and including both the ventral and dorsal noradrenaline bundles as described by Ungerstedt, and
4. the periventricular system.

This latter, previously undescribed, system comprises a dorsal system extending from the medulla oblongata along the dorsal longitudinal fasciculus, and arising from catecholamine-containing cell bodies scattered diffusely along its length as well as receiving fibres from the locus coeruleus; and a ventral component which extends along the periventricular grey of the hypothalamus and innervates mainly the dorsomedial and periventricular hypothalamic nuclei.

C. Adrenaline Systems

On the basis of the development of an immunohistochemical stain for the enzyme phenylethanolamine-N-methyltransferase (PNMT) it has recently been suggested (Hökfelt et al., 1974) that a number of the catecholamine-containing cell bodies in the caudal brain stem are

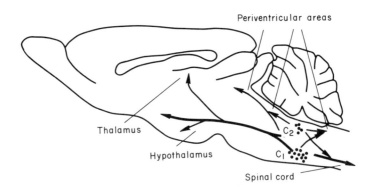

Fig. 5. The distribution of possible adrenaline-containing neurones as revealed by an immunohistochemical technique for PNMT (from Hökfelt et al., 1974). The cell-body groups C_1 and C_2 probably include cells in the rostral parts of the previously described medullary catecholamine-containing cell-body groups, i.e. A_1 and A_2.

adrenaline- rather than noradrenaline-releasing cells. The cells concerned form the anterior parts of the A_1 and A_2 cell-body groups as described by Dahlström and Fuxe and have been labelled C_1 and C_2 by Hökfelt *et al.* (1974). It is suggested that these cells give rise to ascending and descending fibres, although the distribution of terminals is not yet clear (Fig. 5).

IV. 5-Hydroxytryptamine-containing Neurones

Serotonin-containing neuronal systems share many characteristics with catecholamine neurones, but are distinguished by the singular fact that they arise from a series of nuclei situated in the mid-line of the brain stem, the raphé nuclei. With the exceptions that the A_{10} cell-body group of dopamine neurones lies across the mid-line, and the B_9 group of serotonin-containing neurones is paired, and lies above the medial lemniscus on either side, it appears to be a general rule that catecholamine-neuronal cell-body groups are paired, while serotonin-containing groups are unpaired mid-line structures. The significance of this finding has yet to be established.

Serotonergic fibres descend to the spinal cord as do the noradrenergic systems, and the terminals are distributed mainly to the ventral and intermediate horns. Serotonergic terminals are diffusely distributed to the corpus striatum along with the terminals of the nigro-striatal dopamine system, to the neo-, meso-and palaeo-cortices, and the cerebellar cortex along with terminals of the noradrenergic systems, and to various hypothalamic, including particularly the suprachiasmatic, and the amygdaloid, nuclei. In many respects the distribution of serotonergic terminal networks parallels that of the catecholamine systems. However, the detailed anatomy of serotonergic neurones remains much less well described on account of the relative transience of the 5-hydroxytryptamine fluorophore. The recent introduction of neurotoxic dihydroxytryptamines (e.g. 5, 6-and 5, 7-dihydroxytryptamine) which are relatively selective in their effects on 5-hydroxytryptamine neurones, and are able to cause an acute and pronounced build up of transmitter in the axons when administered by local intracerebral injection, has allowed more extensive anatomical mapping with the Falck–Hillarp technique than was previously possible. Fuxe and Jonsson (1974) in particular have developed this technique. The main findings of their work are shown in Fig. 6.

Major ascending pathways arise from cell-body groups situated rostrally in the brain stem, including relatively discrete groups of cell bodies in the floor of the fourth ventricle (B_4 and B_6), in the dorsal raphé nucleus (B_7), in the ventral part of the periacqueductal grey matter, and the more ventrally situated B_5 and B_8 groups (the pontine, and median, or superior central, raphé nuclei). As previously mentioned the B_9 group is a paired bilateral structure lying above, and to a certain extent within, the medial lemniscus as it passes through the ventral mesencephalon. The precise terminal distributions arising from each of these nuclei remain unclear. From the results of studies on the effects of lesions of various raphé nuclei on the content (Lorens

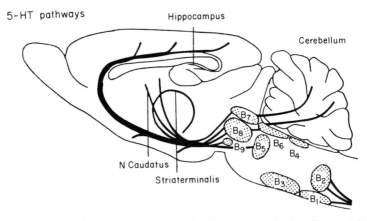

Fig. 6. The major 5-hydroxytryptamine-containing fibres as described by Fuxe and Jonsson (1974) in studies using the neurotoxic dihydroxytryptamines. The B_7 and B_8 groups correspond to the dorsal and median raphé nuclei respectively.

and Guldberg, 1974) and uptake (Fuxe and Jonsson, 1974) of 5-hydroxytryptamine in various forebrain regions it appears that there is considerable overlap in the distribution of terminals from the different raphé nuclei to areas such as the neocortex and corpus striatum. To a certain extent these results may represent the technical difficulties of achieving selective and complete ablations of individual nuclei. On the basis of their studies with neurotoxic dihydroxytryptamines Fuxe and Jonsson suggest that there are two major ascending pathways, a medial pathway innervating mainly hypothalamic and preoptic structures and a lateral pathway which gives rise to the terminals in cortical areas. A smaller far-lateral fibre tract innervates the corpus striatum (Fig. 7).

The caudal cell-body groups (B_1–B_3) which include the relatively large nucleus raphé magnus (B_3) appear to give rise to descending pathways to the spinal cord.

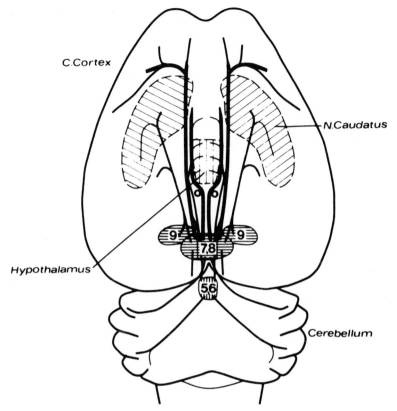

Fig. 7. A dorsal view of the ascending 5-hydroxytryptamine-containing pathways arising from the rostral 5-HT cell-body groups (from Fuxe and Jonsson, 1974).

V. Monoamine Systems in Human Brain

Two recent studies have investigated the structure of monoamine neurones in the human brain by applying the Falck–Hillarp technique to foetal material (Olson *et al.*, 1973; Nobin and Björklund, 1973). The results reveal the same basic features as are seen in the rat. A large complex of catecholamine-containing neurones in the ventral mesencephalon includes the pars compacta of the substantia nigra and sends axons forwards to the corpus striatum. The locus coeruleus complex consists of a principal nucleus of densely packed cells and a number of loosely packed satellite groups (including the nucleus subcoeruleus) which appear somewhat more extensive than the corresponding structures in the rat (Fig. 8).

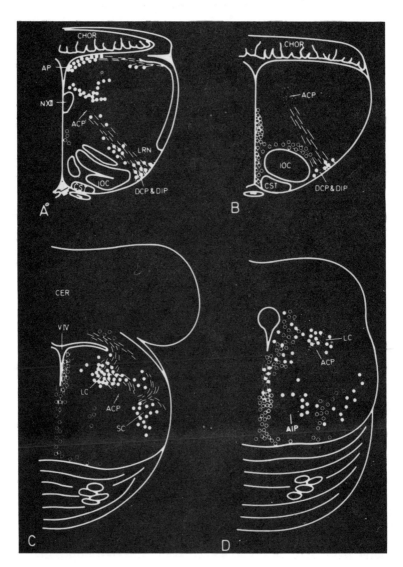

Fig. 8. Monoamine-containing cell-bodies in the human foetal brain stem according to the studies of Nobin and Björklund (1973). Closed circles: catecholamine-containing cell-bodies, open circles: indoleamine-containing cell bodies. Dashed lines: monoamine-containing axons in longitudinal sections, dots: transverse section. The locus coeruleus (LC) and subcoeruleus (SC) complex appears more extensive than the corresponding structure in the adult rat, as also do the indoleamine-containing structures. ACP: ascending catecholamine pathway, AIP: ascending indoleamine pathway, AP: area postrema, CER: cerebellum, CST: corticospinal tract, DCP: descending catecholamine pathway, DIP: descending indoleamine pathway, IOC: inferior olivary complex.

5-Hydroxytryptamine-containing neurones were identified in the mid-line raphé regions of the medulla and pons-mesencephalon including a particularly large group in the area of the nucleus raphé dorsalis (Olson et al., 1973). Other indoleamine-containing cell-bodies were identified in the ventrolateral mesencephalon (corresponding to the B_9 area of Dahlström and Fuxe), and catecholamine-containing systems in the ventral and ventrolateral, and dorsal and dorsomedial, regions of the medulla oblongata, corresponding approximately to the A_1 and A_2 areas described in the rat. A small group of indoleamine-containing cells are described in the roof of the fourth ventricle (Nobin and Björklund, 1973) which have no obvious counterparts in the rat, but in many other respects the anatomical arrangements of mono-amine cell-body groups and fibre systems are similar.

VI. The Ontogeny of Monoamine Systems

From the studies of Seiger and Olson (1972) of the rat embryo from the gestational age of 12–15 days it is clear that monoamine neurones develop their capacity for synthesis and storage of amines at a very early stage. 5-Hydroxytryptamine neurones develop in the 8 mm embryo, dopamine neurones in the 9 mm embryo, and noradrenaline neurones at the 11 mm stage. By the 12 mm stage several axonal projections have developed and are apparently able to synthesize the neurotransmitters.

Catecholamine neurones develop from three primordia—a caudal complex which later gives rise to the A_1–A_3 cell-body groups, a mid-pontine complex which includes the A_4–A_7 cell-body groups, and a ventral mesencephalic constellation of dopamine neurones (the A_8–A_{10} cell-body groups). Serotonin neurones develop from a caudal complex including the B_1–B_3 groups and a ponto-mesencephalic complex giving rise to groups B_4–B_9 (Fig. 9). The later development suggests that the catecholamine cells, at least, subdivide into a dorsal column (A_2, A_4, A_6 and perhaps A_7) and a ventral column of cells (A_1, A_3, A_5, A_8, A_9 and A_{10}).

VII. Functions of Monoamine Neurones

The anatomical characteristics of monoamine neurones, with axonal systems arising from relatively discrete nuclei to give rise to diffusely distributed terminal networks covering large areas of the CNS,

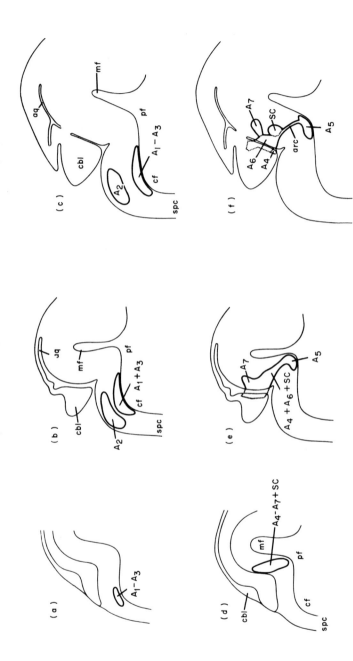

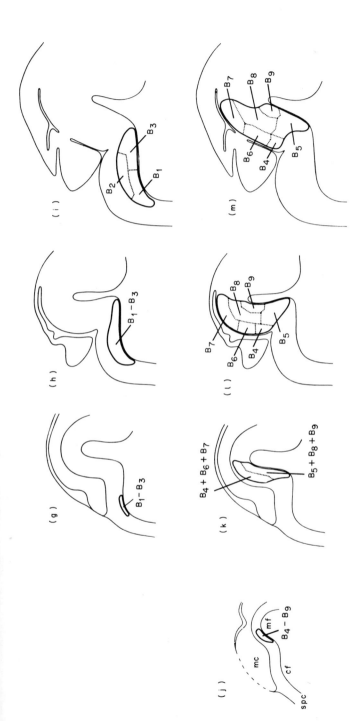

Fig. 9. The ontogeny of noradrenaline (A_1–A_7) and indoleamine (B_1–B_9) cell-body groups in the rat brain stem according to Olson and Seiger (1973). Drawings a to c show the development from a single primordium in the caudal brain stem of cell-body groups A_1–A_3, d to f of cell-body groups of the locus coeruleus complex (A_4–A_7 including the subcoeruleus, SC), drawings g to i the development of the caudal indoleamine cell bodies (B_1–B_3) and j to m the development of the rostral indoleamine groups (B_4–B_9). The stages of development are j—CRL 8 mm; d, g, k—11–12 mm; a—13 mm; b, e, h, l—19 mm; c, f, i, and m—36–38 mm. spc: spinal cord, cf: cervical flexure, pf: pontine flexure, mf: mesencephalic flexure, mc: myelocoele, cbl: cerebellar anlage, aq: aqueductus Sylvii.

suggests that these systems exert a rather general regulatory influence, perhaps performing functions quite distinct from those of the more classical anatomical pathways, which appear better suited for transmitting neural messages of high information content. Before the development of the Falck–Hillarp technique it was clear that drugs such as reserpine which deplete the cerebral stores of all three monoamines, probably by interfering with intracellular storage mechanisms (Andén, 1968), and the amphetamines, which release both catecholamines, and probably 5-hydroxytryptamine also (Fuxe and Ungerstedt, 1970), exert profound effects on behaviour. Because of its apparent ability to induce symptoms closely similar to those occurring in depressive illnesses (Muller *et al.*, 1955; Lemieux *et al.*, 1956) the mechanism of action of reserpine on behaviour attracted particular interest. Carlsson *et al.* (1957), for example, demonstrated that the characteristic inertia and ptosis induced in rabbits by reserpine administration can be reversed by the catecholamine precursor dihydroxyphenylalanine, but not by the serotonin precursor tryptophan. They argued that central catecholaminergic mechanisms must exert an arousing or activating influence on behaviour. More recently it has been recognized that the paranoid psychosis which results from administration of relatively large doses of the amphetamines bears a close resemblance to some aspects of schizophrenic illnesses (Connell, 1958), and this also has stimulated research on the mode of action of amphetamine in relation to monoaminergic mechanisms. Research on the functions of monoamine neurones has been greatly facilitated by studies of the behavioural and physiological effects of drugs acting relatively selectively upon aminergic mechanisms. On the basis of the anatomical knowledge deriving from the Falck–Hillarp technique strategies have been devised for selectively stimulating and ablating particular monoamine systems.

A. Catecholamine Systems

1. Drug studies

α-*Methyl-p-tyrosine.* α-Methyl-p-tyrosine is a relatively selective inhibitor of the enzyme tyrosine hydroxylase (Weissman and Koe, 1965). Following its administration central and peripheral catecholamine stores become depleted over the course of 12–24 h and then recover slowly over two to four days. The behavioural sequelae of α-methyl-p-tyrosine administration closely resemble those following reserpine. The animals are akinetic, show impaired responsiveness to environmental stimuli and eat and drink little. The syndrome can be reversed by administration of L-DOPA (Moore and Rech, 1967).

Amphetamine stereotypies. The amphetamines differ from the catecholamines in lacking the ring hydroxyl groups and, probably for this reason, enter the central nervous system without difficulty. Here they interact with catecholamines by enhancing the release of transmitter from the nerve endings. At low doses this action is probably dependent on nerve impulses, but at higher doses may occur as a result of direct release. Randrup *et al.* (1963) first described in detail the behaviours resulting from amphetamine administration. In a variety of species there is an increase in motor activity and the emergence of a syndrome of repetitive sniffing, licking and gnawing which can include other motor behaviours (Randrup and Munkvad, 1967). A similar syndrome can also be provoked by L-DOPA (Randrup and Munkvad, 1966a). The amphetamine-induced behaviours are antagonized by administration of neuroleptics (Randrup and Munkvad, 1965) and α-methyl-*p*-tyrosine, but not by inhibitors of the enzyme dopamine-β-hydroxylase (Randrup and Munkvad, 1966b), nor by a variety of non-neuroleptic sedative drugs (Munkvad and Randrup, 1966). The expression of the syndrome appears to depend on excess dopamine release, and a number of experiments have been conducted to elucidate the anatomical site at which amphetamine elicits these behaviours. Early experiments suggested that the syndrome was unaffected by electrolytic lesions of the substantia nigra (Simpson and Iversen, 1971). Bilateral injections of the neurotoxic agent 6-hydroxy-dopamine, which relatively selectively destroys catecholamine neurones, into the corpus striatum reducing dopamine to 9.3% of control levels, abolished the sniffing, licking and gnawing behaviour (Creese and Iversen, 1974). Similar lesions of the terminals in the tuberculum olfactorium had no such effect, and neither lesion reduced the effects of amphetamine on motor activity. Bilateral injections of 6-hydroxydopamine into the substantia nigra which resulted in a depletion of over 99% of striatal tyrosine hydroxylase activity abolished both the locomotor effects and the stereotyped behaviours suggesting that "both are dependent on the functional integrity of the nigro-striatal system" (Creese and Iversen, 1975). More recently the locomotor response to amphetamine has been relatively selectively abolished by 6-hydroxydopamine induced lesions of the nucleus accumbens (Kelly *et al.*, 1975). These experiments illustrate the difficulties of determining the functions of central catecholamine systems in lesioning experiments, perhaps because "the survival of a relatively small number of neurones may suffice for conditions where demand is within normal limits" (Vogt, 1973). The results suggest that only when relatively complete ablations of a particular catecholamine system have been achieved do the effects become apparent.

The drug apomorphine can induce a syndrome closely resembling that seen following amphetamine (Ernst, 1970). The syndrome is also seen following direct implantation of crystalline apomorphine into the corpus striatum. The apomorphine effect is not blocked by α-methyl-p-tyrosine, but is effectively inhibited by a variety of neuroleptic drugs. These and other data suggest strongly that apomorphine acts directly to stimulate dopamine receptors in the corpus striatum.

There is evidence that following degeneration of the presynaptic neurone the postsynaptic monoamine receptor develops super-sensitivity (Ungerstedt, 1971b), and, in the case of the dopamine neurone for example, an increased response to apomorphine is seen. The case that the hyperactivity and stereotyped behaviour responses are due to dopamine receptor stimulation in the nucleus accumbens and corpus striatum, respectively, is strengthened therefore by the observation that selective 6-hydroxydopamine lesions in the nucleus accumbens enhance the locomotor response while lesions in the corpus striatum enhance the stereotype response to apomorphine (Kelly *et al.*, 1975).

2. *Electrical stimulation; catecholamine neurones and reward*

Perhaps the most direct approach to the function of monoamine neurones is by activation of these pathways through stereotaxically-implanted electrodes. Such studies often encounter difficulties in defining the behavioural effects of stimulation, and dissociating the effects of activation of the particular monoamine pathway from that of nearby anatomical structures. However there is now a substantial case for regarding some catecholamine systems as "reward pathways" on the basis of studies with the electrical self-stimulation technique of Olds and Milner.

Olds and Milner (1954) discovered that rats with electrodes implanted in certain lateral hypothalamic and septal sites will press a lever to pass trains of electrical stimuli through the implanted electrode. The behaviour presumably reveals the existence of central "reward mechanisms", and it is observed that the behaviour often persists for long periods of time, and contrary to the interests of homoeostasis. These pathways presumably are an integral part of the organism's normal mechanisms for responding to significant environmental stimuli. The pathways involved and their normal functions have for long remained obscure. Stein (1964) first suggested that they might release a catecholamine, noradrenaline, as a neurohumor, on the basis of the observation that this behaviour is remarkably sensitive to enhancement by small doses of drugs of the amphetamine group. It is also inhibited by α-methyl-*p*-tyrosine (Poschel and Ninteman, 1966), and there are grounds for thinking that this inhibition is not merely secondary to impaired motor capacity (Black and Cooper, 1970). Since the lateral hypothalamus, which includes many ascending catecholamine fibres, has been an area from which self-stimulation has been consistently obtained, it is a plausible hypothesis that activation of one or more ascending catecholamine systems is responsible for the reward effect.

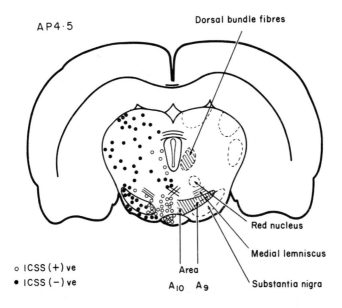

Fig. 10. Electrical self-stimulation sites in the rat mesencephalon (adapted from Crow, 1972a and Anlezark *et al.*, 1973a). ICSS (+) ve: electrode tips positive for intracranial self-stimulation, ICSS (−) ve: negative sites. The A_9 and A_{10} cell-body groups of dopamine neurones and the location of the ascending fibres of the dorsal noradrenaline bundle are shaded.

This question has been investigated by mapping electrical self-stimulation sites in relation to the cell-body groups of origin of catecholamine fibres in the brain stem. A map of self-stimulation sites across the mesencephalon at the level of origin of the dopaminergic A_9 and A_{10} cell bodies (Crow, 1972a; Anlezark *et al.*, 1973a) revealed:

1. a large group of positive sites stretching across the mid-line from one substantia nigra pars compacta to the other, and corresponding quite closely to the distribution of dopamine neurones, but including also the interpeduncular nucleus, and
2. a small group of sites placed further dorsally just lateral to the central grey substance (Fig. 10).

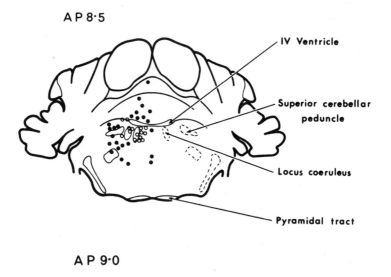

AP 8·5

IV Ventricle

Superior cerebellar peduncle

Locus coeruleus

Pyramidal tract

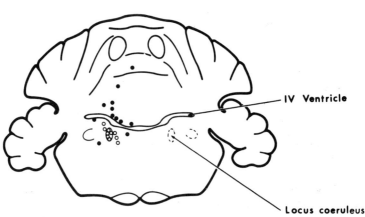

AP 9·0

IV Ventricle

Locus coeruleus

Fig. 11a. Sites positive (open circles) for electrical self-stimulation in the region of the locus coeruleus in the floor of the fourth ventricle in the mid-pontine region. Section AP 9·0 is 0·5 mm behind AP 8·5.

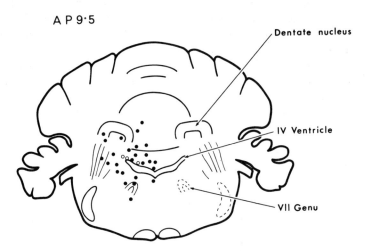

Fig. 11b. Three positive sites behind the level of the locus coeruleus and at the lateral margin of the fourth ventricle. These sites appear to be close to the location of the cell bodies of the A_4 group. (Data taken from Crow et al., 1972, and Anlezark et al., 1973b.)

These latter sites were in the general region in which the noradrenergic fibres of the dorsal bundle were known to pass through the mesencephalon. There is now a considerable body of evidence (Crow, 1976a) consistent with the original hypothesis (Crow, 1972b) that activation of dopamine neurones is the essential element in some forms of self-stimulation behaviour. The second hypothesis suggested by the distribution of self-stimulation sites in the mesencephalon (Fig. 10) was that activation of a second catecholamine system, the dorsal bundle of noradrenaline neurones, also had rewarding effects. The prediction that self-stimulation should also be obtained with electrode tips located close to the cell-bodies of origin of this system, the locus coeruleus (A_6 area) in the mid-pontine region, was tested and verified in a subsequent series of experiments (Crow et al., 1972; Anlezark et al., 1973b) (Fig. 11).

The results showed that the behaviour could be obtained with electrode tips either within, or in close proximity to, the cells of the locus coeruleus, but could not be obtained with electrodes within the cerebellum, or at various brain stem sites lateral, ventral and medial to the locus coeruleus. At this level of the brain stem self-stimulation sites appear to be highly localized. Further evidence that the positive electrodes were activating the cells of the locus coeruleus was obtained by the demonstration that the turnover of noradrenaline in the ipsilateral cortex was increased by stimulation in animals who had self-stimulated, but was unchanged relative to the contralateral cortex following such stimulation in animals who had not self-stimulated, and whose electrode tips were found not to be in close proximity to the nucleus (Anlezark *et al.*, 1975). A third series of investigations (Anlezark *et al.*, 1973b) (Fig. 12) established that self-stimulation could not be obtained with electrodes implanted in the cell-body groups of origin of the ventral bundle, the A_1 and A_2 areas.

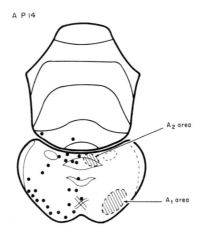

A P 14

A_2 area

A_1 area

Fig. 12. Electrode sites tested for intracranial self-stimulation in relation to cell-body groups A_1 and A_2 in the caudal brain stem. None of these electrodes supported self-stimulation. (From Anlezark *et al.*, 1973b.)

These findings suggested that two of the three major ascending catecholamine systems might function as reward pathways in the sense that electrical activation of the neurones of these systems will support self-stimulation responding (Crow, 1972b). The behaviour seen in either case seems, however, to be somewhat different. With electrodes located amongst the ventral mesencephalic dopamine neurones quite marked activation of motor behaviour is seen. The animals appear excited, are easily trained to lever press, and often sniff, lick and gnaw at the lever in an energetic manner. Rats with electrodes positioned in the locus coeruleus show no such activation of behaviour and often take much longer to train.

3. Lesioning studies

Dopamine neurones. Ungerstedt (1971c) first described the behavioural effects of lesioning the ascending dopaminergic pathways using 6-hydroxydopamine. With bilateral lesions animals become akinetic, aphagic and adipsic, and while some animals show recovery if force-fed, it appears likely that those with the most complete lesions do not. Ungerstedt drew attention to the similarity of this picture to the previously described "lateral hypothalamic syndrome" (Anand and Brobeck, 1951), and to the fact that many of the lesions previously shown to produce the syndrome will have interrupted dopaminergic pathways in their course through the lateral hypothalamus. Rats with 6-hydroxydopamine lesions of ascending dopaminergic systems who recover from the initial stages of the syndrome, who may therefore have less than complete destruction of the systems, show impaired responsiveness to glucoprivation, and challenges to body water regulation (Zigmond and Strickler, 1973; Marshall, Richardson and Teitelbaum, 1974). In these respects, as in several others, the animals resemble those recovering from the lateral hypothalamic syndrome.

It has also been recognized that "sensory neglect" to contralateral stimuli in various modalities is a component of the lateral hypo-thalamic syndrome (Marshall et al., 1971), and similar sensory or "attentional" deficits have been demonstrated after lesions of dop-aminergic pathways (Ungerstedt and Ljungberg, 1975). The extent to which these various elements of the syndrome resulting from lesions to dopamine neurones can be dissociated from each other by selective lesions of, say, the mesolimbic dopamine pathway, is not yet clear. In the literature most of the defects have been attributed to the demonstrated interruption of the nigro-striatal tract. In many cases, however, particularly when 6-hydroxydopamine has been injected into the ventral tegmental area, the mesolimbic neurones will also have been damaged.

The dorsal bundle of noradrenaline neurones. In marked contrast to the effect of lesions of dopamine neurones on motor and motivational behaviours, are the effects of lesions of the dorsal bundle of noradre-naline neurones. In spite of the very widespread distribution of the terminals of this system, lesions have so far been shown to have no unequivocal effects on behaviour. Most investigations indicate that lesions, whether induced by electrolysis of the cell bodies in the locus coeruleus, or by 6-hydroxydopamine injection into the fibres of the dorsal bundle, cause no significant change in motor activity, or food and water intake.

On the basis of the hypothesis that the locus coeruleus system constitutes a "reinforcement" mechanism necessary for establishing the changes in synaptic conductivity underlying learning (see below), it was predicted that lesions of the system would impair the organism's ability to acquire new behaviours. The increase in running speed for a food reward in a simple runway was taken as an index of learning. Normal rats and rats with brain stem and cerebellar lesions, as well as rats with partial lesions of the locus coeruleus showed no impairment, but rats with relatively complete and bilateral electrolytic ablations of the locus coeruleus showed deficits in this experimental situation (Anlezark *et al.*, 1973). However, no such deficit is reported after bilateral 6-hydroxydopamine induced lesions of the ascending fibres of the dorsal bundle (Mason and Iversen, 1976; Roberts *et al.*, 1976). There appear to be two possible explanations of this discrepancy; either that the behavioural effects of the electrolytic lesions are due to damage to some structure in the mid-pontine region other than the cells of the locus coeruleus, or that the function of the locus coeruleus system is revealed only when both its ascending axons to the cerebral cortex (the dorsal bundle) and its fibre system to the cerebellar cortex are eliminated. In an experiment in which 6-hydroxydopamine was injected close to the locus coeruleus impairments in learning were seen in a quite different behavioural task—a one-trial passive avoidance test (Crow and Wendlandt, 1976). There has also been interest in the question of whether the coerulocortical system may be involved in sleep mechanisms. Lidbrink (1974) demonstrated a decrease in total waking time shortly after lesions of locus coeruelus, but the sleep rhythm returned to normal within a few days. The possible role of the locus coeruleus in REM, or paradoxical, sleep (Jouvet, 1972) is the subject of current investigation (see p. 293).

The ventral bundle of noradrenaline neurones. Two recent investigations (Ahlskog and Hoebel, 1973; Kapatos and Gold, 1973) agree in finding that following lesions of the ventral bundle of noradrenaline neurones, whether induced electrolytically or by 6-hydroxydopamine injections into the fibres, rats show increased food intake and weight gain. Some fibres of the bundle pass close to the ventromedial nucleus of the hypothalamus, and whether or not lesions of these fibres have contributed substantially to the behavioural effects previously observed after lesions of this nucleus, sometimes referred to as the "ventromedial satiety centre", has been discussed (Gold, 1973). The results of the ventral bundle lesioning experiments suggest, however, that the ventral bundle, or some part of this bundle, may itself function as a component of a "satiety mechanism".

4. *An integrated view of catecholamine pathways*

Table 1 summarizes the above findings relating to the possible functions of catecholamine neuronal systems.

Table 1

Summary of studies of the effects of lesioning and electrically-stimulating ascending catecholamine systems

CA pathway	Cell-body groups	Effects of lesions	Electrical self-stimulation	Acquisition of e.ss. responding	Behaviour associated with e.ss.
Dopamine neurones	A_8, A_9, A_{10}	Bilateral: akinesia aphagia adipsia Unilateral: contralateral sensory neglect	Yes	Fast	Motor excitation: elements of the sniffing, licking gnawing syndrome
Dorsal bundle of noradrenaline neurones	A_6, A_4	?Learning deficits	Yes	Slow	
Ventral bundle of noradrenaline neurones	A_1, A_2	Increased food intake and weight gain	No	—	Motor excitation absent —

Electrical self-stimulation: e.ss.

Dopamine neurones may function as an "activating mechanism" which mediates the organism's response to significant environmental stimuli. Its function, in the rat at least, appears to be closely related to ingestive behaviours.

The dorsal bundle also appears to function as a reward pathway, although of a rather different type.

The ventral bundle may function as a "satiety mechanism" concerned with some aspects of limiting food intake. Its activation does not have rewarding effects.

It has been suggested that rewarding stimuli may have two quite different effects on the organism:

1. to energize or activate behaviour towards possible primary biological rewards (e.g. sources of food). This is sometimes referred to as the "incentive" effect, and
2. to reinforce or "stamp-in" some neural record of situations or behaviours associated with reward. This function was described as the "confirming reaction" by Thorndike (1933), the "results of action signal" by Young (1964), and the "now-print" mechanism by Livingston (1967).

The above findings suggest strongly that the dopamine pathways may function as part of an "incentive" mechanism, perhaps as the final common pathway for mediating the effects of incentive stimuli on behaviour. By contrast, in view of its lack of activating effects, and, perhaps especially, on account of its terminal distribution to the cerebral and cerebellar cortices, and locus coeruleus system, including the dorsal bundle, appears an attractive candidate as a reinforcement system.

Very little work has been done on afferent connections of mono-amine systems. It may be instructive, however, to consider the possibility that ascending catecholamine systems have a particular association with specific sensory pathways. There appear to be interesting relationships between the three catecholamine systems and the three modalities particularly concerned with food intake— olfaction, gustation and gastro-intestinal sensation. The relationships are listed below.

1. Olfactory connections reach the ventral tegmental area of the dopamine neurones both by way of the medial forebrain bundle, and via the habenular nuclei and habenulo-peduncular tracts. Tulloch (1975) has recently shown that dopamine neurones respond to stimulation of the olfactory bulbs.

2. The locus coeruleus lies at the head of the visceral afferent column (Russell, 1955) directly ahead of the nucleus tractus solitarius, the rostral part of which receives the primary gustatory endings.

3. The A_2 area, one of the origins of the ventral bundle, lies in close relationship to the caudal end of the tractus solitarius, and to the nucleus intercalatus of Staderini, both of which may receive ascending visceral fibres.

It has been suggested (Crow and Arbuthnott, 1972; Crow, 1973; Crow, 1976b) that these relationships may illuminate the functions of catecholamine neurones. Olfaction is a distance receptor, and the appropriate response to an olfactory stimulus associated with food is activation of the organism's responses toward the source of the stimulus (cf. the incentive effect). Gustatory receptors are stimulated only when food is actually in the mouth. It is at this point that the "confirming reaction" or "results of action signal" might register the successful outcome of the behavioural sequence. Finally when the stomach is distended with food it may be expected that a gastrointestinal satiety signal will play some role in reducing further intake.

These relationships are summarized in Table 2. It is suggested that the three ascending catecholamine systems may have their phylogenetic origins in relation to the three afferent pathways concerned with food intake. In the course of evolutionary development other afferent modalities have come to influence these systems but their functions with respect to behaviour may have remained fundamentally the same. According to this hypothesis central catecholamine neurones were originally concerned primarily with the detection of food, and the three major systems were distinguished from each other by the domain to which their respective receptors were orientated.

B. Serotonergic Systems

Partly because our present anatomical knowledge of serotonergic systems is less precise than our knowledge of catecholamine systems functional studies of the role of serotonin in the CNS have focussed rather more upon the effects of drugs than upon lesioning and stimulation experiments.

1. Drug studies

p-Chlorophenylalanine. The drug *p*-chlorophenylalanine is a relatively selective inhibitor of tryptophan hydroxylase and depletes the brain of 5-hydroxytryptamine over a period of several days (Koe and

Table 2

Hypothesis relating the three ascending catecholamine systems to food-related afferent pathways and their postulated behavioural functions

Catecholamine pathway	Cell-body groups	Terminals	Associated afferent pathway	Behavioural function
Dopamine neurones	A_8, A_9, A_{10}	Corpus striatum nucleus accumbens etc.	Olfaction	"Incentive" drive induction
Noradrenaline neurones (dorsal bundle)	A_6, A_4 ($?A_5$, A_7)	Cerebral and cerebellar cortices	Gustation	"Reinforcement" "Confirming reaction" "Results of action signal"
Noradrenaline neurones (ventral bundle)	A_1, A_2	Hypothalamic nuclei	Gastric sensation	Satiety mechanism

Weissman, 1966). There is also a reduction of the brain content of noradrenaline but this is less marked and much shorter in duration. *p*-Chlorophenylalanine has proved an extremely important tool in studying the central functions of 5-hydroxytryptamine.

The behavioural effects of *p*-chlorophenylalanine are quite distinct from those of reserpine and α-methyl-*p*-tyrosine. The decrease in activity following these latter two drugs is not seen, and in some circumstances there is an increase in activity (Fibiger and Campbell, 1971). In various species *p*-chlorophenylalanine administration is followed by the development of marked insomnia, and this can be reversed by administration of the serotonin precursor 5-hydroxytryptophan (Jouvet, 1969; Koella, 1969). The drug also increases pain sensitivity and can reduce the analgesic effects of morphine (Tenen, 1967). Animals generally show increased responsiveness to most types of sensory stimulation, and this is accompanied in many species by increased irritability and aggressiveness (Weissman and Harbert, 1972). Tagliamonte *et al.* (1969) and Hoyland *et al.* (1970) demonstrated an increase in sexual activity, and although to a certain extent dependent upon hormonal status, this finding has been confirmed in most species in which it has been examined (Weissman and Harbert, 1972). Increased social interaction has also been described (Shillito, 1970) and like the enhanced irritability and aggressiveness, this may be interpreted as an increased responsiveness to environmental stimuli. In many of these cases the changes have been shown to be reversible by administration of 5-hydroxytryptophan.

These data suggest strongly that the general action of serotonin with respect to behaviour is an inhibitory one, and that a relative lack of 5-hydroxytryptamine results in hypersensitivity to environmental cues. In view of the well-marked similarities between catecholaminergic and serotonergic systems, and the evidence for interconnections between them, it is tempting to speculate that the serotonin systems function in some way in opposition to the catecholamine systems.

For example some workers have suggested that the serotonin systems may include one or more "punishment" systems. Geller and Blum (1970) demonstrated that *p*-chlorophenylalanine disinhibited the response suppression induced by an auditory stimulus which signalled that the response would be punished by shock, but did not influence baseline responding for food reward. This disinhibition was reversed by 5-hydroxytryptophan administration. Wise *et al.* (1970) showed that the suppressive effects of prior shock-conditioning on a drinking response were attenuated by *p*-chlorophenylalanine, and increased by pargyline and 5-hydroxytryptophan.

Tryptophan and monoamine oxidase inhibition. In view of the apparently inhibitory influences of serotonin on behaviour as revealed by experiments with *p*-chlorophenylalanine it is somewhat surprising to find that a number of drug treatments which might be expected to induce increased serotonin release produce signs of behavioural excitation. Hess and Doepfner (1961) first described the effects of administration of tryptophan and a monoamine oxidase inhibitor, and these have recently been studied in detail by Grahame-Smith (1971) and Green and Grahame-Smith (1974). Rats treated with this drug combination show hyperactivity, tremor, rigidity, hindlimb abduction, lateral head weaving, forepaw treading, and the Straub tail phenomenon. The syndrome is blocked by *p*-chlorophenylalanine administration, and can be reproduced by *N, N*-dimethyl-tryptamine, a drug which may stimulate the serotonin receptor directly.

The apparent paradox of this syndrome has recently been elucidated somewhat by Jacobs and Klemfuss (1975), who demonstrated that some of these behaviours can still be elicited after a transverse cut through the brain at the level of the caudal mesencephalon. Presumably therefore the syndrome depends on an action of tryptophan on descending serotonergic neurones. It seems likely that many of the behaviourally inhibitory actions of serotonin inferred from experiments with *p*-chlorophenylalanine are associated with systems ascending from the anterior raphé nuclei.

Lesions of serotonin neurones. Consistent with this interpretation are observations that lesions of the median raphé nucleus which cause substantial reductions in forebrain 5-hydroxytryptamine content lead to increases in locomotor activity similar to those seen after *p*-chlorophenylalanine administration (Steranka and Barrett, 1974; Jacobs *et al.*, 1975). No such changes are seen after lesions of the dorsal raphé nucleus (Jacobs *et al.*, 1975).

Combined lesions of the dorsal and median raphé nuclei produced transient increases in food and water intake, and faster acquisition of an active two-way conditioned avoidance response (Lorens *et al.*, 1971). Animals with these lesions show increased running wheel and open-field activity, and enhanced reactivity to novel stimuli and environmental change, and are also deficient in the acquisition and retention of a one-way avoidance response (Srebro and Lorens, 1975). Steranka and Barrett (1974) suggest that the facilitation of active avoidance observed following raphé lesions is attributable to the fact that such lesions attenuate the behavioural suppression or "freezing" commonly observed following shock administration. The lesions may thus result in a behavioural baseline which is more compatible with the acquisition of an avoidance response.

These observations are consistent with the hypothesis that the 5-hydroxytryptamine system arising from the median raphé (B_8) nucleus exerts inhibitory effects on motor behaviour and may mediate some of the behaviourally suppressive effects of aversive stimuli. No specific behavioural disturbance has yet been observed following discrete lesions of the dorsal raphé nucleus (Srebro and Lorens, 1975), and few investigations have yet extended to the other 5-hydroxytryptamine-containing cell-body areas giving rise to ascending fibres.

VIII. Functions of Monoamine Neurones at the Cellular Level

The existence of neuronal systems with the anatomical characteristics of the monoamine pathways poses a conceptual problem. While it is very plausible that systems which arise from relatively discrete nuclei of origin, and "fan out" to innervate large areas of the CNS, function by delivering some generalized message "to whom it may concern", it is difficult to imagine that this message is received by the postsynaptic cell in terms of the usual excitatory or inhibitory postsynaptic potential. If such a change occurred simultaneously across, say, the entire cerebral cortex the effect would surely be to disrupt on-going activity if not, in the case of an excitatory potential, to induce an epileptic fit. Such theoretical consequences encourage the consideration of other forms of postsynaptic effect. Descarries *et al.* (1975) have argued on the basis of quantitative electron microscopic studies that many monoamine terminal varicosities do not in any case make postsynaptic contacts of the previously recognized type.

McIlwain (1970) has suggested that metabolic adaptation may be a common function of various neurohumoral agents at the postsynaptic cell, arguing from evidence from various studies for transmitter-stimulated increases in cyclic nucleotide production, and possible consequent activations of phosphorylase kinase, protein kinase and peptide formation. The existence of a dopamine-sensitive adenylate cyclase in the caudate nucleus is now well established (Clement-Cormier *et al.*, 1975) and it seems likely that other monoamines may act in a similar way. The problem is to understand how such a quasi-hormonal mode of action, with possible metabolic consequences, may be related to on-going nerve activity in the postsynaptic field.

One speculative concept has been advanced in relation to the adrenergic innervation of the cerebral cortex. Crow (1968) and Kety (1970) have proposed that the noradrenergic input acts selectively upon recently active cells and has the ability to promote the growth of recently-active synaptic connections. According to this concept the "to whom it may concern" message is received only by cells in a particular state of neuronal activity and acts upon these cells in a trophic or growth-promoting way. Such a concept would be consistent with a role for a noradrenergic reinforcement system in establishing the neural traces underlying learning such as that reviewed on p. 161. The evidence is at present equivocal, but such a concept may be taken as a particular version of the more general hypothesis that monoamine neurones are part of the mechanism whereby significant environmental stimuli come to modify the neural connections which determine behaviour.

IX. Summary

The development of histochemical techniques has greatly advanced the study of monoamine-containing neurones in the central nervous system. Neuronal systems containing catecholamines and indoleamines arise from relatively small groups of cell bodies, mainly within the brain stem, and give rise to terminal networks distributed to wide areas of the central nervous system. These systems arise early in phylogeny and ontogeny, and presumably serve fundamental behavioural and physiological functions.

Three major ascending catecholamine-containing systems are described: the dopamine neurones arising from the ventral mesencephalon giving rise to terminals in the corpus striatum, nucleus accumbens and frontal cortex; the dorsal bundle of noradrenaline neurones arising mainly from the locus coeruleus with a terminal distribution to cortical areas and the ventral bundle of noradrenaline neurones arising from the caudal medulla with terminals distributed mainly to the hypothalamus. Experiments with stereotaxically-implanted electrodes suggest that the two former systems, but not the ventral bundle, are reward pathways in the sense that electrical activation of these systems will support self-stimulation responding. Self-stimulation behaviour with electrodes in the region of the dopamine-containing cell bodies is accompanied by marked activation of behaviour, but with electrodes in the region of the locus coeruleus has no such concomitants. This suggests that the functions of these two pathways are quite different.

Bilateral lesions of dopamine neurones cause profound motor and motivational deficits similar to those seen in the "lateral hypothalamic syndrome", and unilateral lesions appear to result in attentional deficits toward stimuli in the contralateral sensory field. Lesions of the system of noradrenaline neurones arising from the locus coeruleus appear to cause no motor or motivational impairments but some experiments suggest that such lesions may interfere with the organism's ability to learn. Lesions of the ventral bundle of noradrenaline neurones have been reported to cause increased food intake and weight gain.

The anatomical relationships between the ascending catecholamine systems and olfactory, gustatory and ascending visceral afferent pathways suggest the possibility that there is a fundamental relationship between catecholamine neurones and the sensory mechanisms for detecting food. Perhaps catecholamine neurones originally developed as pathways mediating the behavioural response to stimulation of food-related afferent pathways, but in the course of evolution have developed to mediate similar responses to a wider range of afferent stimuli. The hypothesis is proposed that dopamine neurones mediate the "incentive" or activating response to rewarding environmental stimuli whereas the locus coeruleus noradrenaline system mediates the "reinforcing" or behaviour-modifying aspects of such stimuli. Thus dopamine neurones may be expected to be active in appetitive, and the locus coeruleus in consummatory, behaviours. The ventral bundle of noradrenaline neurones is envisaged as a satiety mechanism which can terminate a positively-rewarded behavioural sequence.

Indoleamine neuronal systems arise mainly from the mid-line raphé nuclei. Experiments with the tryptophan hydroxylase inhibitor *p*-chlorophenylalanine suggest that these neurones exert an inhibitory or restraining influence on a variety of motor, social and sexual behaviours. Some findings are consistent with the hypothesis that serotonin-containing neurones mediate some aspects of the effects of punishing stimuli on behaviour. Lesions of the median raphé nucleus suggest that the system of fibres arising from this nucleus exert an inhibitory influence on motor behaviour.

The concept that monoamine neurones exert their effects on behaviour not by an excitatory or inhibitory influence on cell-firing in the classical electrophysiological manner, but by a metabolic or trophic effect on postsynaptic elements is consistent with the anatomical characteristics of these neurones and with some biochemical actions of monoamines at the cellular level. It is suggested that monoamine systems may contribute to the plasticity of behaviour with respect to differing environments by allowing a general message of the "reward" or "punishment" type to be delivered to a large area of neuronal elements e.g. the cortex, so that an interaction between the monoamine and certain recently-active postsynaptic elements can take place. The effects of this interaction may be to modify certain synaptic connections and thus to influence the course of learning and unlearning.

References

Amin, A. H. T., Crawford, T. B. B. and Gaddum, J. H. (1954). *J. Physiol. (London)* **126**, 596–618.

Ahlskog, J. E. and Hoebel, B. G. (1973). *Science* **182**, 166–169.

Anand, B. K. and Brobeck, J. R. (1951). *Yale J. Biol. Med.* **24**, 123–140.

Andén, N.-E. (1968). *Ann. Med. Exp. Biol. Fenn.* **46**, 361–366.

Andén, N. E., Dahlström, A., Fuxe, K., Larsson, K., Olson, L. and Ungerstedt, U. (1966). *Acta Physiol. Scand.* **67**, 313–326.

Anlezark, G. M., Arbuthnott, G. W., Christie, J. E. and Crow, T. J. (1973a). *J. Physiol. (London)* **234**, 103–104P.

Anlezark, G. M., Arbuthnott, G. W., Christie, J. E., Crow, T. J. and Spear, P. J. (1973b). *J. Physiol. (London)* **237**, 31–32P.

Anlezark, G. M., Crow, T. J. and Greenway, A. P. (1973). *Science* **181**, 682–684.

Anlezark, G. M., Walter, D. S., Arbuthnott, G. W., Crow, T. J. and Eccleston, D. (1975). *J. Neurochem.* **24**, 677–681.

Björklund, A., Ehinger, B. and Falck, B. (1968). *J. Histochem. Cytochem.* **16**, 263–270.

Black, W. C. and Cooper, B. R. (1970). *Physiol. Behav.* **5**, 1405–1409.

Carlsson, A. (1965). *In* "Handbook of Experimental Pharmacology", Vol. 19, 5-Hydroxytryptamine and related indole-alkylamines. (O. Eichler and A. Farah, eds). Springer-Verlag, Berlin, pp. 529–592.

Carlsson, A., Lundqvist, M. and Magnusson, T. (1957). *Nature* **180**, 1200.

Clement-Cormier, Y., Parrish, R. C., Petzold, G. L., Kebabian, J. W. and Greengard, P. (1975). *J. Neurochem.* **25**, 143–149.

Connell, P. H. (1958). "Amphetamine Psychosis", Maudsley Monograph, No. 5, Chapman and Hall, London.

Creese, I. and Iversen, S. D. (1974). *Psychopharmacologia* **39**, 345–357.

Creese, I. and Iversen, S. D. (1975). *Brain Res.* **83**, 419–436.

Crow, T. J. (1968). *Nature* **219**, 736–737.

Crow, T. J. (1972a). *Brain Res.* **36**, 265–273.

Crow, T. J. (1972b). *Psychol. Med.* **2**, 414–421.

Crow, T. J. (1973). *Psychol. Med.* **3**, 66–73.

Crow, T. J. (1976a). *In* "Brain Stimulation Reward" (A. Wauquier and E. T. Rolls, eds). Elsevier, Amsterdam, pp. 211–237.

Crow, T. J. (1976b). *In* "Brain-Stimulation Reward" (A. Wauquier and E. T. Rolls, eds). Elsevier Press, Amsterdam, pp. 587–591.

Crow, T. J. and Arbuthnott, G. W. (1972). *Nature New Biol.* **238**, 245–246.

Crow, T. J., Spear, P. J. and Arbuthnott, G. W. (1972). *Brain Res.* **36**, 275–287.

Crow, T. J. and Wendlandt, S. (1976). *Nature* **259**, 42–44.

Dahlström, A. and Fuxe, K. (1964). *Acta Physiol. Scand.* **62**, *Suppl.* 232.

Descarries, L., Beaudet, A. and Watkins, K. C. (1975). *Brain Res.* **100**, 563–588.

Eränkö, O. (1955). *Acta Endocrinol. (Copenhagen)* **18**, 174–179.

Ernst, A. M. (1970). "Excerpta Med. Int. Congr.", Series no. 220, pp. 18–23.

Falck, B., Hillarp, N.-A., Thieme, G. and Torp, A. (1962). *J. Histochem. Cytochem.* **10**, 348–354.

Feldberg, W (1950). *Brit. Med. Bull.* **6**. 312–321.

Fibiger, H. C. and Campbell, B. A. (1971). *Neuropharmacology* **10**, 25–32.

Fuxe, K. and Jonsson, G. (1974). *Advan. Biochem. Psychopharmacol.* **10**, 1–12.

Fuxe, K. and Ungerstedt, U. (1970). In "Amphetamines and Related Compounds" (E. Costa and S. Garratini, eds). Raven Press, New York, pp. 257–288.

Fuxe, K., Hökfelt, T. and Nilsson, O. (1969). *Neuroendocrinology* **5**, 257–270.

Geller, I. and Blum, K. (1970). *Eur. J. Pharmacol.* **9**, 319–324.

Gold, R. M. (1973). *Science* **182**, 488–490.

Grahame-Smith, D. G. (1971). *J. Neurochem.* **18**, 1053–1066.

Green, A. R. and Grahame-Smith, D. G. (1974). *Neuropharmacology* **13**, 949–959.

Hess, S. M. and Doepfner, W. (1961). *Arch. Int. Pharmacodyn. Ther.* **134**, 89–99.

Hökfelt, T., Fuxe K., Goldstein, M. and Johansson, O. (1974). *Brain Res.* **66**, 235–251.

Hoyland, V. J., Shillito, E. E. and Vogt, M. (1970). *Brit. J. Pharmacol.* **40**, 659–667.

Jacobs, B. L. and Klemfuss, H. (1975). *Brain Res.* **100**, 450–457.

Jacobs, B. L., Trimbach, C., Eubanks, E. E. and Trulson, M. (1975). *Brain Res.* **94**, 253–261.

Jonsson, G. (1971). *Progr. Brain Res.* **34**, 53–61.

Jouvet, M. (1969). *Science* **163**, 32–41.

Jouvet, M. (1972). *Ergebn. Physiol.* **64**, 166–307.

Kapatos, G. and Gold, R. M. (1973). *Pharmacol. Biochem. Behav.* **1**, 81–87.

Kelly, P. H., Seviour, P. W. and Iversen, S. D. (1975). *Brain Res.* **94**, 507–522.

Kety, S. S. (1970). In "The Neurosciences: Second Study Program" (F. O. Schmitt, ed.). Rockefeller University Press, New York, pp. 324–336.

Koe, B. K. and Weissman, A. (1966). *J. Pharmacol. Exp. Ther.* **154**, 499–516.

Koella, W. P. (1969). *Biol. Psychiat.* **1**, 161–177.

Lemieux, G., Davignon, A. and Genest, J. (1956). *Can. Med. Ass. J.* **74**, 522–526.

Lidbrink, P. (1974). *Brain Res.* **74**, 19–40.

Lindvall, O. and Björklund, A. (1974). *Acta Physiol. Scand. Suppl.* 412.

Livingston, R. B. (1967). "The Neurosciences", (G. C. Quarton, T. Melnechuk and F. O. Schmitt, eds). Rockefeller University Press, New York, pp. 568–577.

Loewi, O. (1921). *Pflügers Arch. Gesamte. Physiol. Menschen.* **189**, 239–242.

Lorens, S. A. and Guldberg, H. C. (1974). *Brain Res.* **78**, 45–56.

Lorens, S. A., Sorensen, J. P. and Yunger, L. M. (1971). *J. Comp. Physiol. Psychol.* **77**, 48–52.

McIlwain, H. (1970). *Nature* **226**, 803–806.

Marshall, J. F., Turner, B. H. and Teitelbaum, P. (1971). *Science* **174**, 523–525.

Marshall, J. F., Richardson, J. S. and Teitelbaum, P. (1974). *J. Comp. Physiol. Psychol.* **87**, 808–830.

Mason, S. T. and Iversen, S.D. (1976). *J. Comp. Physiol. Psychol.* (*in press*).

Moore, K. E. and Rech, R. H. (1967). *J. Pharm. Pharmacol.* **19**, 405–407.

Muller, J. C., Pryor, W. W., Gibbons, J. E. and Orgain, E. S. (1955). *J. Amer. Med. Ass.* **159**, 836–839.

Munkvad, I. and Randrup, A. (1966). *Acta Psychiat. Scand.* **42**, *Suppl.* 191, 178–187.

Nobin, A. and Björklund, A. (1973). *Acta Physiol. Scand. Suppl.* 388, 1–40.

Olds, J. and Milner, P. (1954). *J. Comp. Physiol. Psychol.* **47**, 419–427.

Olson, L., Boréus, L. O. and Seiger, Å. (1973). *Z. Anat. Entwicklungsgesch* **139**, 259–282.

Poschel, B. P. H. and Ninteman, F. W. (1966). *Life Sci.* **5**, 11–16.

Randrup, A. and Munkvad, I. (1965). *Psychopharmacologia* **7**, 416–422.

Randrup, A. and Munkvad, I. (1966a). *Acta Psychiat. Scand. Suppl.* 191, **42**, 193–199.

Randrup, A. and Munkvad, I. (1966b). *Nature* **211**, 540.

Randrup, A. and Munkvad, I. (1967). *Psychopharmacologia* **11**, 300–310.

Randrup, A., Munkvad, I. and Usden, P. (1963). *Acta Pharmacol. (Kbh)* **20**, 145–157.

Roberts, D. C. S., Price, M. H. T. and Fibiger, H. C. (1976). *J. Comp. Physiol. Psychol.* **90**, 363–372.

Russell, G. V. (1955). *Tex. Rep. Biol. Med.* **13**, 939–988.

Seiger, Å. and Olson, L. (1973). *Z. Anat. Entwicklungsgesch* **140**, 281–318.

Shillito, E. E. (1970). *Brit. J. Pharmacol.* **38**, 305–315.

Simpson, B. A. and Iversen, S. D. (1971). *Nature (London)* **230**, 30–32.

Srebro, B. and Lorens, S. A. (1975). *Brain Res.* **89**, 303–325.

Stein, L. (1964). *Fed. Proc.* **23**, 836–850.

Steranka, L. R. and Barrett, R. J. (1974). *Behav. Biol.* **11**, 205–213.

Tagliamonte, A., Tagliamonte, P., Gessa, G. and Brodie, B. (1969). *Science* **166**, 1433–1435.

Tenen, S. S. (1967). *Psychopharmacologia* **10**, 204–219.

Thorndike, E. L. (1933). *Psychol. Rev.* **40**, 434–439.

Tulloch, I. (1975). *J. Physiol. (London)* **248**, 47–48P.

Ungerstedt, U. (1971a). *Acta Physiol. Scand. Suppl.* **367**, 1–48.

Ungerstedt, U. (1971b). *Acta Physiol. Scand. Suppl.* **367**, 69–93.

Ungerstedt, U. (1971c). *Acta Physiol. Scand. Suppl.* **367**, 95–122.

Ungerstedt, U. and Ljungberg, T. (1975). *In* "Catecholamines and Schizophrenia" (S. Matthysse and S. S. Kety, eds). Pergamon Press, Oxford, pp. 149–150.

Vogt, M. (1954). *J. Physiol. (London)* **123**, 451–481.

Vogt, M. (1973). *Brit. Med. Bull.* **29**, 168–171.

Weissman, A. and Harbert, C. A. (1972). *Ann. Rep. Medicin. Chem.* **7**, 47–58.

Weissman, A. and Koe, B. K. (1965). *Life Sci.* **4**, 1037–1048.

Wise, C. D., Berger, B. D. and Stein, L. (1970). *Dis. Nerv. Syst. GWAN Suppl.* **31**, 34–37.

Young, J. Z. (1964). A model of the brain. Oxford University Press, Oxford.

Zigmond, M. J. and Stricker, E. M. (1973). *Science* **182**, 717–719.

Chapter 6

Physiological Aspects of Brain Energy Metabolism

B. K. SIESJÖ

*Research Department 4, E-Blocket, University Hospital,
S-221 85 Lund, Sweden*

I. Introduction

This chapter is intended to give a brief account of the coupling between function, metabolism and blood flow in the brain. The objectives require that information is drawn mainly from studies on the intact brain. However, in order to provide a necessary background to events occurring at cellular level, we will briefly consider results obtained on isolated tissues. Readers interested in the detailed aspects of the metabolism of nervous tissues, as these can be studied *in vitro*, and of the metabolism of radioactive substrates, should consult available reviews and textbooks (e.g. McIlwain, 1963; Balázs, 1970; McIlwain and Bachelard, 1971). Recent textbook chapters and reviews have been devoted to aspects of brain metabolism in hypoxia and ischemia (Maker and Lehrer, 1971; Siesjö and Plum, 1972; Siesjö *et al.*, 1974, 1975a). A more detailed and exhaustive account of the subjects considered in the present chapter will be given in a forthcoming textbook on brain energy metabolism (Siesjö, 1977). Presently, we will attempt to bring together information obtained in a variety of conditions, emphasizing the coupling between functional activity, metabolism and blood flow. By necessity, the number of references quoted must be restricted and, to facilitate access to the literature, recent articles will be favoured. A more detailed list of references is published elsewhere (Siesjö, 1977).

II. Methods for Blood Flow and Metabolism

In the brain, measurements of blood flow, metabolic rate and metabolic state present some special problems, and it seems warranted to discuss shortly the characteristics of those methods that may be used for quantitative studies.

A. *Blood Flow and Oxygen Consumption*

With few exceptions, methods for cerebral metabolic rate (CMR) are based on measurements of cerebral blood flow (CBF) and appropriate arteriovenous differences (AVD), i.e. values are calculated from the equation

$$CMR = CBF \times AVD.$$

Due to the complex anatomical arrangement of its vascular supply, the brain does not easily lend itself to direct measurements of arterial inflow or venous outflow. The methods that have been described (e.g. Schmidt *et al.*, 1945; Geiger and Magnes, 1947; Gilboe and Betz, 1973; Gilboe *et al.*, 1973) necessitate such extensive surgery that there is the risk of tissue damage. Some of these models have shown characteristics that are not normally encountered in intact animals, e.g. reduced or abolished response of CBF to high CO_2 or low O_2, loss of vascular reaction to changes in blood pressure, lack of metabolic reaction to convulsant drugs, and passive relationship between perfusion rate and oxygen uptake. Thus, although useful for many purposes such methods may not be ideal for studies of coupling between function, metabolism and blood flow. Less trauma is involved in those methods that are based on venous outflow from normally perfused brains (Rapela and Green, 1964; Michenfelder et al., 1968). Although these methods have yielded important information on CBF and CMR_{O_2}, it is not clear that the values are always quantitative. This is due to the fact that blood is drained both via the sampling catheter(s) and other venous channels, and the proportion between these volumes of blood must depend on the outflow resistances.

For all these reasons, the inert gas technique described by Kety and Schmidt (1948a) is preferred to those subsequently described when the objective is to measure both CBF and CMR_{O_2}. The method is an ingenious application of the law of conservation of matter to a non-steady-state situation in which a subject is made to inhale an inert, diffusible substance. CBF is calculated from the equation

$$CBF = \frac{100\lambda \; C_v'}{\int_0^T (C_a - C_v) \, dt}$$

where C_a and C_v are the tracer concentrations in arterial and cerebral venous blood, C_v' is the tracer concentration in venous blood at the end of the saturation period (usually 10–15 min), and λ is a partition coefficient (tissue/blood) for the tracer. It is usually more practical to measure CBF during desaturation, and use a radioactive gas (e.g. [133]xenon) instead of nitrous oxide. In man, venous blood is usually obtained from the jugular bulb to give the CBF value for the whole of the brain. In experimental animals, venous blood can be sampled from the superior sagittal sinus (Homburger et al., 1946) and the CBF value reflects mainly cortical flow.

It is important that the requirements of the Kety and Schmidt technique can be shown to be fulfilled. The most important of these are: 1. CBF must be constant during the measurement, 2. the tissue should not contain masses with very slow perfusion rates, and 3. the venous blood sampled must not be contaminated with blood from extracerebral tissues (skin, bone or muscles). In comparison to brain, such tissues have slow perfusion rates. It can usually be ascertained that the first requirement is fulfilled by performing repeated determinations of AVD_{O_2}. If requirements 2. and 3. are not fulfilled there will be a lingering difference in tracer activity between arterial and cerebral venous blood. In the rat, and when venous blood is sampled from the superior sagittal sinus, none of the potential errors complicate the measurements (Norberg and Siesjö, 1974) and the values obtained should be quantitative measures of CBF (Fig. 1). It is also possible to measure whole brain CBF if special precautions are taken to exclude extracerebral contamination (Nilsson and Siesjö, 1976).

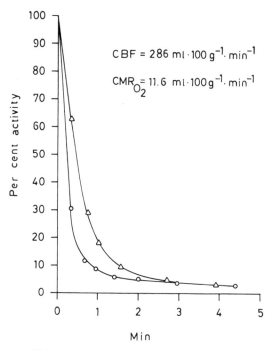

$$CBF = 286 \ ml \cdot 100 \ g^{-1} \cdot min^{-1}$$

$$CMR_{O_2} = 11.6 \ ml \cdot 100 g^{-1} \cdot min^{-1}$$

Fig. 1. Representative [133]Xenon desaturation curves in the rat, allowing calculation of CBF according to the principle of Kety and Schmidt (1948a). The animal was saturated with [133]Xenon for 20 min, whereafter the [133]Xenon supply was discontinued and repeated samples were taken from a peripheral artery (circles) and from the superior sagittal sinus (triangles). All values given as a percentage of venous activity at the end of the saturation period. CBF was calculated with the trapezoid rule and CMR_{O_2} was derived by multiplying CBF with the arteriovenous difference in oxygen content.

Much information has been obtained from measurements of regional CBF (rCBF). The two most important methods are based on the equations described by Kety (1960). The residue detection method requires that the tracer is added to the arterial inflow of the brain; flow is then calculated from the externally recorded clearance of tracer

(Ingvar and Lassen, 1962). With ^{85}Kr as a tracer, the method allows measurements of rCBF in the superficial cortical layers (in animal experiments), and with ^{133}xenon the method can be used to measure rCBF in man. The tissue uptake method, which is applicable only to animals, requires that a diffusible tracer is continuously infused into the blood stream and that the uptake into the tissue is measured after a period of e.g. 30 or 60 sec (Landau et al., 1955; Reivich et al., 1969). Its usefulness depends on the fact that the tissue concentration can be measured autoradiographically, allowing measurements in any cerebral structure.

As usually applied, both rCBF methods are based on two assumptions the validity of which is not always known: 1. there is "instantaneous" diffusion of tracer between blood and tissue, and 2. the tissue under study is homogenously perfused. At high flow values, these assumptions are not necessarily valid (see Eklöf et al., 1974). Besides, the methods are not well suited for studies of CMR_{O_2} since there is considerable uncertainty about the appropriate venous source. However, both methods have given most valuable information on the coupling between function and rCBF.

B. Glucose Consumption

In the past, glucose consumption (CMR_{gl}) has been obtained from CBF and arteriovenous differences (AVD_{gl}), but at high flow values and normal or increased plasma glucose concentrations, this is not sufficiently sensitive. Besides, regional CMR_{gl} has been inaccessible. It is, therefore, of importance that two new methods for glucose consumption have been developed, one of which is truly regional. Based on a procedure described by Gaitonde (1965) a method for glucose consumption, applicable to animal experiments, was described by Hawkins et al. (1974). The basic equation is similar to that already mentioned

$$CMR_{gl} = \frac{\Delta[^{14}C](T)}{\int_0^T (GSA)\,dt}$$

where $\Delta[^{14}C](T)$ is the amount of ^{14}C accumulated in tissue metabolites (other than glucose) from ^{14}C-glucose injected into the circulation, and $\int_0^T(GSA)\,dt$ is the integral of the specific activity of glucose in the tissue during time T. If the ^{14}C-glucose used is labelled in the 2-position, any radioactivity lost as CO_2 during 5–10 min is small. Hawkins et al. (1974) derived specific activity in tissue from that in the blood, allowing measurements in individual animals. A minor modification of the method with direct measurements of specific activity in tissue has been described (Borgström *et al.*, 1976). Although this necessitates that groups of animals are studied it allows measurements of CMR_{gl} in short periods (e.g. 2 min).

The other regional CMR_{gl} method, developed in Sokoloff's laboratory, is one in which glucose consumption is derived from the rate of accumulation of radioactive 2-deoxyglucose in the tissue, following parenteral administration (Reivich *et al.*, 1975; Sokoloff, 1975, 1976). Most importantly, the method allows autoradiographic estimation of CMR_{gl} and, since a similar technique is used for $rCBF$, flow and metabolic rate can be measured in any cerebral region provided that the conditions of the experiments allow a steady-state period of about 40 min.

C. *High Energy Phosphate Utilization*

In a pioneering study, Lowry *et al.* (1964) delineated the metabolic changes that occur following interruption of circulation in mouse brain. The authors assumed that, when circulation ceases, metabolic rate continues for some time (e.g. 15 sec) at the predecapitation rate. Since oxygen is unavailable the tissue can only obtain energy by utilizing its own high energy phosphate stores (phosphocreatine and ATP), or by degrading glucose and glycogen to lactic acid. Accordingly, high energy phosphate ($\sim P$) utilization can be calculated from the equation:

$$\Delta \sim P = \Delta PCr + 2\Delta ATP + \Delta ADP + 2\Delta glucose + 2 \cdot 9\Delta glycogen.$$

For short ischemic periods, the equation can be simplified into

$$\Delta \sim P = \Delta PCr + 2\Delta ATP + \Delta lactate$$

(Gatfield *et al.*, 1966). In their studies on mice, Lowry *et al.* (1964) obtained a $\sim P$ use of 27 $\mu mol.g^{-1}.min^{-1}$. This can be interpreted as follows. If glucose is completely oxidized to CO_2 and water the following equation applies:

$$glucose + 6O_2 + 38ADP + 38P_i \rightarrow 6CO_2 + 44H_2O + 38ATP.$$

Allowing for about 5% of the glucose extracted to be converted to lactic acid, each mole of glucose consumed corresponds to the formation of about 36 moles of ATP. Thus, the $\sim P$ utilization measured is synonymous with a glucose consumption of 0·75 $\mu mol.g^{-1}.min^{-1}$,

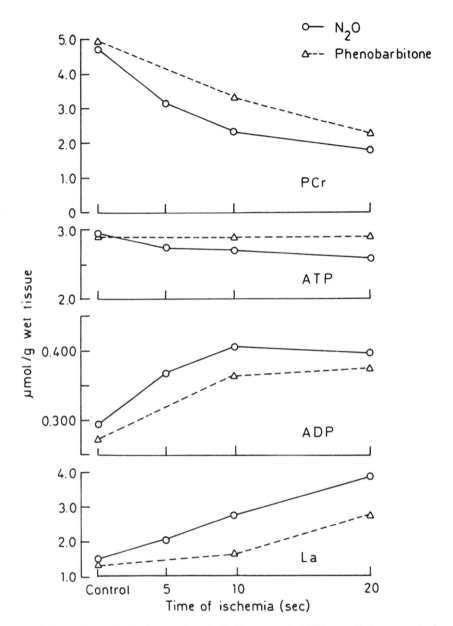

Fig. 2. Illustration of "closed system" method of Lowry *et al.* (1964) as applied to rat cerebral cortex. The data show the rate of changes in phosphocreatine (PCr), ATP, ADP and lactate following decapitation. The tissue was frozen either without decapitation, or after 5, 10 and 20 sec of ischemia. The animals were anaesthetized either with 70% N_2O or with phenobarbital, dosage 150 mg.kg^{-1}. (Data from Nilsson *et al.*, 1975a.)

and an oxygen consumption of $4 \cdot 5$ $\mu mol.g^{-1}.min^{-1}$. We recognize that these figures are about three times as high as those obtained from CBF and the appropriate AVDs in man (see below).

Using a freezing method allowing short, accurately defined periods of ischemia to be studied, Nilsson et al. (1975a) compared values obtained with the method of Lowry et al. (1964) to CMR_{O_2} in rat cerebral cortex. Figure 2 shows the changes occurring in PCr, ATP, ADP and lactate. After five seconds of ischemia, calculated $\sim P$ use in N_2O and phenobarbitone anaesthesia was 30 and 12 $\mu mol.g^{-1}.min^{-1}$, respectively. These values compare favourably with those derived from measured CMR_{O_2} (29 and 15 $\mu mol.g^{-1}.min^{-1}$, respectively), supporting the original assumption of Lowry et al. (1964). However, in N_2O anaesthesia the calculated $\Delta \sim P$ values gradually declined and the data indicate that, at normal metabolic rate, the method gives accurate values only if very short ischemic periods are used (e.g. 5 sec). It was tentatively assumed that postdecapitation metabolic rate falls off as soon as there is a decrease in ATP concentration. It is doubtful that the method can be successfully applied to situations with an increased metabolic rate.

D. Fixation of Tissue for Metabolite Analyses

It has been known for a long time that, due to the high metabolic rate of brain tissues, special precautions must be taken to avoid autolytic artefacts during the fixation of the tissue for metabolite analyses. In the rat cerebral cortex, $\sim P$ utilization is about $0 \cdot 5$ $\mu mol.g^{-1}.sec^{-1}$. Since glucose consumption is $0 \cdot 8$ $\mu mol.g^{-1}.min^{-1}$ (see below) pyruvate is produced at a rate of $1 \cdot 6$ $\mu mol.g^{-1}.min^{-1}$. During ischemia, the rate of glycolysis may increase about five times (Lowry et al., 1964, see also Nilsson et al., 1975a). Accordingly, $\sim P$ production from anaerobic glycolysis ($\Delta \sim P = \Delta La$) is maximally $0 \cdot 16$ $\mu mol.g^{-1}.sec^{-1}$, or less than a third of the initial $\sim P$ use. Thus, about $0 \cdot 35$ $\mu mol.g^{-1}$ of high energy phosphate groups must be tapped off the available energy stores (PCr plus ATP) per second. These figures emphasize that the concentrations of labile substances are seriously distorted if there is a delay between interruption of circulation and fixation of tissue.

In unanaesthetized small animals the most common method is to immerse the whole animal into a suitable coolant (Stone, 1938; Lowry et al., 1964). In mice, the freezing of the brain is so rapid that any autolytic artefacts may be assumed to be small but, in rats, this seems less clear. The advantage of the immersion method is that unanaesthetized animals can be used. However, the procedure carries a risk of misinterpretation of data since physiological parameters have seldom been controlled.

For anaesthetized animals, the classical procedure is that of Kerr (1935) who fixed the tissue by pouring a coolant onto the surface of the exposed dura. The method has been adapted to artificially ventilated, small animals—freezing through the intact skull bone—and the results on labile cerebral metabolites indicate that more optimal conditions are obtained than by immersion of either rats (Pontén *et al.*, 1973a) or mice (Pontén *et al.*, 1973b). The crucial point is that still unfrozen parts of the tissue are supplied with well-oxygenated blood (cf. Richter and Dawson, 1948). If very quick freezing of the cortical surface is desirable, the tissue can be frozen through the intact dura after removal of the bone (Nilsson *et al.*, 1975a).

Recently, two new methods have been described for ultra-rapid freezing of brains in unanaesthetized rats. In one (freeze-blowing) two hollow probes are forced into the skull and the supratentorial parts of the brain are blown out and frozen to a thin wafer in a chamber at liquid nitrogen temperature (Veech *et al.*, 1973). In the other (freeze-clamping) a circular section is cut out of the brain and instantly clamped between two cooled metal blocks (Quistorff, 1975).

In the last few years, several studies have appeared in which tissue fixation has been achieved by microwave irradiation (MWI). A comparison with freeze-blowing showed that MWI gave less optimal values for labile metabolites (Veech *et al.*, 1973). Previously, it was assumed that the tissue concentrations of PCr and AMP provided the most sensitive indicators of autolysis but it now appears that the concentration of cyclic 3'5'—AMP (cAMP) and the ratio of phosphorylase *a* activity to total phosphorylase activity (percentage phosphorylase *a*) are even more sensitive. Lust *et al.* (1973) found that cAMP was lower after MWI than after freeze-blowing but since PCr was lower, and the percentage phosphorylase *a* was higher, it was concluded that the low cAMP values on MWI did not indicate that the method gives rapid inactivation of enzyme activities.

It appears that no fixation method described is superior to all others. Rather, the choice of method must be dictated by the requirements of the experiments. The highest values of PCr and the lowest values for AMP are obtained with surface-freezing in paralysed animals (Pontén *et al.*, 1973a and b) and, with freezing through the dura, the method also gives the lowest values for percentage phosphorylase *a* (less than 15%, Folbergrová *et al.*, in preparation). Freeze-blowing and freeze-clamping give somewhat less optimal values. This may not only be due to the (admittedly short) period of ischemia before freezing. Possibly, the "explosive" trauma involved could accelerate metabolic rate in the tissue. Several of the methods mentioned allow studies on un-anaesthetized animals. However, it would be a mistake to conclude that it is always an advantage to avoid anaesthesia. First, some forms of anaesthesia (e.g. 70% N_2O) do not measurably lower cerebral metabolic rate (Carlsson et al., 1976b). Second, as the following discussion will bear out, restraining of unanaesthetized animals carries the risk of a stress-induced increase in metabolic rate.

E. Species Differences

The ultimate objective of most animal studies is to increase knowledge about events occurring in man. When inferences are drawn from experimental work it is essential to keep in mind that there are species differences in cerebral blood flow and metabolism. Early in vitro studies showed that oxygen uptake of cerebral cortex slices varied inversely with the size of the animal. Recently, complementary data were obtained for the elephant and the whale. The combined data indicate that the brains from small animals have a higher oxygen uptake because they contain more densely packed neurones, and have a lower glia to neurone ratio (Tower and Young, 1973).

Results obtained in vivo corroborate the conclusions drawn from the in vitro studies. Table 1 shows CBF and CMR_{O_2} values for the human and rat brain, and for the dog and rat cerebral cortex. All results were obtained with the Kety and Schmidt technique (or were validated against this technique) and apply either to the unanaesthetized state, or to such superficial anaesthesia that unanaesthetized values were approached. As can be seen, the rat has CBF and CMR_{O_2} values approximately twice as high as in man. Furthermore, CBF and CMR_{O_2} in rat cerebral cortex are twice as high as those measured in the dog.

The most complete results on cerebral blood flow and metabolism exist for rats. As can be seen, CMR_{O_2} for cerebral cortex and whole brain are 4·6 and 3·4 $\mu mol.g^{-1}.min^{-1}$, respectively. Since any influence of the N_2O anaesthesia used should be less than 10% (Carlsson et al., 1976b) we may assume that the values are representative of the unanaesthetized state. If 95% of the glucose taken up is oxidized to CO_2 and H_2O, the figures given would correspond to CMR_{gl} values of 0·79 and 0·6 $\mu mol.g^{-1}.min^{-1}$, respectively. The values directly determined, using the method of Hawkins et al. (1974) are for the

Table 1

Cerebral oxygen consumption (CMR_{O_2}) and cerebral blood flow (CBF) in man, dog and rat

Species (anaesthesia)	Source of venous blood	CBF (ml.g^{-1}.min^{-1})	CMR_{O_2} (μmol.g^{-1}.min^{-1})	Reference
Man (awake)	Jugular bulb	0·54 ± 0·12	1·47 ± 0·18	Kety and Schmidt (1948a)
Dog (spinal)	Sup. sag. sinus	0·57 ± 0·03	2·50 ± 0·12	Theye and Michenfelder (1968)
Rat (70% N_2O)	Retroglenoid vein	0·80 ± 0·02	3·38 ± 0·08	B. Nilsson and Siesjö (1976)
Rat (70% N_2O)	Sup. sag. sinus	1·08 ± 0·05	4·60 ± 0·09	Hägerdal et al. (1975a)

The values are means ± S.E.M. (± S.D. in case of data from man). All values were obtained with the inert gas technique of Kety and Schmidt (1948a), or were validated against this technique (Theye and Michenfelder, 1968).

cerebral cortex $0.77\ \mu mol.g^{-1}.min^{-1}$ (Borgström *et al.*, 1976) and for the supratentorial parts of the brain $0.62\ \mu mol.g^{-1}.min^{-1}$ (Hawkins *et al.*, 1974). Since also the $\sim P$ use rate, measured according to Lowry *et al.* (1964), is comparable (see above), three independent methods have given very similar results. Besides, data exist for rCBF and rCMR$_{gl}$ in a great number of brain regions (Reivich *et al.*, 1975).

It seems clear that there are species differences also for levels of metabolites. In the rat cerebral cortex, the concentrations for PCr, ATP, ADP and AMP are about 5, 3, 0.3 and $0.03\ \mu mol.g^{-1}$, respectively. In larger animals and in man, the ATP concentration and the size of the adenine nucleotide pool are lower (see e.g. Schmahl *et al.*, 1965, Schmiedek *et al.*, 1974). Such differences exist for many other metabolites. In other words, results obtained in different species are not directly comparable.

III. General Coupling of Function, Metabolism and Blood Flow in Neuronal Systems

It has been known for a long time that increased neuronal activity is accompanied by an increased oxygen consumption. The coupling between function and metabolism has been shown most clearly under *in vitro* conditions. Gerard (1932) reported that when the sciatic nerve of the frog was electrically stimulated it practically doubled its oxygen consumption (see also Baker and Conelly, 1966; Ritchie, 1967; Greengaard and Ritchie, 1971). A close correlation between functional activity and metabolic rate has been demonstrated for perfused sympathetic ganglia (Larrabee and Klingman, 1962). Finally, extensive data on brain slices (for reviews, see McIlwain, 1963; Harvey and McIlwain, 1969) have shown that electrical stimulation approximately doubles their oxygen uptake.

A relationship between increased neuronal activity and increased blood flow has been established both in experimental animals, and in man. The classical experiments of Schmidt and Hendrix (see Reivich, 1974) showed that when the visual pathways were activated by light, the blood flow of the occipital cortex, as measured with thermocouples, increased. Comparable data exist in man. For example, it has been shown that when the hand muscles are activated, there is an increased blood flow in the region of the specific projection area (Olesen, 1971).

In the experiments quoted there has been a coupling between, on one hand, functional activity and metabolic rate, and on the other hand, between functional activation and blood flow. It has been more difficult to obtain direct evidence that activation of specific neuronal pathways leads to increases in both metabolic rate and blood flow, and the coupling factors have proved even more elusive. Recent experiments in which rCBF has been measured with the tissue uptake method, and regional metabolic rate with the deoxyglucose method, have given direct proof that e.g. visual stimuli do not only cause increased rCBF in the appropriate projection or association areas, but also increased glucose consumption (Sokoloff, 1975; Kennedy et al., 1975). These results strongly indicate that, locally, increased neuronal firing is associated with an elevated metabolic rate. Simultaneously, or as a result of the functional activity, blood flow increases. These interrelationships appear valid since they only express what has been considered a general biological principle (see Sokoloff, 1969). However, as we will see, there are difficulties of proving this principle at the level of the whole brain.

There is agreement that an appreciable proportion of the metabolism of the brain is required for ion pumping, i.e. to maintain the concentration gradients for Na^+ and K^+ across the excitable membranes. In fact, the influx of Na^+ and efflux of K^+ that occur during depolarization are considered to be the pacemakers of metabolism (see e.g. Ritchie, 1973). A plausible coupling is the following. When Na^+ enters the cell during depolarization it activates the Na^+-K^+-dependent, membrane-bound, ATPase, and when the enzyme achieves vectorial translocation of ions, ATP is hydrolysed to ATP and P_i. The change in the ratio ATP/ADP, or (ATP)/(ADP$\cdot P_i$) (phosphate potential) then triggers an increased oxidative phosphorylation and, possibly in conjunction with Ca^{2+} that enters during depolarization, also an increased glycolytic rate. This explanation is supported by results showing that during electrical stimulation of tissue slices (see McIlwain, 1963; Harvey and McIlwain, 1969) or isolated nerves (Greengaard and Straub, 1959; Chmouliosky et al., 1969) breakdown of PCr and ATP, and accumulation of ADP, AMP and P_i occurs.

In spite of considerable experimentation and speculation it is still not known how an increased functional activity leads to increased blood flow. The most prevalent hypothesis is a metabolic one according to which products of an increased activity or an increased metabolism are assumed to achieve feedback relaxation of resistance vessels. During recent years, there has been a tendency to favour H^+, emanating either from CO_2 or lactic acid, as the coupling factor (e.g. Lassen, 1968). However, it cannot be excluded that an increase in extracellular K^+ activity contributes (see Betz, 1972), and lately, adenosine has received considerable interest (Rubio *et al.*, 1975). If adenosine is a coupling factor, as it may be in the coronary circulation (Rubio and Berne, 1975), it must be assumed that there is increased degradation of AMP during functional activity and that adenine quickly leaks through cell membranes. At the present time, there is no conclusive evidence in favour of any of these alternatives. Recent results suggest that neurogenic factors contribute in regulating CBF (e.g. Harper *et al.*, 1975) also that there may be control of CBF from extracerebral sites, e.g. the carotid and aortic chemoreceptors (see Purves, 1972; James, 1975). It is clear that if neurogenic mechanisms are involved it is not necessary to assume that increased CBF is the consequence of an increased metabolic rate; conceivably, the two phenomena may occur in parallel.

IV. Conditions with a Primary Decrease in Functional Activity

A corollary of the assumed coupling between function, metabolism and blood flow is that when there is a primary decrease in functional activity, metabolic rate and blood flow should also decrease. We will consider two such conditions—anaesthesia and hypothermia—and discuss possible coupling factors. To simplify the discussion, we will confine ourselves to barbiturate anaesthesia.

A. *Barbiturate Anaesthesia*

There is considerable evidence that, *in vitro*, barbiturates and some other anaesthetics block election transfer between NADH and flavo-proteins (for review, see Cohen, 1973). If this were the only effects of the anaesthetics one could assume that unconsciousness resulted because energy production was curtailed. There is now extensive *in vivo* data on labile phosphates which show that anaesthesia does not derange cerebral energy state (e.g. Goldberg *et al.*, 1966; MacMillan and Siesjö, 1973a; Nilsson and Siesjö, 1974). Therefore, the primary physiological action of barbiturates is probably to depress functional activity. Secondarily, there is reduction in metabolic rate and blood flow. Results reported from Kety's group show that the reduction in CBF and CMR_{O_2} is dose-dependent and, in deep anaesthesia, CMR_{O_2} is reduced to about 50% of control (for review see Sokoloff, 1972). These results have been confirmed in animal experiments and, if the

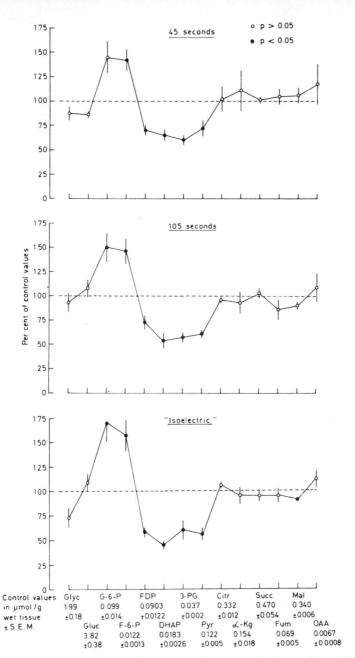

Control values in μmol/g wet tissue ±S.E.M.	Glyc 1.99 ±0.18	G-6-P 0.099 ±0.014	FDP 0.0903 ±0.0122	3-PG 0.037 ±0.002	Citr 0.332 ±0.012	Succ 0.470 ±0.054	Mal 0.340 ±0.006
	Gluc 3.82 ±0.38	F-6-P 0.0122 ±0.0013	DHAP 0.0183 ±0.0026	Pyr 0.122 ±0.005	α-Kg 0.154 ±0.018	Fum 0.069 ±0.005	OAA 0.0067 ±0.0008

Fig. 3. Changes in glycolytic metabolites and citric acid cycle intermediates following intravenous injection of thiopental in doses that caused a reduction of cerebral oxygen uptake to about 60% of control (70% N_2O). The tissue was frozen for analyses either 45 or 105 sec after the start of the infusion. In a third group enough thiopental was given to induce marked burst supression in the EEG (isoelectric) after 1·5–2 min. Each value is a percentage of control ±S.E.M. In all groups the tissue concentrations of ATP, ADP and AMP were unchanged. glyc: glycogen, gluc: glucose, G-6-P: glucose-6-phosphate, F-6-P: fructose-6-phosphate, FDP: fructose-1,6-diphosphate, DHAP: dihydroxyacetone phosphate, 3-PG: 3-phosphoglycerate, pyr: pyruvate, citr: citrate, α-KG: α-ketoglutarate, succ: succinate, fum: fumarate, mal: malate, OAA: oxaloacetate. (Data from Carlsson *et al.*, 1975c.)

CO_2 tension is maintained constant, it can be shown that CMR_{O_2} and CBF are reduced by proportional amounts (L. Nilsson and Siesjö, 1975).

Results reported by Goldberg et al. (1966) showed that, following administration of barbiturate to mice, there was accumulation of glucose-6-phosphate (G-6-P) and reduction in pyruvate concentration and of several citric acid cycle metabolites. Furthermore, there were moderate increases in PCr and ATP, and reductions in ADP and AMP. It is tempting to conclude from these results that secondary to the changes in labile phosphates, there is a reduction in rate of oxidative phosphorylation (e.g. due to the elevated phosphate potential), and retardation of glycolytic rate due to inhibition of phosphofructokinase (PFK) activity. Clear evidence of PFK inhibition has later been obtained in rats following intravenous (i.v.) administration of thiopental (Carlsson et al., 1975c). The most straightforward way of interpreting such results is from the Krebs postulate which states that, when there is a reduction in flux rate, there must be an increase in the concentration of the substrate of a regulatory enzyme (see Rolleston, 1972; Newsholme and Start, 1973). As can be seen in Fig. 3, there was accumulation of fructose-6-phosphate, F-6-P (and G-6-P), demonstrating inhibition of PFK. The triggering factors are less obvious. It was stressed by Goldberg et al. (1966) that their results on PCr, ATP, ADP and AMP could have been influenced by autolytic artefacts. Later results have also shown that, when a freezing technique is used that minimizes autolytic artefacts, the concentrations of ATP, ADP and AMP remain unchanged (MacMillan and Siesjö, 1973a; L. Nilsson and Siesjö, 1974; Carlsson et al., 1975c). The only phosphate change is a minor increase in PCr but, since barbiturate anaesthesia induces intracellular alkalosis and since the creatine kinase equilibrium is pH-dependent, at least part of this increase could have been due to intracellular alkalosis (MacMillan and Siesjö, 1973a). Thus, the expected signals causing inhibition of glycolysis, and decrease in rate of oxidative phosphorylation, cannot be detected by tissue analyses. This problem, which is encountered also in other tissues, has been extensively discussed by Newsholme and Start (1973).

B. Hypothermia

Like barbiturate anaesthesia, induced hypothermia leads to reductions in CMR_{O_2} and CBF (Rosomoff and Holaday, 1954; Bering, 1961; Michenfelder and Theye, 1968) at unchanged tissue concentrations of

ATP, ADP and AMP (Hägerdal *et al.*, 1975b). When plasma pH is maintained constant, both CMR_{O_2} (Fig. 4) and CBF vary linearly with body temperature. The results show that for 1° change in body temperature there is a 5% change in CMR_{O_2} (Hägerdal *et al.*, 1975a). The alterations occurring in glycolytic metabolites and citric acid cycle intermediates are somewhat more difficult to interpret than those occurring in anaesthesia. Thus, there were decreases in concentration of all glycolytic and citric acid cycle intermediates except G-6-P and citrate (Hägerdal *et al.*, 1975b). The relative increases in G-6-P and citrate make it tempting to conclude that inhibition occurs at the PFK and the isocitrate dehydrogenase steps.

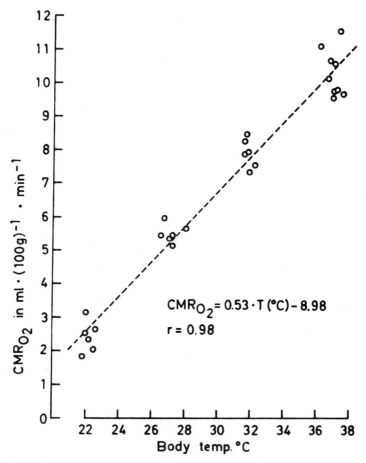

$$CMR_{O_2} = 0.53 \cdot T \, (°C) - 8.98$$
$$r = 0.98$$

Fig. 4. Relationship between body temperature and cerebral oxygen uptake as measured in rats under N_2O anaesthesia. (Data from Hägerdal *et al.*, 1975a.)

We observe that in both barbiturate anaesthesia and in hypothermia, there are parallel reductions in CMR_{O_2} and CBF. In neither of these situations are the coupling factors known, and direct measurements have failed to indicate that the extracellular H^+ or K^+ activities change in barbiturate anaesthesia. Thus, there is presently no satisfactory explanation for how metabolic rate is depressed to match the reduced demands, or for how CBF is adjusted to the metabolic requirements.

V. Conditions With a Primary Increase in Functional Activity

Until very recently, three basic concepts about cerebral metabolism have been stressed in a number of articles and reviews. 1. The brain is exclusively dependent on glucose for its oxidative requirements. 2. A decrease in metabolic rate occurs in anaesthesia, in hypothermia, and in coma of varying etiology and, in these conditions, there is a relatively strict relationship between level of consciousness and metabolic rate. 3. Brain metabolism is constant in a variety of conditions that seemingly differ in degree or intensity of mental activity and, with the possible exceptions of grave apprehension and anxiety, an increased cerebral metabolic rate is encountered only in epileptic seizures. It is now clear that all these concepts must be modified. First, as originally observed by Owen et al. (1967) in man, and later confirmed in animal experiments (Hawkins et al., 1971; Ruderman et al., 1974), starvation is accompanied by significant cerebral oxidation of ketone bodies that may amount to 50% of normal CMR_{O_2}. Second, some drugs, e.g. ketamine and diazepam, induce unconsciousness and/or anaesthesia without a corresponding decrease in CMR_{O_2} (Dawson et al., 1971; Takashita et al., 1972; Carlsson et al., 1976c). Third, recent animal experiments demonstrate that there are conditions, not involving seizure activity, which are associated with marked increases in CMR_{O_2} and CBF. In this paragraph, we will briefly discuss these hyper-metabolic conditions. In order to give some perspective on the quantitative relationships we will start by considering epileptic seizures and hyperthermia.

A. Epileptic Seizures

Almost all quantitative data on CMR_{O_2} and CBF stem from experiments on animals. The two classical studies are those of Schmidt et al.

(1945) and Geiger and Magnes (1947) which demonstrate that CMR_{O_2} increases by 50–100% during seizures induced by pentylenetetrazol (PTZ) or picrotoxin. A similar increase (to about 160% of control) was reported by Plum *et al.* (1968). For methodological reasons it has remained unsettled whether or not these figures represent those maximally obtained during seizures. Recent studies during bicuculline-induced status epilepticus in rats demonstrate that a 2·5-fold increase in CMR_{O_2} is upheld for at least two hours of continuous seizure activity (Chapman *et al.*, 1975; Meldrum and Nilsson, 1976). In absolute figures, this corresponds to a CMR_{O_2} of more than 20 ml.$100g^{-1}$.min^{-1}. Under these circumstances there is a severalfold increase in CBF but, due to the pressure-passive flow, the actual value depends on the level of cerebral perfusion pressure.

It is of interest that during continuous seizure activity, and in spite of adequate oxygenation of blood and tissue (see Jöbsis *et al.*, 1971, 1975), there are moderate but significant decreases in PCr and ATP, and increases in ADP, AMP and P_i, as well as a relatively marked increase in lactate concentration (Duffy *et al.*, 1975, Chapman *et al.*, 1977). It would seem that at this excessive increase in metabolic rate the previously missing signals, i.e. the factors responsible for accelerating glycolytic rate and oxidative phosphorylation, are present. However, it has been suggested by Balázs (1970) that the rate of oxidative metabolism in the brain can only increase threefold. Thus, the perturbation of cerebral energy state during seizures could reflect the rate-limiting nature of oxidative phosphorylation.

If we are in some difficulty when trying to define the factors that couple the increase in neuronal activity to the augmented metabolic rate there is an even larger uncertainty about the mechanisms behind the decrease in cerebrovascular resistance. In seizures induced by PTZ, Howse *et al.* (1974, see also Plum and Duffy, 1975) obtained some evidence that lactic acid production and increase in extracellular H^+ activity were responsible. In bicuculline-induced seizures this does not seem to be the case since dilatation occurs before extracellular acidosis has developed or, in fact, when there is a transient increase in pH (Astrup *et al.*, 1976). It certainly cannot be excluded that a decisive role is played by neurogenic influences.

B. *Hyperthermia*

There is a paucity of data on the effect of hyperthermia on CMR_{O_2} and CBF in man but two experimental studies show that, up to a temperature of 42°, hyperthermia is associated with increases in CMR_{O_2} and CBF (Nemoto and Frankel, 1970; Carlsson *et al.*, 1976a). At still higher temperatures (43–44°) Goldberg *et al.* (1966) observed increases in the tissue concentrations of pyruvate, malate and fumarate. Since these experiments were conducted on unanaesthetized animals the results could have been influenced by heat-induced hyperventilation. Thus, when arterial P_{CO_2} was kept constant in rats there were no consistent changes in any glycolytic or citric acid cycle intermediate measured (Carlsson *et al.*, 1976a). Furthermore, since PCr, ATP, ADP and AMP remained constant we once again lack the appropriate signals to an increased metabolic rate. Equally undefined are the factors leading to cerebral hyperemia.

C. *Amphetamine Intoxication*

When the effect of hyperthermia was studied in our laboratory, a means of increasing CMR_{O_2} at normal temperature was sought. Although previous studies in man had indicated that amphetamine in moderate doses (20 mg total dose) did not affect CMR_{O_2} or CBF, a study by Nahorski and Rogers (1973) suggested that larger doses (5 mg.kg^{-1}) were effective in rats. These authors reported that $\sim P$ utilization, as measured according to Lowry *et al.* (1964), decreased initially, returned to normal after about 30 min, and subsequently increased by 20–30%. Later measurements in rats under nitrous oxide anaesthesia, using the modified Kety and Schmidt (1948a) technique, gave unexpected results (Fig. 5, data from Carlsson *et al.*, 1975a, and unpublished results). Thus, following intraperitoneal (i.p.) injection of amphetamine sulphate in a dose of 5 mg.kg^{-1} CMR_{O_2} increased to 140% of control at 30 min and to 180% of control at 60 min. In spite of the fact that mean arterial blood pressure did not increase by more than 10–20 mm Hg, CBF rose to 400% of control at 30 min and to 600% of control at 60 min. In view of the technical difficulties of measuring such high CBF values the results might be regarded as tentative. However, it appears probable that amphetamine augments both CBF and CMR_{O_2}.

Since amphetamine does not induce seizure activity it may represent a more "physiological", functional activation than that occurring in epileptic seizures. It is therefore of interest to consider results on cerebral metabolic state. However, apart from its well known glycogenolytic effect (Estler and Ammon, 1967; Hutchins and Rogers, 1970) amphetamine did not cause changes in glycolytic metabolites, citric

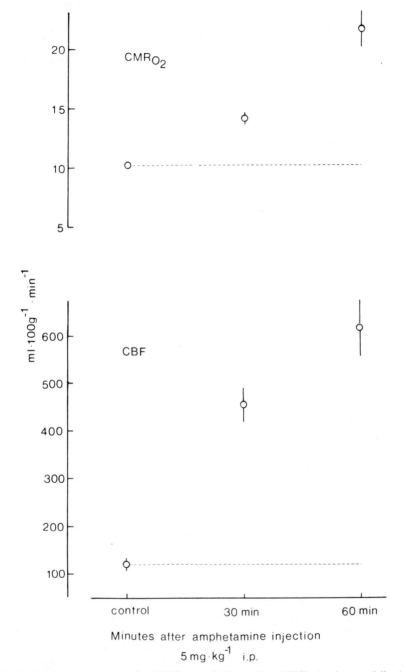

Fig. 5. Cerebral oxygen uptake (CMR_{O_2}) and blood flow (CBF) in the rat following amphetamine sulphate in a dose of 5 mg.kg^{-1}. The values are means $\pm$ S.E.M. (Data from Carlsson *et al.*, 1975a, and unpublished.)

acid cycle intermediates, associated amino acids or organic phosphates (Carlsson *et al.*, 1975a, and unpublished results). Furthermore, there were no changes in H^+ or K^+ activities in extracellular fluid in a direction that might cast light on the mechanisms causing this pronounced increase in CBF.

D. *Anxiety and Stress*

Since many years, it has been held possible that grave apprehension and anxiety may give rise to an increase in cerebral metabolic rate. Kety (1950) quotes observations in one subject suggesting that one unusually high CMR_{O_2} value ($5\cdot4$ ml.100 $g^{-1}.min^{-1}$) was correlated to grave apprehension, but a larger series reported by Scheinberg and Stead (1949) did not support the conclusion. In 1952, King *et al.* reported that intravenous (i.v.) infusion of large doses of adrenaline (but not of noradrenaline) was accompanied by a 20% increase in CMR_{O_2} and CBF. It was concluded that the increase in CMR_{O_2} (and CBF) was caused by apprehension and anxiety. However, Sensenbach *et al.* (1953) failed to observe changes in oxygen uptake and blood flow following intramuscular administration of comparable doses of adrenalin, although the symptoms experienced by the subjects appeared similar.

Recent results from the present laboratory seem to demonstrate beyond doubt that stressful situations may considerably increase CMR_{O_2}. In the course of a study of drug effects on the brain, it was deemed necessary to evaluate the effect of 70% nitrous oxide on CMR_{O_2} and CBF in rats (Carlsson *et al.*, 1975b). The animals were operated upon under anaesthesia (halothane-nitrous oxide) whereafter all operative wounds were infiltrated with local anaesthetic and measures were taken to minimize discomfort. Nitrous oxide was then withdrawn for either 5 or 30 min during maintained immobilization and artificial ventilation. As the results show (Fig. 6) CMR_{O_2} increased to 140% of control at 5 min and to 180% of control at 30 min, with a comparable elevation of CBF. Since the increase in CMR_{O_2} (and CBF) was prevented by previous adrenalectomy, or by prior administration of a β-adrenergic-receptor blocker (propranolol) it seemed to represent an effect mediated by catecholamines.

It is of considerable interest that both amphetamine administration and immobilization stress are known to increase turnover of the central catecholamine pools (see Costa and Garratini, 1970). Therefore, the increase in CMR_{O_2} and CBF may occur by related mechanisms. The

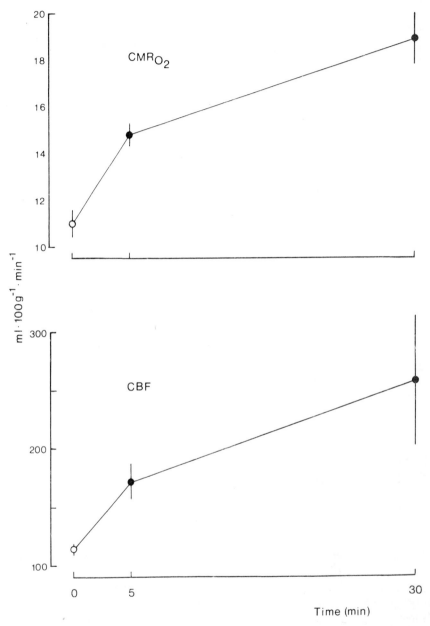

Fig. 6. Cerebral oxygen uptake (CMR_{O_2}) and blood flow (CBF) 5 and 30 min, respectively, after withdrawal of nitrus oxide in paralysed and artificially ventilated rats. Means, $\pm$ S.E.M. Since the increase in CMR_{O_2} and CBF was prevented by adrenalectomy, or by previous administration of propranolol, it seemed to represent an effect of catecholamines. (Data from Carlsson *et al.*, 1975b, and unpublished.)

results on metabolite levels are also similar although immobilization stress does not lead to glycogen breakdown. In general, the pronounced increases in CMR_{O_2} and CBF occur at unchanged tissue concentrations of glycolytic and citric acid cycle intermediates, of labile phosphates, or of amino acids belonging to the glutamate group (i.e. glutamate, glutamine, aspartate, GABA and alanine). Thus, there is an increase in cerebral metabolic rate without perturbation of cerebral metabolic state.

VI. Conditions with a Primary Decrease in Oxygen or Glucose Supply

When sufficiently severe, or sufficiently prolonged, both hypoxia and hypoglycemia encrouch upon energy production in the brain and ultimately lead to irreversible neuronal damage. However, before this stage is reached compensatory mechanisms come into play that involve both changes in CBF and in intermediary metabolism.

A. *Hypoxia*

Hypoxia is a somewhat ambiguous term. At tissue level, it may result either from a decrease in arterial oxygen tension (hypoxic hypoxia) or content (anaemic hypoxia), or from a reduction in perfusion rate (ischemia or venous hypoxia). Since ischemia often involves a reduced supply of both oxygen and exogenous substrate (glucose) we will confine the discussion to arterial hypoxia (hypoxic or anaemic). In many experiments on unanaesthetized animals, this distinction is not possible since, when sufficiently severe, arterial hypoxia is accompanied by cardiovascular failure, and thus by ischemia.

In man, consciousness is usually lost when arterial P_{O_2} is reduced to about 30 mm Hg but symptoms of oxygen lack appear at much higher P_{O_2} values (Luft, 1965). The relationships between these functional changes, and those affecting cerebral energy metabolism, are illustrated by two kinds of observations. First, Kety and Schmidt (1948b) observed that when arterial P_{O_2} was reduced to about 40 mm Hg in human subjects there was an increase in CBF but no significant change in CMR_{O_2}. These observations were later confirmed and shown to apply to arterial P_{O_2} values of 35 mm Hg (Cohen *et al.*, 1967). Second, experiments on dogs (Gurdjian *et al.*, 1944) demonstrated that although a lowering of P_{O_2} to below about 50 mm Hg gave rise to an increase in brain lactate and a decrease in PCr content, the ATP content appeared unchanged. In view of these results, it was speculated by many authors that below arterial P_{O_2} values of about 50 mm Hg tissue hypoxia induces anaerobic glycolysis which, through an effect of extracellular H^+ activity on cerebrovascular resistance, leads to a compensatory increase in CBF. In this way, gross energy failure is prevented until very low P_{O_2} values are reached.

Recent animal experiments have extended the results quoted and provided evidence that physiological compensation occurs by other mechanisms than those suggested. Results on rats showed that the tissue concentrations of ATP, ADP and AMP did not change significantly even if arterial P_{O_2} was reduced to about 20 mm Hg, unless there was a fall in blood pressure (Siesjö and Nilsson, 1971; Duffy et al., 1972; MacMillan and Siesjö, 1972). Since tissue lactate concentration increased when arterial P_{O_2} was reduced below about 50 mm Hg, the fall in PCr content could tentatively be ascribed to a H^+-dependent shift in the creatine kinase equilibrium. Derivation of cytoplasmic NADH to NAD^+ ratios indicated that a redox change occurred at P_{O_2} values of 50, and lower (see Siesjö et al., 1975b). Thus, at P_{O_2} levels that are associated with symptoms of oxygen lack there are clear signs of a redox change, and stimulation of anaerobic glycolysis, but no signs of overt energy failure.

There is some controversy about the homeostatic mechanisms involved. On the basis of calculated $\sim P$ use, Duffy et al. (1972) suggested that, when threatened by energy failure, the tissue may decrease its energy use rate. However, the results may have been influenced (or caused) by concomitant hypothermia. Direct measurements of CMR_{O_2} in rats at arterial P_{O_2} values of below 25 mm Hg have failed to demonstrate reduced oxygen uptake (Jóhannsson and Siesjö, 1975), and the results suggest that the main (or sole) homeostatic mechanism is the increase in CBF. At very low oxygen tensions, CBF increases four- to fivefold. However, if this increase is curtailed or prevented by concomitant hypotension, or by unilateral clamping of the carotid artery, there is energy failure at tissue level with resulting neuronal change (Siesjö and Nilsson, 1971; Salford et al., 1973a and b), even though CBF has not been reduced below control levels (Salford and Siesjö, 1974).

Recent observations indicate that the homeostatic increase in CBF during hypoxia is unrelated to extracellular acidosis. First, Ponte and Purves (1974) produced evidence that the response of the cerebral circulation to hypoxia is reflexly elicited from the carotid chemoreceptors. Second, following induction of hypoxia in rats, CBF was

B. K. SIESJÖ

increased before cellular or extracellular acidosis developed (Borgström et al., 1975; Norberg and Siesjö, 1975a; Nilsson et al., 1975b). Thus, rather than providing the stimulus for an increase in CBF the lactic acidosis may just reflect the fact the compensation by hyperemia is insufficient to maintain a completely adequate oxygenation.

Unlike many of the conditions discussed above, hypoxia is accompanied by marked perturbation of metabolite levels in the tissue. The glycolytic events are dominated by increased glycolytic rate and reduction of the $NADH/NAD^+$ system. For some time, there were difficulties in explaining the increased glycolytic rate (Duffy et al., 1972; Bachelard et al., 1974). However, subsequent studies showed that shortly following reduction of P_{O_2} there were decreases in F-6-P and G-6-P (Norberg and Siesjö, 1975a) and an increased glycolytic flux (Borgström et al., 1976). These results are compatible with activation of PFK, possibly triggered by small changes in labile phosphates (see Norberg and Siesjö, 1975a). At steady-state this pattern disappears, possibly because other regulatory enzymes (hexokinase, pyruvate kinase) catch up with the enhanced PFK activity.

Citric acid cycle changes (Fig. 7) are initially dominated by a fall in α-ketoglutarate (α-KG) and later by a progressive rise in the size of the citric acid cycle pool. The predominant changes in amino acids are a rise in alanine, a fall in aspartate and a (late) rise in GABA (see Duffy et al., 1972; Norberg and Siesjö, 1975b). The mechanisms behind these changes will be discussed below.

B. Hypoglycemia

Like hypoxia, hypoglycemia gives signs of energy failure and, if sufficiently severe, it causes neuronal damage (Brierley et al., 1971). However, there are obvious differences. In hypoxia, there is lack of oxygen but substrate is supplied in excess. In hypoglycemia, there is shortage of exogenous substrate but since oxygen is available the tissue has to resort to its own endogenous substrate to maintain oxidative phosphorylation. We will discuss three main questions. 1. How are CMR_{O_2}, CMR_{gl} and CBF affected during moderate and severe hypoglycemia? 2. Are the signs and symptoms of hypoglycemia caused by failing energy production? 3. What endogenous substrates are utilized?

The classical study of Kety et al. (1947–1948) established that during hypoglycemic coma there is proportionally larger reduction in CMR_{gl} than in CMR_{O_2}, suggesting that endogenous substrates were

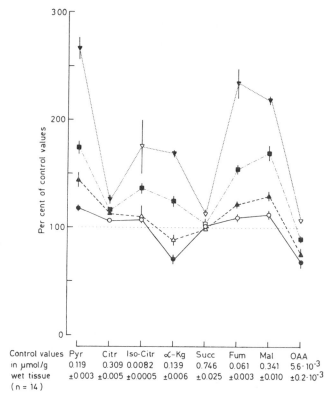

Fig. 7. Influence of hypoxia (arterial P_{O_2} of about 25 mm Hg) of 1–30 min (O 1 min, △ 2 min, □ 15 min, ▽ 30 min) duration upon cerebral cortical concentrations of pyruvate and of citric acid cyclic intermediates. The values (means ± S.E.M.) are given as a percentage of controls. Filled symbols denote values significantly different from controls (p < 0.05). For abbreviations, see Fig. 3. (From Norberg and Siesjö, 1975b.)

consumed. This basic observation has been confirmed in man (Della Porta *et al.*, 1964) and in experimental animals (Pappenheimer and Setchell, 1973; Norberg and Siesjö, 1976). However, all these studies showed that CMR_{O_2} was barely affected, if at all, even at very low blood glucose concentrations, and two have shown an increase in CBF (Della Porta *et al.*, 1964; Norberg and Siesjö, 1976). Although there may not be general agreement on these latter findings it should be recalled that Geiger *et al.* (1952) observed a near-normal CMR_{O_2} when cat brains were perfused with a glucose-free fluid.

There has been some controversy regarding changes in cerebral energy state in hypoglycemia (see Hinzen and Müller, 1971; Ferrendelli and Chang, 1973; Lewis *et al.*, 1974a; Norberg and Siesjö,

1976). However, it seems established that when blood glucose concentrations are reduced below 1 µmol.g^{-1} in normothermic animals, and when there is an isoelectric EEG, there are marked reductions in the tissue concentrations of PCr and ATP, and increases in ADP and AMP. Such changes are observed even if tissue oxygenation is adequately maintained. However, although this means that "coma" is invariably associated with energy failure many of the less severe symptoms of hypoglycemia (e.g. somnolence, lethargy and convulsive activity) cannot be explained by failing energy production. It is possible, however not established, that changes in amino acids (see below) may underlie such symptoms.

In the perfused cat brain, aglycemia leads to breakdown of proteins, nucleic acids and lipids (Abood and Geiger, 1955). Subsequent animal studies have failed to corroborate that a significant breakdown of proteins or nucleic acids occurs, and interest has centred on endogenous carbohydrate stores, amino acids and phospholipids. It has been clearly established that, in severe hypoglycemia, there is not only depletion of tissue levels of glucose and glycogen but also a reduction of the concentrations of glycolytic metabolites and citric acid cycle intermediates (see Tews et al., 1965; Goldberg et al., 1966; Norberg and Siesjö, 1976). However, once glycogen and glucose have disappeared, additional carbohydrate stores are quantitatively of little importance. Pioneering studies by Dawson (1950) and by Cravioto et al. (1951) demonstrated that hypoglycemia is accompanied by decreases in tissue concentrations of glutamate, glutamine, GABA and alanine, and by a rise in aspartate. These results have subsequently been repeatedly confirmed and it has also been shown that ammonia accumulates. Figure 8 illustrates changes observed in rats after 5–15 min of isoelectricity in the EEG. Three aspects should be stressed. First, there was massive accumulation of ammonia. Second, the pool of amino acids decreased by about 4 µmol.g^{-1}. Third, since the changes observed were manifest already after 5 min of isoelectric EEG, with no obvious further changes in the following ten minutes period, since glucose and glycogen were depleted at an earlier stage, and since CMR$_{O_2}$ was far in excess of what could be accounted for in terms of glucose extraction, it seems obvious that non-carbohydrate, non-amino acid substrate was oxidized.

These results allow the conclusion that substrate carbon is made available for oxidation from amino acids by both transamination and deamination mechanisms. Subsequent studies have given relatively clear evidence that the missing substrate is provided by breakdown of phospholipids (Knauff and Böck, 1961; Knauff et al., 1961; Hinzen et *al.*, 1970). Oddly enough, although there is some evidence that CMR_{O_2} is upheld even in coma (Norberg and Siesjö, 1976) there is extensive breakdown of high energy phosphate compounds. Two tentative explanations can be offered. Thus, either there is an increased energy demand during extreme hypoglycemia or there is a deficient coupling

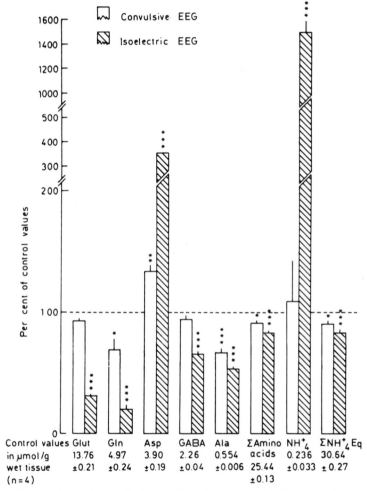

Fig. 8. Influence of profound insulin-induced hypoglycemia upon amino acids and ammonia in rat cerebral cortex. The tissue was frozen for analyses either when the EEG showed slow wave-polyspike activity (convulsive) or when the EEG was isoelectric for 5–15 min (isoelectric). The values, which are given as percentage of controls, are means with S.E.M. indicated $* = p < 0.05$, $** = p < 0.01$, $*** = p < 0.001$. glut: glutamate, Gln: glutamine, Asp: aspartate, Ala: alanine, NH_4^+ Eq: sum of ammonia equivalents (ammonia plus amino acids with glutamine taken twice). (From Norberg and Siesjö, 1976.)

between oxygen consumption and ATP production when endogenous lipids are being burned. It is possible that when a stage of hypoglycemia has been reached, at which oxidation of lipid occurs, structural degradation of membranes begins.

VII. Coupling Mechanisms

It may now be appropriate to summarize information concerning the coupling of functional activity, metabolic rate and blood flow. In addition, we will discuss the relationship between metabolic rate and metabolic state.

A. *Coupling of Functional Activity and Metabolic Rate*

It is a truism to state that there is a mutual relationship between function and metabolism. On the one hand, any increase in functional activity is associated with an increased metabolic rate. On the other, any interference with metabolic rate, e.g. due to oxygen or substrate deficiency, leads to symptoms of functional derangement.

As we have discussed, *in vitro* results give clear evidence of a direct relationship between intensity of neuronal activity and metabolic rate. This concept can be applied in a relatively straightforward way to the intact brain in conditions of a primary decrease in functional activity (e.g. barbiturate anaesthesia and hypothermia) mainly because these conditions give, when sufficiently severe, overt signs of neuronal depression. It is more difficult to define increased activity in the brain unless we consider the excessive, synchronous discharge of masses of neurones occurring during seizure states. Thus, it is mostly by inference from the increased metabolic rate we conclude that hyperthermia, amphetamine intoxication and stressful situations involve an increased neuronal activity.

In vitro results suggest that increased neuronal activity is accompanied by changes in high energy phosphate compounds. Results obtained *in vivo* show that, with an intact circulation, production of energy is so closely matched to consumption that the system remains in tight balance (see below). However, we are then at a loss in trying to define the appropriate signals, coupling metabolic rate to function. If the appropriate signals to changes in metabolic rate involve changes in concentration of PCr, ATP, ADP, AMP and P_i it seems necessary to invoke compartmentation, i.e., to assume changes in concentration gradients within the microenvironment of the energy-transducing systems.

B. Coupling of Metabolism and Blood Flow

In spite of considerable effort, the factors that adjust local circulation to the metabolic rate remain undefined. Of the various metabolic factors proposed (e.g. H^+, K^+ and adenosine) none can satisfactorily explain the vasodilation occurring in all conditions presently discussed. In four situations (hypoxia, hypoglycemia, amphetamine intoxication and induced status epilepticus) CBF has been studied in the present laboratory. In all of them, vasodilation occurs either before the extracellular fluid has become acidified or without any accompanying acidosis, and in only one (seizures) is there a rise in extracellular K^+ activity of sufficient magnitude to help explaining the hyperemia (Astrup et al., 1976). It remains to be proven if adenosine fulfils the requirements of a general coupling factor. However, it may not be only fruitless but also conceptually wrong to look for a single factor. Thus, although it has been speculated that neural mechanisms of extracerebral origin may be involved in the vascular response to hypoxia and hypercapnia (Ponte and Purves, 1974) such mechanisms, if they exist, may not suffice to explain the coupling between regional metabolism and blood flow.

C. Relationships Between Metabolic Rate and Metabolic State

It now seems clear that the cerebral metabolic rate may vary from 25% normal (reduction in body temperature to 22°) to 200% normal (immobilization stress) without any perturbation of cerebral energy state, as this can be evaluated from tissue concentration of ATP, ADP and AMP. It is only under special hypermetabolic conditions (epileptic seizures) that the energy state is altered but, if oxygenation is upheld, even this alteration is relatively moderate. Obviously, determinations of adenine nucleotide levels are of very restricted value in assessing the functional state of the tissue, and they become useful only in conditions of oxygen or substrate deficiency.

The results quoted suggest that there may be at least a twofold change in metabolic rate without any accompanying alteration of the tissue concentrations of glycolytic metabolites, of citric acid cycle intermediates, of associated amino acids, or of ammonia (amphetamine intoxication, immobilization stress). It is thus not possible to draw conclusions about metabolic flux rate from levels of individual metabolites. However, changes in metabolic levels occur in several conditions, four of which have been discussed (barbiturate anaesthesia, hypothermia, hypoxia and hypoglycemia). It will be proposed that these changes are caused mainly by two mechanisms, namely, a mismatch between glycolytic rate and citric acid cycle flux, and an accompanying redox change. The results obtained suggest a coherent sequence of events that links glycolysis to the metabolism of citric acid cycle intermediates and amino acids.

Consider the sequence of a redox change as it occurs during hypoxia, (see Duffy et al., 1972; Norberg and Siesjö, 1975b). An increase in cytoplasmic NADH to NAD^+ ratio will cause a rise in malate to oxaloacetate (OAA) ratio, and lead to a fall in OAA. The latter will shift the aspartate aminotransferase (Asp-AT) reaction

$$\text{Glutamate} + \text{OAA} \rightleftharpoons \text{Aspartate} + \alpha\text{-KG}$$

to the left, explaining the fall in α-ketoglutarate (α-KG) and aspartate. Moreover, lack of mitochondrial NAD^+ may cause inhibition of the further metabolism of GABA (via oxidation of succinic semialdehyde) and thus provide a plausible explanation for the rise in GABA. The other mechanism, the increase in glycolytic rate, which as we have discussed is secondary to activation of PFK. The resulting increase in pyruvate will have two consequences. First, it will accelerate CO_2 fixation at the pyruvate carboxylase step (Patel, 1974; Mahan et al., 1975). Second, it will cause a shift in the alanine aminotransferase (Ala-AT) reaction

$$\text{Glutamate} + \text{Pyruvate} \rightleftharpoons \text{Alanine} + \alpha\text{-KG}$$

towards formation of alanine. The latter reaction explains the rise in alanine concentration, and both reactions contribute to the increase in the size of the citric acid pool. Unaccounted for is why there is no change in glutamate. Two explanations seem plausible. 1. Some glutamate will be lost in the Ala-AT reaction. 2. Since there is an increase in NH_4^+ in the absence of a fall in ATP, glutamate may be amidated to glutamine (which rises significantly with prolonged hypoxia).

If the above explanation is correct, the same sequence of events should occur in other conditions associated with an increase in anaerobic glycolysis and a reduction of cytoplasmic (and mitochondrial) NAD^+. This has been shown to be the case with pronounced hypocapnia, which leads to an increase in the size of the citric acid cycle pool, and to similar changes in amino acids (see MacMillan and Siesjö, 1973b; Norberg, 1976).

Changes affecting citric acid cycle intermediates and associated amino acids during hypoglycemia offer an interesting insight into mechanisms linking glycolysis, citric acid cycle metabolism and amino acid metabolism. Tentatively, we may assume that some of these mechanisms, as in hypoxia, involve changes in redox state and in pyruvate concentration, both being caused by an insufficient supply of exogenous carbohydrate substrate. Essential to our discussion is that both endogenous carbohydrate stores (e.g. citric acid cycle intermediates) and amino acids are used as alternative substrates. We can distinguish between two series of events, namely, those leading to transamination and those making citric acid cycle intermediates and amino acids available for oxidation. In all probability, the shift in the Asp-AT reaction towards formation of aspartate is driven by a rise in OAA concentration. This can have two causes: 1. due to the reduced concentration of pyruvate there will be less acetyl-CoA available for condensation to citrate (Dawson, 1950), and 2. reduced substrate availability gives rises to oxidation of the cytoplasmic (and mitochondrial?) $NADH/NAD^+$ system (Lewis et al., 1974b). This, by lowering the malate to OAA ratio, should increase the concentration of OAA.

The Asp-AT reaction, delivering one carbon atom for oxidation in the citric acid cycle, is limited by the availability of glutamate. However, three other reactions deliver additional glutamate. These are the glutaminase reaction (which may proceed because there is insufficient glutamate and insufficient ATP available to drive glutamine synthesis), the GABA transaminase reaction (which may be accelerated by excess of NAD^+ for the subsequent oxidation of succinic semialdehyde) and the Ala-AT reaction (which proceeds towards pyruvate formation when the latter is at low concentration). In this way, carbon skeletons are mobilized from glutamine, GABA and alanine for transamination to aspartate.

Accumulation of NAD^+ favours oxidative deamination of glutamate

$$\alpha\text{-KG} + NH_3 + NADH + H^+ \rightleftharpoons \text{Glutamate} + NAD^+$$

and this may be the mechanism whereby part of the amino acid pool is oxidized. Alone, this reaction should increase the citric acid cycle pool size but since this pool is reduced in size, other reactions must accomplish a loss of carbon skeletons from the cycle. One such reaction is that catalysed by Ala-AT but others must contribute, e.g. those which, when driven in the opposite direction, cause CO_2 fixation. In this way, amino acids and citric acid cycle intermediates may be delivered to the glycolytic chain for further, complete oxidation.

Again, if the explanation is correct, similar changes should occur, whenever there is a primary decrease in pyruvate availability and/or a redox change in the direction of oxidation. There are results to show that this is so. Thus, in hypercapnia there are reductions in glycolytic metabolites from fructose diphosphate and onwards, reductions in all citric acid cycle metabolites except succinate, a fall in glutamate, a transient rise in aspartate followed by a return to normal, and subsequently to subnormal values, an increase in NH_4^+ and a delayed rise in glutamine concentration (Folbergrová et al., 1972a and b, 1974, 1975). On the basis of these results, it was concluded that hypercapnia gives rise to a condition of relative substrate deficiency in which the reduced availability of pyruvate from exogenous glucose leads to oxidation of glycolytic and citric acid cycle intermediates, and to mobilization of amino acids as alternative substrates (Folbergrová et al., 1975). Miller et al. (1975), who could confirm the changes occurring in carbohydrate intermediates and amino acids, arrived at a similar conclusion on the basis of direct measurements of glucose consumption (see also Borgström et al., 1976). We recognize that the pattern of changes observed in hypercapnia is similar to that occurring in hypoglycemia. The differences that exist may largely be due to the absence of a measurable redox change in hypercapnia (for discussion, see Norberg and Siesjö, 1976). In hypoglycemia, the reduced availability of pyruvate is caused by a fall in glucose delivery to the tissue. In hypercapnia, there is a fall in glucose consumption (Miller et al., 1975; Borgström et al., 1976) and an initial accumulation of G-6-P and F-6-P (Folbergrová et al., 1975), indicating that the reduction in pyruvate availability is due to PFK inhibition.

In summary, there is now considerable evidence to suggest that many of the changes affecting citric acid cycle intermediates and associated amino acids in a variety of conditions are secondary to glycolytic events, the most important of which are a change in glycolytic rate and an alteration of the redox state.

Acknowledgements

Most of the work from the author's own laboratory was supported by grants from the Swedish Medical Research Council (Project No. 14X-00263-12) and from U.S. PHS Grant No. RO1 NSO7838-07 from NIH.

References

Abood, L. G. and Geiger, A. (1955). *Amer. J. Physiol.* **182**, 557–560.

Astrup, J., Heuser, D., Lassen, N. A., Nilsson, B., Norberg, K. and Siesjö, B. K. (1976). *In* "Ionic Actions on Vascular Smooth Muscle" (E. Betz, ed.). Springer-Verlag, Berlin, Heidelberg, pp. 110–115.

Bachelard, H. S., Lewis, L. D., Pontén, U. and Siesjö, B. K. (1974). *J. Neurochem.* **22**, 395–401.

Baker, P. F. and Conelly, C. M. (1966). *J. Physiol. (London)* **185**, 270–297.

Balázs, R. (1970). *In* "Handbook of Neurochemistry" (A. Lajtha, ed.), Vol. 3. Plenum Press, New York, pp. 1–36.

Bering, E. A., jun. (1961). *Amer. J. Physiol.* **200**, 417–419.

Betz, E. (1972). *Physiol. Rev.* **52**, 595–630.

Borgström, L., Jóhannsson, H. and Siesjö, B. K. (1975). *Acta Physiol. Scand.* **93**, 423–432.

Borgström, L., Norberg, K. and Siesjö, B. K. (1976). *Acta Physiol. Scand.* **96**, 569–574.

Brierley, J. B., Brown, A. W. and Meldrum, B. S. (1971). *Brain Res.* **25**, 483–499.

Carlsson, C., Hägerdal, M. and Siesjö, B. K. (1975a). *Acta Physiol. Scand.* **94**, 128–129.

Carlsson, C., Hägerdal, M. and Siesjö, B. K. (1975b). *Acta Physiol. Scand.* **95**, 206–208.

Carlsson, C., Harp, J. R. and Siesjö, B. K. (1975c). *Acta Anaesthesiol. Scand. Suppl.* **57**, 7–17.

Carlsson, C., Hägerdal, M. and Siesjö, B. K. (1976a). *J. Neurochem.* **26**, 1001–1006.

Carlsson, C., Hägerdal, M. and Siesjö, B. K. (1976b). *Acta Anaesthesiol. Scand.* **20**, 91–95.

Carlsson, C., Hägerdal, M., Kaasik, A. E. and Siesjö, B. K. (1976c). *Anesthesiology* **45**, 319.

Chapman, A. G., Meldrum, B. S. and Siesjö, B. K. (1975). *J. Physiol.* **254**, 61–62p.

Chapman, A. G., Meldrum, B. S. and Siesjö, B. K. (1977). *J. Neurochem.* (in press).

Chmouliovsky, M., Shorderet, M. and Straub, R. W. (1969). *J. Physiol. (London)* **202**, 90P–92P.

Cohen, P. J. (1973). *Anesthesiology* **39**, 153–164.

Cohen, P. J., Alexander, S. C., Smith, T. C., Reivich, M. and Wollman, H. (1967). *J. Appl. Physiol.* **23**, 183–189.

Costa, E. and Garattini, S. (eds) (1970). "Amphetamine and related compounds". Raven Press, New York.

Cravioto, R. O., Massieu, G. and Izquierdo, J. J. (1951). *Proc. Soc. Exp. Biol. Med.* **78**, 856–858.

Dawson, R. M. C. (1950). *Biochem. J.* **47**, 386–395.

Dawson, B., Michenfelder, J. D. and Theye, R. A. (1971). *Anesth. Analg. Curr. Res.* **50**, 443.

Della Porta, P., Maiolo, A. T., Negri, V. V. and Rossella, E. (1964). *Metabolism* **13**, 131–140.

Duffy, T. E., Nelson, S. R. and Lowry, O. H. (1972). *J. Neurochem.* **19**, 959–977.

Duffy, T. E., Howse, D. C. and Plum, F. (1975). *J. Neurochem.* **24**, 925–934.

Eklöf, B., Lassen, N. A., Nilsson, L., Norberg, K., Siesjö, B. K. and Torlöf, P. (1974). *Acta Physiol. Scand.* **91**, 1–10.

Elliott, K. A. C. and Henderson, N. (1948). *J. Neurophysiol.* **11**, 473–484.
Estler, C.-J. and Ammon, H. P. T. (1967). *J. Neurochem.* **14**, 799–805.
Ferrendelli, J. A. and Chang, M. M. (1973). *Arch. Neurol.* **28**, 173–177.
Folbergrová, J., MacMillan, V. and Siesjö, B. K. (1972a). *J. Neurochem.* **19**, 2497–2505.
Folbergrová, J., MacMillan, V. and Siesjö, B. K. (1972b). *J. Neurochem.* **19**, 2507–2517.
Folbergrová, J., Pontén, U. and Siesjö, B. K. (1974). *J. Neurochem.* **22**, 1115–1125.
Folbergrová, J., Norberg, K., Quistorff, B. and Siesjö, B. K. (1975). *J. Neurochem.* **25**, 457–462.
Gaitonde, M. K. (1965). *Biochem. J.* **95**, 803–810.
Gatfield, P. D., Lowry, O. H., Schultz, D. W. and Passonneau, J. V. (1966). *J. Neurochem.* **13**, 185–195.
Geiger, A. and Magnes, J. (1947). *Amer. J. Physiol.* **149**, 517–537.
Geiger, A., Magnes, J. and Geiger, R. S. (1952). *Nature* **170**, 754–755.
Gerard, R. W. (1932). *Physiol. Rev.* **12**, 469–592.
Gilboe, D. D. and Betz, A. L. (1973). *Amer. J. Physiol.* **224**, 588–595.
Gilboe, D. D., Betz, A. L. and Langebartel, D. A. (1973). *J. Appl. Physiol.* **34**, 534–537
Goldberg, N. D., Passonneau, J. V. and Lowry, O. H. (1966). *J. Biol. Chem.* **241**, 3997–4003.
Greengaard, P. and Ritchie, J. M. (1971). *In* "Handbook of Neurochemistry" (A. Lajtha, ed.), Vol. 5. Plenum Press, New York, pp. 317–335.
Greengaard, P. and Straub, R. W. (1959). *J. Physiol. (London)* **148**, 353–361.
Gurdjian, E. S., Stone, W. E. and Webster, J. E. (1944). *Arch. Neurol.* **51**, 472–477.
Hägerdal, M., Harp, J., Nilsson, L. and Siesjö, B. K. (1975a). *J. Neurochem.* **24**, 311–316.
Hägerdal, M., Harp, J., Siesjö, B. K. (1975b). *J. Neurochem.* **24**, 743–748.
Harper, M., Jennett, B., Miller, D. and Rowan, J. (eds.) (1975). "Blood flow and metabolism in the brain". Churchill Livingstone, London.
Harvey, J. A. and McIlwain, H. (1969). *In* "Handbook of Neurochemistry" (A. Lajtha, ed.), Vol. II. Plenum Press, New York, pp. 115–136.
Hawkins, R. A., Williamson, D. H. and Krebs, H. A. (1971). *Biochem. J.* **122**, 13–18.
Hawkins, R. A., Miller, A. L., Cremer, J. E. and Veech, R. L. (1974). *J. Neurochem.* **23**, 917–923.
Hinzen, D. H. and Müller, U. (1971). *Pfluegers Arch. Gesamte Physiol.* **322**, 47–59.
Hinzen, D. H., Becker, P. and Müller, U. (1970). *Pfluegers Arch. Gesamte Physiol.* **321**, 1–14.
Homburger, E., Himwich, W. A., Etsten, B., York, G., Maresca, R. and Himwich, H. E. (1946). *Amer. J. Physiol.* **147**, 343–345.
Howse, D. C., Caronna, J. C., Duffy, T. E. and Plum, F. (1974). *Amer. J. Physiol.* **227**, 1444–1451.
Hutchins, D. A. and Rogers, K. J. (1970). *Brit. J. Pharmacol.* **39**, 9–25.
Ingvar, D. H. and Lassen, N. A. (1962). *Acta Physiol. Scand.* **54**, 325–338.
James, I. M. (1975). *In* "Advan. Neurology" (B. S. Meldrum and C. D. Marsden, eds), Vol. 10. Raven Press, New York, pp. 167–180.
Jöbsis, F. F., O'Connor, M., Vitale, A. and Vreman, H. (1971). *J. Neurophysiol.* **36**, 735–749.
Jöbsis, F., Rosenthal, M., Lamanna, J., Lothman, E., Cordingly, G. and Somjen, G. (1975). *In* "Brain Work", Alfred Benzon Symp. 8 (D. H. Ingvar and N. A. Lassen, eds). Munksgaard, Copenhagen, pp. 185–196.

Jóhannson, H. and Siesjö, B. K. (1975). *Acta Physiol. Scand.* **93**, 269–276.
Kennedy, C., Des Rosiers, M. H., Jehle, J. W., Reivich, M., Sharpe, F. and Sokoloff, L. (1975). *Science* **187**, 850–853.
Kerr, S. E. (1935). *J. Biol. Chem.* **110**, 625.
Kety, S. S. (1950). *Amer. J. Med.* **8**, 205.
Kety, S.S. (1960). *In* "Methods in Medical Research". Year Book Publ., Chicago, pp. 223–227.
Kety, S. S. and Schmidt, C. F. (1948a). *J. Clin. Invest.* **27**, 476–483.
Kety, S. S. and Schmidt, C. F. (1948b). *J. Clin. Invest.* **27**, 484–492.
Kety, S. S., Woodford, R. B., Harmel, M. H., Freyhan, F. A., Appel, K. E. and Schmidt, C. F. (1947–48). *Amer. J. Psychiat.* **104**, 765–770.
King, B. D., Sokoloff, L. and Wechsler, R. L. (1952). *J. Clin. Invest.* **31**, 273–279.
Knauff, H. G. and Böck, F. (1961). *J. Neurochem.* **6**, 171–182.
Knauff, H. G., Marx, D. and Mayer, G. (1961). *Hoppe-Seylers Z. Physiol. Chem.* **326**, 227–234.
Landau, W. M., Freygang, W. H., Jr., Rowland, L. P., Sokoloff, L. and Kety, S. S. (1955). *Trans. Amer. Neurol. Ass.* **80**, 125–129.
Larrabee, M. G. and Klingman, J. D. (1962). *In* "Neurochemistry" (K. A. C. Elliott, I. H. Page and J. H. Quastel, eds). C. C. Thomas, Springfield, Illinois, pp. 150–176.
Lassen, N. A. (1968). *Scand. J. Clin. Lab. Invest.* **22**, 247.
Lewis, L. D., Ljunggren, B., Ratcheson, R. A. and Siesjö, B. K. (1974a). *J. Neurochem.* **23**, 673–679.
Lewis, L. D., Ljunggren, B., Norberg, K. and Siesjö, B. K. (1974b). *J. Neurochem.* **23**, 659–671.
Lowry, O. H., Passonneau, J. V., Hasselberger, F. K. and Schultz, D. W. (1964). *J. Biol. Chem.* **239**, 18–30.
Luft, U. C. (1965). *In* "Handbook of Physiology—Respiration" (W. O. Fenn and K. Rahn, eds), Vol. 2. American Physiological Soc., Washington, D.C., pp. 1099–1145.
Lust, W. D., Passonneau, J. V. and Veech, R. L. (1973). *Science* **181**:1, 280–282.
MacMillan, V. and Siesjö, B. K. (2972). *Scand. J. Clin. Lab. Invest* **30**, 127–136.
MacMillan, V. and Siesjö, B. K. (1973a). *J. Neurochem.* **20**, 1669–1681.
MacMillan, V. and Siesjö, B. K. (1973b). *J. Neurochem.* **21**, 1283–1299.
Mahan, D. E., Mushawar, I. K. and Koeppe, R. E. (1975). *Biochem. J.* **145**, 25–35.
Maker, H. S. and Lehrer, G. M. (1971). *In* "Handbook of Neurochemistry" (A. Lajtha, ed.), Vol. 6. Plenum Press, New York, pp. 267–310.
McIlwain, H. (ed.) (1963). "Chemical Exploration of the Brain". Elsevier Press, Amsterdam.
McIlwain, H. and Bachelard, H. S. (1971). "Biochemistry and the Central Nervous System". Churchill Livingstone, London.
Meldrum, B. S. and Nilsson, B. (1976). *Brain* **99**, 523–542.
Michenfelder, J. D. and Theye, R. A. (1968). *Anesthesiology* **29**, 1107–1112.
Michenfelder, J. D., Messick, J. M., jun. and Theye, R. A. (1968). *J. Surg. Res.* **8**, 475–481.
Miller, A. L., Hawkins, R. A. and Veech, R. L. (1975). *J. Neurochem.* **25**, 553–558.
Nahorski, S. R. and Rogers, K. J. (1973). *J. Neurochem.* **21**, 679–686.
Nemoto, E. M. and Frankel, H. M. (1970). *Amer. J. Physiol.* **219**, 1784–1788.
Newsholme, E. A. and Start, C. (1973). "Regulation in Metabolism". John Wiley and Sons, London.
Nilsson, L. and Siesjö, B. K. (1974). *J. Neurochem.* **23**, 29–36.
Nilsson, L. and Siesjö, B. K. (1975). *Acta Anaesthesiol. Scand. Suppl.* **57**, 18–24.
Nilsson, B. and Siesjö, B. K. (1976). *Acta Physiol. Scand.* **96**, 72–82.

Nilsson, B., Norberg, K., Nordström, C.-H. and Siesjö, B. K. (1975a). *Acta Physiol. Scand.* **93**, 569–571.

Nilsson, B., Norberg, K., Nordström, C.-H. and Siesjö, B. K. (1975b). *In* "Blood Flow and Metabolism in the Brain", Proc. of 7th Int. Symp., Aviemore (M. Harper, B. Jennett, D. Miller and J. Rowan, eds). Churchill Livingstone, London, pp. 9.19–9.23.

Norberg, K. (1976). *J. Neurochem.* **26**, 353–359.

Norberg, K. and Siesjö, B. K. (1974). *Acta Physiol. Scand.* **91**, 154–164

Norberg, K. and Siesjö, B. K. (1975a). *Brain Res.* **86**, 31–44.

Norberg, K. and Siesjö, B. K. (1975b). *Brain Res.* **86**, 45–54.

Norberg, K. and Siesjö, B. K. (1976). *J. Neurochem.* **26**, 345–352.

Olesen, J. (1971). *Brain* **94**, 635–646.

Owen, O. E., Morgan, A. P., Kemp, H. G., Sullivan, J. M., Herrera, M. G. and Cahill, G. F., jun. (1967). *J. Clin. Invest.* **46**, 1589.

Pappenheimer, J. R. and Setchell, B. P. (1973). *J. Physiol.* **223**, 529–551.

Patel, M. S. (1974). *J. Neurochem.* **22**, 717–724.

Plum, F. and Duffy, T. E. (1975). *In* "Brain Work", Alfred Benzon Symp. 8 (D. H. Ingvar and N. A. Lassen, eds). Munksgaard, Copenhagen, pp. 197–214.

Plum, F., Posner, J. B. and Troy, B. (1968). *Arch. Neurol.* **18**, 1–13.

Ponte, J. and Purves, M. J. (1974). *J. Physiol.* **237**, 315–340.

Pontén, U., Ratcheson, R. A., Salford, L. G. and Siesjö, B. K. (1973a). *J. Neurochem.* **21**, 1127–1138.

Pontén, U., Ratcheson, R. A. and Siesjö, B. K. (1973b). *J. Neurochem.* **21**, 1121–1126.

Purves, M. J. (ed.) (1972). "The Physiology of the Cerebral Circulation". Cambridge University Press, London.

Quistorff, B. (1975). *Anal. Biochem.* **68**, 102–118.

Rapela, C. E. and Green, H. D. (1964). *Circ. Res.* **14**, 205–211.

Reivich, M. (1974). *In* "Brain Dysfunction in Metabolic Disorders" (F. Plum, ed.), Vol. 53. Raven Press, New York, pp. 125–140.

Reivich, M., Jehle, J., Sokoloff, L. and Kety, S. S. (1969). *J. Appl. Physiol.* **27**, 296–300.

Reivich, M., Sokoloff, L., Kennedy, C. and Des Rosiers, M. (1975). *In* "Brain Work", Alfred Benzon Symp. 8 (D. H. Ingvar and N.A. Lassen, eds). Munksgaard, Copenhagen, pp. 377–384.

Richter, D. and Dawson, R. M. C. (1948). *Amer. J. Physiol.* **154**, 73.

Ritchie, J. M. (1967). *J. Physiol. (London)* **188**, 309–329.

Ritchie, J. M. (1973). *In* "Progress in Biophysics and Molecular Biology" (J. A. V. Butler and D. Noble, eds), Vol. 26. Pergamon Press, Oxford, pp. 149–187.

Rolleston, F. S. (1972). *In* "Current Topics in Cellular Regulation" (B. K. Horecker and E. R. Stadtman, eds), Vol. 5. Academic Press, New York and London, pp. 47–75.

Rosomoff, H. L. and Holaday, D. A. (1954). *Amer. J. Physiol.* **179**, 85–88.

Rubio, R. and Berne, R. M. (1975). "Progress in Cardiovascular Diseases", Vol. 18, No. 2, pp. 105–122.

Rubio, R., Berne, R. M., Bockman, E. L. and Curnish, R. R. (1975). *Amer. J. Physiol.* **228**, 1896–1902.

Ruderman, N. B., Ross, P. S., Berger, M. and Goodman, M. N. (1974). *Biochem. J.* **138**, 1–10.

Salford, L. G. and Siesjö, B. K. (1974). *Acta Physiol. Scand.* **92**, 130–141.

Salford, L. G., Plum, F. and Siesjö, B. K. (1973a). *Arch. Neurol.* **29**, 227–233.

Salford, L. G., Plum, F. and Brierley, J. B. (1973b). *Arch. Neurol.* **29**, 234–238.

Scheinberg, P. and Stead, E. A. (1949). *J. Clin. Invest.* **28**, 1163–1171.
Schmahl, F. W., Betz, E., Talke, H. and Hohorst, H. J. (1965). *Biochem. Z.* **342**, 518–531.
Schmidt, C. F., Kety, S. S. and Pennes, H. H. (1945). *Amer. J. Physiol.* **143**, 33–52.
Schmiedek, P., Baethman, A., Sippel, G., Oettinger, W., Enzenback, R., Marguth, F. and Brendel, W. (1974). *J. Neurosurg.* **40**, 351.
Sensenbach, W., Madison, L. and Ochs, L. (1953). *J. Clin. Invest.* **32**, 226–232.
Siesjö, B. K. (1977). "Brain Energy Metabolism". John Wiley and Sons, London (to be published).
Siesjö, B. K. and Nilsson, L. (1971). *Scand. J. Clin. Lab. Invest.* **27**, 83–96.
Siesjö, B. K. and Plum, F. (1972). *In* "Biology of Brain Dysfunction" (G. E. Gaull, ed.), Vol. 1. Plenum Press, New York, pp. 319–372.
Siesjö, B. K., Jóhannsson, H., Ljunggren, B. and Norberg, K. (1974). *In* "Brain Dysfunction in Metabolic Disorders" (F. Plum, ed.), Vol. 53. Raven Press, New York, pp. 75–112.
Siesjö, B. K., Norberg, K., Ljunggren, B. and Salford, L. G. (1975a). *In* "A Basis and Practice of Neuroanaesthesia" (E. Gordon, ed.). Excerpta Medica, Amsterdam, pp. 47–82.
Siesjö, B. K., Jóhansson, H., Norberg, K. and Salford, L. (1975b). *In* "Brain Work", Alfred Benzon Symp. 8 (D. H. Ingvar and N. A. Lassen, eds). Munksgaard, Copenhagen, pp. 101–119.
Sokoloff, L. (1969). *In* "Psychochemical Research in Man" (A. J. Mandell and M. P. Mandell, eds). Academic Press, New York and London.
Sokoloff, L. (1972). *In* "Basic Neurochemistry" (R. W. Albers, G. J. Siegel, R. Katzman and B. W. Agranoff, eds). Little, Brown and Co., Boston, pp. 299–325.
Sokoloff, L. (1975). *In* "Brain Work", Alfred Benzon Symp. 8 (D. H. Ingvar and N. A. Lassen, eds). Munksgaard, Copenhagen, pp. 385–388.
Sokoloff, L. (1976). Proc. of 4th World Congress of Psychiatric Surgery. University Park Press.
Stone, W. E. (1938). *Biochem. J.* **32**, 1908–1918.
Takeshita, H., Okuda, Y. and Sari, A. (1972). *Anesthesiology*, **36**, 69.
Tews, J. K., Carter, S. H. and Stone, W. E. (1965). *J. Neurochem.* **12**, 679–693.
Theye, R. A. and Micheufelder, J. D. (1968). *Anesthesiology* **29**, 1119–1124.
Tower, D. B. and Young, O. M. (1973). *J. Neurochem.* **20**, 253–267.
Veech, R. L., Harris, R. L., Veloso, D. and Veech, E. H. (1973). *J. Neurochem.* **20**, 183–188.

Chapter 7

The Physiology of the Neurohypophysial System and its Relation to Memory Processes

TJ. B. VAN WIMERSMA GREIDANUS AND D. DE WIED

Rudolf Magnus Institute for Pharmacology, Medical Faculty, University of Utrecht, Vondellaan 6, Utrecht, The Netherlands

I. Introduction

A. *Synthesis, Storage and Release of Vasopressin*

Vasopressin is known as one of the hormones that is secreted by the pars nervosa of the neurohypophysis. It is synthesized in cell bodies of neurosecretory neurones which are situated in the anterior hypothalamus and in particular, in the nucleus supraopticus and nucleus paraventricularis (Sachs *et al.*, 1969). It is also found in the nucleus suprachiasmaticus (Burlet and Marchetti, 1975; Swaab *et al.*, 1975). The perikarya of these neurones in the hypothalamus synthesize the vasopressin peptide and the carrier proteins which then are transported, either singly or as aggregates to the nerve terminals from where they are released. These nerve terminals are generally situated in the posterior pituitary which functions as a storage organ for vasopressin. The transport of the hormone from their hypothalamic sites of synthesis to the nerve terminals takes place by protoplasmatic axonal flow through the neurones. Those axons comprise the so called tractus supraoptico-hypophyseos or tractus paraventriculo-hypophyseos. This intraneuronal transport occurs at rates of several mm per h (Pickering *et al.*, 1971). It appears that the neurohypophysial hormone

Table 1

Amino acid sequence of several vasopressin analogues and their presence in the subclasses of the vertebrates

Vasopressin analogues	Vertebrate subclasses
Arginine vasotocin	Mammals
	Birds
CyS—Tyr—Ile—Gln—Asn—CyS—Pro—Arg—Gly(NH$_2$) 1 2 3 4 5 6 7 8 9	Reptiles
	Amphibians
	Fishes
Oxytocin	Mammals
	Birds
CyS—Tyr—Ile—Gln—Asn—CyS—Pro—Leu— Gly(NH$_2$)	Reptiles
	Amphibians
	Cartilagenous fishes
Arginine vasopressin	
CyS—Tyr—Phe—Gln—Asn—CyS—Pro— Arg—Gly(NH$_2$)	Mammals
Lysine vasopressin	
	Mammals
CyS—Tyr—Phe—Gln—Asn—CyS—Pro— Lys—Gly(NH$_2$)	(Suiformes)

vasopressin is bound to a specific protein, neurophysin II, with a molecular weight of approximately 10 000. Neurophysin is present throughout the entire neurosecretory neurone: cell body, axon and posterior pituitary terminals. This suggests that it is intimately associated with vasopressin from its locus of synthesis to the site of its secretion (Zimmerman *et al.*, 1973a). The hormone–protein complex is packed in special neurosecretory granules. The release of vaso-pressins from these granules and from cells of the hypothalamo–neurohypophysial complex has been extensively studied. The essential features of this process of exocytosis involve fusion of the neurosec-retory granule with the plasma membrane and rupture of the membrane at the fusion site, followed by an expulsion of the granular contents (Douglas, 1974).

On the basis of their studies in which they showed that high quantities of vasopressin and neurophysin are present in hypophysial portal blood of monkeys Zimmerman and coworkers (1973b) propose two secretory pathways and two hormonal functions for vasopressin. The secretion into the general circulation from the posterior pituitary for the antidiuretic action in the kidney and the discharge into the hypophysial portal vessels to affect the release of anterior pituitary hormones. Data to be presented in the second part of this chapter point to a third route of secretion with respect to central nervous system effects of vasopressin. This effect of vasopressin probably results from a direct release of the peptide into the cerebrospinal fluid.

B. *Structure and Phylogeny of Vasopressin and Vasopressin-like Peptides*

Vasopressin is a nonapeptide containing a ring structure of six amino acids and a tail of three amino acids. The ring structure is closed by a disulphide link between two half-cystine residues in positions 1 and 6. For this reason vasopressin can also be regarded as an octapeptide, because the two half-cystine residues with the S—S bridge can be considered as one cysteine residue.

Among the mammalian species two types of vasopressin occur. The most common structure of vasopressin among these species is arginine-8-vasopressin, AVP (Table 1). In the group of suiformes the arginine residue in position 8 is replaced by lysine (lysine-8-vasopressin, LVP). A structurally related peptide is oxytocin. This hormone, which is synthesized, transported and stored in the same way as vasopressin, causes contraction of the myoepithelial elements in the alveolar walls in the mammae, to induce milk ejection. Besides this mammotropic effect, oxytocin has also an uterotropic action by stimulating contractions of the myometrium. The precursor of the mammalian hormones oxytocin and vasopressin which generated these peptides during evolution is arginine-8-vasotocin (AVT). This uniquitous peptide occurs in the neurohypophyses of all non-mammalian vertebrates, and has also been found in the pineal gland of mammals (Pavel, 1965; Rosenbloom and Fisher, 1975). AVT combines the effects of AVP and oxytocin. Only a few substitutions in the basic nonapeptide molecule appear to have had adaptive value and have survived among the living vertebrates. These substitutions only occur in positions 3, 4 and 8. Cystine is the only natural amino acid that contains a covalent bridge that can close the ring structure of the molecule. Thus, no other natural amino acid in position 1 or 6 could be substituted for these half-cystines in a biologically active analogue (Sawyer and Manning, 1973).

During evolution a single mutation may have taken place in the base sequence of triplets coding for the incorporation of a certain amino acid into the peptide chain during synthesis of the neurohypophysial hormones (Vliegenthart and Versteeg, 1967). Some of the naturally occurring peptides were synthesized in the laboratory before their existence in nature was discovered. In almost all vertebrae classes two neurohypophysial hormones occur. It is suggested that two peptide series have evolved after doubling of the gene controlling the synthesis of vasotocin, which is thought to be the developmentally oldest peptide (Sawyer, 1964; Vliegenthart and Versteeg, 1965). In the first series vasotocin remain unchanged until the appearance of the primitive Mammalia. In the other series a variety of oxytocin principles were derived from vasotocin by consecutive mutations. This latter series is beyond the scope of this chapter.

In the primitive Mammalia, vasotocin seems to have been converted to arginine vasopressin by the substitution of phenylalanine for isoleucine in position 3. Lysine vasopressin is an aberrant hormone, specific for Suiformes, which originated from AVP by the replacement of arginine by lysine in position 8. In Table 1 the structures of several vasopressin analogues are depicted and their appearance in the vertebrate classes and subclasses are indicated.

II. Peripheral Actions of Vasopressin*

A. *Physiological Effects of Vasopressin*

The name vasopressin is based on the action of the hormone on blood pressure. This effect is caused by constriction of peripheral blood vessels, with a resulting rise in blood pressure. In much lower amounts vasopressin acts as the mammalian antidiuretic principle. Therefore, this nonapeptide is also known as antidiuretic hormone (ADH). It acts to conserve body water by concentrating the urine and thus reducing the water required to excrete the waste solutes. This conservation of body water is also enhanced by the effect of the hormone on various amphibian membranes, such as the frog and toad skin as well as urinary bladders.

B. *Mode of Action of Vasopressin*

Because the antidiuretic effect of vasopressin is the most extensively studied action *in vivo* as well as *in vitro*, the mode of action of vasopressin on toad bladder and mammalian kidney will be briefly discussed here as an example.

1. Toad bladder

The toad bladder serves as a reservoir for water. Vasopressin has been found to affect the permeability of isolated toad bladder epithelium to water, to urea and to a group of hydrophilic amides. In addition, the hormone stimulates the active transport of sodium (Leaf *et al.*, 1958). Vasopressin increases the passive permeability of the tissue to water. Water movement across the tissue only occurs in the presence of vasopressin and of a transepithelial osmotic gradient. Then the net water movement is directly related to the transepithelial osmotic gradient which is the driving force for water movement.

Two more or less contradictory hypotheses of how the hormone modifies the tissue to effect these permeability changes to water have been proposed. Koefoed-Johnson and Ussing (1953) suggested that the action of vasopressin is to enlarge the individual pores so that they can accommodate the flow of water. Hays and Franki (1970) and Hays

---

* For a recent review on the physiology of vasopressin, including the factors involved in formation, storage, release, action and metabolism of the hormone and its physiological and pharmacological effects on water and electrolyte transport see Kurtzman and Boonjarern (1975).

et al. (1971), however, have initially proposed that water movement occurs only by diffusion. Further studies will be needed to determine whether vasopressin affects water transport by increasing the size of individual porous channels or whether it simply increases diffusion permeability in the tissue. Although the permeability change induced by vasopressin occurs in the plasma membrane at the apical surface, the hormonal effects are elicited only when the hormone is brought into contact with the serosal surface. This phenomenon is related to the site of adenyl cyclase with which the hormone interacts. The 3'5'-cyclic AMP then produced, mediates the permeability changes in the plasma membrane at the opposite surface of the cell (Orloff and Handler, 1971; Hynie and Sharp, 1971; Jard, 1971). Recent studies indicate that the action of vasopressin on transcellular water movement in the toad bladder involves a mechanism in which microtubules and/or microfilaments participate (Taylor *et al.*, 1973). It was also suggested recently that vasopressin induces changes in the distribution of intramembraneous particles of granular cell luminal membranes and that these changes may underlie vasopressin-induced changes in the transport function of the toad-bladder membrane (Kachadorian *et al.*, 1975).

2. Mammalian kidney

Vasopressin increases the osmolality of urine through its action on the distal convoluted tubule and on the collecting ducts. Under the influence of vasopressin the permeability of the distal convoluted tubule to water is greatly increased. As the, now isotonic, urine traverses the collecting ducts, it is further concentrated by the reabsorption of water by the action of vasopressin and potentiated by the presence of hypertonic interstitial fluid in the renal medulla (Sawyer, 1974; Berliner and Bennett, 1967). The physiological effect of the reabsorption of water under the influence of vasopressin is to conserve free water to the body. This hydro-osmotic effect of vasopressin is mediated by 3'5'-cyclic AMP (Orloff and Handler, 1967). The initial steps in the action of vasopressin involve stimulation of cyclic AMP formation from ATP (Dousa, 1973). The vasopressin receptor within the plasma membrane is assumed to be associated with adenylate cyclase. From studies on isolated perfused collecting ducts it has been concluded that the vasopressin receptor is located on the basilar and lateral plasma membranes of the tubule cell (Grantham and Burg, 1966), whereas the changes in water and urea permeability occur at the luminal plasma membrane (Grantham, 1971).

The mechanism by which cyclic AMP acts to produce a change in membrane permeability is unknown. Studies on isolated tubules have revealed that vasopressin and subsequently cyclic AMP, increases the size or number of existing aqueous channels in the luminal plasma membrane, which is the basis for osmotic water permeability (Grantham and Burg, 1966). The effect of cyclic AMP is also accompanied by an increased mechanical deformability of the membrane (Grantham, 1970). Since changes in permeability of the membrane to water is a highly specific function, it is assumed that this function is associated with membrane proteins that are specifically modified by cyclic AMP (Dousa, 1973). Cyclic AMP, formed under the influence of vasopressin, activates protein kinase which in turn catalyses the phosphorylation of a specific membrane protein involved in the regulation of membrane permeability to water.

C. Regulation of the Secretion of Vasopressin

The regulation of vasopressin secretion involves a complex system with multiple inputs to the hypothalamic centres concerned with synthesis and release of the hormone. The physiological stimuli affecting the release of vasopressin from the posterior pituitary gland are those concerned with the regulation of blood composition and blood volume. In 1947 Verney showed that a rise in plasma osmolality in dogs resulted in an antidiuresis due to the secretion of vasopressin from the pituitary. The osmoreceptors for this response appeared to be situated in the internal carotid artery and subsequently further localized in the hypothalamus (Jewell and Verney, 1957).

Much evidence has accumulated that volume-sensitive mechanism might also be involved in the regulation of vasopressin secretion (Rydin and Verney, 1938; Nash, 1971; Moore, 1971; Dunn et al., 1973; Smith, 1957; Share, 1961, 1967). The volume receptors seem to be located in the left atrium (stretch receptors) (Bonjour and Malvin, 1970; Share, 1965, 1967) and in the carotid sinus and the aortic arch (baro-receptors). The impulses from the left atrial volume receptors are transmitted via the vagal nerve to the diencephalon where a change in the release of vasopressin is effected (Moore, 1971). According to Moore (1971) neither receptor system of the sensitive osmoreceptor and volume receptor systems is dominant over the other. In normal circumstances they act in synchrony to maintain extracellular fluid osmolality and volume via their effect on vasopressin secretion. Dunn et al. (1973) however, conclude that vasopressin secretion is regulated principally by blood osmolality but that the responsiveness of this mechanism may be significantly altered by modest changes in blood volume.

Furthermore it is tempting to believe that an integration exists between the systems controlling the secretion of the adrenocortical hormones and of vasopressin. Renin and angiotensin on the one hand and vasopressin on the other may be involved in a complex feedback control system. Vasopressin release is partly controlled by the plasma angiotensin levels (Malvin, 1971), whereas administration of vasopressin results in an inhibition of renin secretion (Vander, 1968).

Finally, vasopressin release can apparently be increased by a variety of stimuli which can be loosely grouped together as psychogenic. In 1938 Rydin and Verney reported experiments which were interpreted in terms of a significant role for psychogenic factors in the regulation of vasopressin secretion. More recent data point to an increase of vasopressin release by psychogenic stimuli (Nash, 1970). These stimuli include emotional upset or fear (O'Connor and Verney, 1942; Chalmers and Lewis, 1951) pain (Kelsall, 1949; Chalmers and Lewis, 1951; Barnett, 1954), etc.

III. Adenohypophysiotropic Actions of Vasopressin

Exposure of the animal organism to noxious stimuli, or to stimuli which affect the emotions results in an activation of pituitary function. These activities are readily reflected in the release of adrenocorticotrophic hormone (ACTH) from the anterior pituitary and the discharge of vasopressin from the posterior pituitary into the general circulation (Rydin and Verney, 1938; Verney, 1947; Mirsky *et al.*, 1954; De Wied, 1961). Almost forty years ago indirect evidence was produced that stimuli which affect emotionality provoke the release of antidiuretic principles from the posterior lobe of the pituitary (Rydin and Verney, 1938). Later work by O'Connor and Verney (1942) confirmed these results and led to the conclusion that during emotional stress an antidiuretic substance is released from the posterior pituitary. These authors showed that the inhibition of water diuresis by emotional stress in the dog is largely reduced after removal of the posterior lobe of the pituitary gland. Vasopressin release in response to emotional stress and nociceptive stimuli has now been reported for animals and man (Corson and O'Leary Corson, 1967) and even influences on learning processes by manipulating antidiuretic hormone have been suggested (Miller *et al.*, 1968).

Sensory stimuli such as pain, intense light and sound as well as emotions (e.g. fear and anxiety), mild pain or strange environment all induce ACTH release. Since there are no demonstrable nervous connections between the anterior pituitary and the central nervous system Harris (1955) postulated that stress stimuli excite the liberation of ACTH by way of a humoral agent from hypothalamic origin which is released into the hypophysial portal system. A few years later more direct proof of the existence of a specific neurohumor was provided by the demonstration that hypothalamic extracts stimulate the release of ACTH. The term corticotrophin releasing factor (CRF) was subsequently devised for this agent by Saffran et al. (1955).

Several authors proposed that vasopressin was the CRF (Martini and Morpurgo, 1955; Sobel et al., 1955; MacDonald et al., 1956; McCann, 1957). The fact that stimuli which cause a release of ACTH and an activation of the adrenal cortex also induce antidiuresis (Mirsky et al., 1954) and the appearance of increased antidiuretic activity in the blood in situations of high ACTH release presented additional support for this hypothesis and was best explained by the assumption that the same chemical substance is responsible for both antidiuresis and the release of ACTH. However, under certain circumstances a dissociation between the release of vasopressin and the release of ACTH could occur, which suggested that at least one other substance capable of stimulating ACTH release from the pituitary existed in the hypothalamus distinct from vasopressin. The work of Guillemin et al. (1957), Saffran et al. (1955) and of Schally et al. (1958) revealed that posterior lobe preparations contained several ACTH-releasing substances, among which one resembling to or identical with vasopressin and one related to the intermediate lobe hormone: MSH. Although much work has been done to clarify the identity of the physiological CRF its nature remains to be elucidated. A marked resemblance between CRF and vasopressin exists with respect to storage and release (Mulder et al., 1970). Destruction of vasopressin and CRF, however, does not always run parallel indicating structural differences between these two entities (Mulder et al., 1970). Crude extracts of posterior pituitary origin stimulated the release of ACTH in intact rats and in rats which had been made unresponsive to non-specific stimuli by an extensive lesion in the median eminence of the hypothalamus (McCann and Brobeck, 1954; McCann, 1957). From these and additional experiments it was concluded that vasopressin has a direct effect on the anterior pituitary and therefore acts as a CRF. Vasopressin also stimulated the release of ACTH in man (MacDonald et al., 1956; Clayton et al., 1965; Gwinup, 1965; van der Wal, 1965).

Structure–activity relationship studies performed by Doepfner *et al.* (1963) and recently by Pearlmutter *et al.* (1974) again point to an association between the pressor potency of various peptides related to vasopressin and their ACTH-releasing capacity. The ring structure of vasopressin is virtually inactive which implies that the tail portion of the molecule which is essential for the effect on blood pressure is also important for the ACTH-releasing activity of vasopressin. Although it has been reported that pressinoic acid exhibits ACTH-releasing activities *in vitro* and therefore might be regarded as a physiologically functioning CRF (Saffron *et al.*, 1972), the data obtained with this ring-structure analogue of vasopressin appeared to be conflicting. The results obtained were not constant and seemed irreproducable (Saffran *et al.*, 1972; Pearlmutter *et al.*, 1974). Moreover, it seems that vasopressin induces a stimulation of both release and synthesis of ACTH (De Wied *et al.*, 1968, Buckingham and van Wimersma Greidanus, 1977). Despite the fact that vasopressin stimulates the release of ACTH and under certain conditions restores the disturbed ACTH release, the exact role of vasopressin in ACTH release has as yet not been clarified and the physiological role of vasopressin in this respect remains to be elucidated.

Hedge *et al.* (1966) demonstrated that vasopressin has a much more marked effect on ACTH release upon implantation into the median eminence of the hypothalamus than after implantation into the anterior pituitary. Yates *et al.* (1971) have demonstrated that vaso-pressin releases CRF from the hypothalamus and ACTH from the pituitary and that it also potentiates the action of endogenous CRF in releasing ACTH. That vasopressin probably plays a role in the functioning of the pituitary adrenal system is also supported by data on the deficient stress response found in homozygous Brattleboro rats which lack vasopressin (Yates *et al.*, 1971; McCann *et al.*, 1966; Wiley *et al.*, 1974; Bohus *et al.*, 1975). In addition the release of ACTH following neurogenic stimuli or to emotional stress is diminished in posterior lobectomized rats, whereas the ACTH response to somatic stress appeared to be normal. Posterior lobectomized rats, subjected to a strange environment, to sound or to pain, respond less to these stresses with their plasma corticosterone levels than sham-operated controls (Smelik, 1960; De Wied, 1961; Smelik *et al.*, 1962). However, administration of vasopressin to posterior lobectomized rats failed to induce a significant rise in pituitary–adrenal activity. Chronic adminis-tration of pitressin tannate in oil restored the pituitary adrenal response to emotional stress and to vasopressin in these animals (De Wied, 1961; 1968).

Other authors (Miller *et al.*, 1974) reported that the hypothalamic–

anterior-pituitary–adrenal system functions normally in the absence of the posterior pituitary gland, as studied under different conditions of anterior pituitary stimulation: such as the basal state, after altered negative feedback and under different types and intensities of stress. Hypothalamic vasopressin is still present in posterior lobectomized rats whereas homozygous Brattleboro rats, with a hereditary hypothalamic diabetes insipidus, completely lack vasopressin. This may be the reason for the difference in adrenocortical responsiveness between these groups of animals. On the other hand it has been reported (Wiley *et al.*, 1974) that homozygous diabetes insipidus rats respond with a significant rise in corticosterone following stress but the response is lower than that of normal or heterozygous controls. The lower peripheral plasma corticosterone concentration in homozygous diabetes insipidus rats in response to stress can, in part, be explained by a diminished sensitivity of the adrenal glands to ACTH.

In addition these animals contain less growth hormone, GH, in their pituitaries and vasopressin has been implicated as influencing GH secretion (Arimura *et al.*, 1968). Posterior pituitary principles may under certain conditions induce the release of TSH and LH also (Martini and Morpurgo, 1955). However, there is no proof that vasopressin stimulates secretion of these anterior pituitary hormones under physiological conditions.

Recent experiments by Zimmerman *et al.* (1973b) provided new evidence for a physiological role of vasopressin in anterior pituitary activation. These authors demonstrated high vasopressin levels in hypophysial portal blood of monkeys. Using a specific immunocytochemical technique they also showed the existence of neurosecretory nerve endings situated in the capillary loops of hypophysial portal vessels in the median eminence suggesting the expulsion of vasopressin into portal blood from neurone terminals (Zimmerman, 1976). Moreover, they have shown that adrenalectomy selectively stimulates vasopressin and vasopressin neurophysin in neurosecretory pathways to the hypophysial portal system in rats, which lends support to the concept that vasopressin plays a role in the activation of the hypothalamic–pituitary–adrenal system (Seif *et al.*, 1975).

IV. Central Actions of Vasopressin; its Role in Memory Processes

The first evidence that vasopressin is involved in memory processes was obtained in posterior lobectomized rats which were trained in a shuttle-box (De Wied, 1965). Although the removal of the posterior lobe was associated with normal acquisition of the conditioned avoidance response (CAR), the rate of extinction was much faster than that of controls. Posterior lobectomized rats therefore are unable to maintain the response for a considerable period of time. Running speed in response to an unescapable footshock in a straight runway was similar in both posterior lobectomized and sham-operated rats, indicating normal locomotor capacities in posterior lobectomized rats.

Pitressin administered every other day as a long acting tannate preparation in oil, normalized the water intake of the mildly diabetic posterior lobectomized rat and the rate of extinction of the CAR. Purified lysine vasopressin (LVP), administered as a long acting preparation had a similar effect (De Wied, 1965). Restoration of extinction behaviour towards normal in posterior lobectomized rats appeared to be independent of the time of administration of pitressin or LVP. Treatment with pitressin tannate in oil or with purified LVP either during acquisition or during extinction had the same beneficial effect on the rate of extinction.

A. *Vasopressin, Vasopressin Analogues and Avoidance and Approach Behaviour of Intact Rats*

1. *Active avoidance behaviour*

Pitressin also induced marked behavioural effects in intact animals. Subcutaneous injection of 1 iU of the long acting pitressin tannate in oil every two days either during acquisition or during extinction markedly increased resistance to extinction of shuttle-box avoidance behaviour (De Wied and Bohus, 1966). In contrast to control treated animals, rats treated with pitressin maintained a high level of responding during the 14 day period of extinction. Even if extinction behaviour of the rats was studied again three weeks after termination of the first extinction period, the pitressin treated animals still made 60–70% avoidances in response to the presentation of the conditioned stimulus (De Wied *et al.*, 1974). Similar effects were obtained in one way active avoidance behaviour with synthetic posterior pituitary principles. A single injection of 0·6 or 1·8 μg LVP exhibited a long-term, dose-dependent, effect on extinction of the pole-jumping avoidance response which extended beyond the actual presence of the peptide in the organism indicating that vasopressin triggers a long-term effect on the maintenance of avoidance behaviour, probably by facilitating consolidation (De Wied, 1971; van Wimersma Greidanus *et al.*, 1973). Other

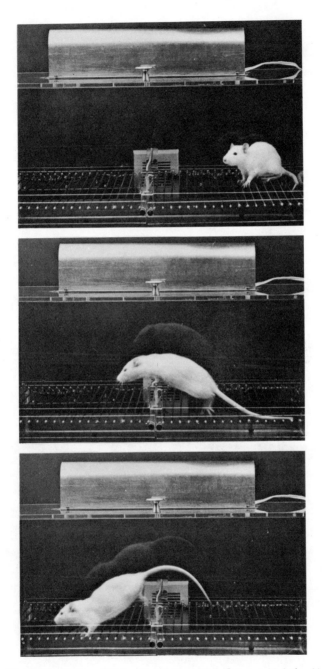

Fig. 1. Shuttle-box. (With acknowledgement to Organon Nederland.)

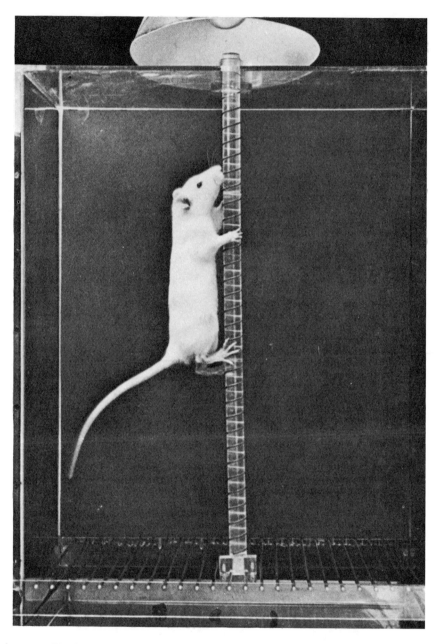

Fig. 2. Pole-jumping test. (With acknowledgement to Organon Nederland.)

structurally and physiologically related peptides like oxytocin, angiotensin II, insulin or growth hormone failed to affect the rate of extinction of the CAR following administration of comparable amounts (De Wied, 1971). Vasopressin analogues such as arginine-8-vasopressin (AVP), the rats natural occurring posterior pituitary hormone, and desglycinamide-lysine vasopressin (DG-LVP), the octapeptide which lacks the antidiuretic, pressor, oxytocic and ACTH releasing activities (De Wied *et al.*, 1972), have a similar behavioural effect to that of LVP (De Wied *et al.*, 1974). These findings indicate that the behavioural effect of vasopressin is not due to its effects on classical target tissues like the kidney, the blood vessel, the uterus and the anterior pituitary.

2. Structure–activity relationship studies

In an attempt to determine the active core of the vasopressin molecule in memory consolidation, the potency of a number of vasopressin analogues was assayed on extinction of the avoidance response in the pole-jumping test (De Wied *et al.*, 1975). Briefly, rats were trained to jump onto a pole in response to the conditioned stimulus (CS) which was a light on top of the box, to avoid the unconditioned stimulus (US) of electric footshock. Ten trials a day were given with an intertrial interval of 60 sec presented in a predetermined sequence for three consecutive days. Peptides were injected subcutaneously at the end of the third acquisition session. Extinction sessions in which the CS was presented only were run on days 4, 5 and 8 of the experiment. Of every peptide tested, the amount needed to induce six or more positive responses on day 8 (third extinction session) was determined. Saline treated rats never scored more than two positive responses in this extinction session. If the criterion was not reached with a dose of 5 µg of the peptide per rat, it was considered inactive. AVP appeared to be the most potent peptide followed by LVP. Removal of the glycinamide (DG-LVP and DG-AVP) decreases the potency to approximately 50%. Oxytocin and vasotocin are equally effective and possess *c.* 20% of the activity of AVP. Pressinamide (PA) has retained only 10% of the behavioural potency.

$$\frac{\text{AVP}}{\text{LVP}} \quad \text{H—Cys—Tyr—Phe—Gln—Asn—Cys—Pro—} \begin{matrix} \text{Arg} \\ \text{Lys} \end{matrix} \text{—Gly—NH}_2$$

$$\text{DG} \frac{\text{AVP}}{\text{LVP}} \quad \text{H—Cys—Tyr—Phe—Gln—Asn—Cys—Pro—} \begin{matrix} \text{Arg} \\ \text{Lys} \end{matrix} \text{—OH}$$

$$\text{PA} \quad \text{H—Cys—Tyr—Phe—Gln—Asn—Cys—NH}_2$$

Thus removal of the C-terminal part leads to a drastic decrease in potency. It may be that it protects the active moiety against metabolic degradation en route to the central nervous system (CNS). Indeed, if PA is administered via one of the lateral ventricles only twice as much AVP is needed for an equipotent effect on extinction of the pole-jumping avoidance response. In addition, AVP is 200 and PA 1000 times more active when given through the cerebro-ventricular route as compared with subcutaneous administration. This suggests that the receptor in the brain interacts with only a part of the molecule presumably located in the ring structure. The isolation of these receptors may eventually reveal the essential requirements for the behavioural effect of vasopressin analogues. The potency of in-traventricularly administered vasopressin suggests that its behavioural effect results from release from its production sites in the anterior hypothalamus into the CSF (see also p. 241) (De Wied, 1976).

In order to determine the critical period for the effect of vasopressin to occur, LVP was injected at 6, at 3 and at 1 h before, or immediately, 1 and 6 h after the first extinction session. Vasopressin was administered within 1 h before or after the first extinction session in order to be completely effective in inhibiting the extinction of the CAR (De Wied, 1971). Since the inhibitory effect of vasopressin and vasopressin analogues on extinction of active avoidance behaviour might be explained by a general increase in locomotor activity, the effect of vasopressin was also studied in a so called open field. No difference in rearing, grooming or ambulation were observed following adminis-tration of LVP, as compared with saline treatment.

3. Passive avoidance behaviour

Moreover, it appeared that vasopressin not only affects active avoid-ance behaviour, but passive behaviour as well, as studied in a single "step-through" passive avoidance situation (Ader et al., 1972). This situation uses the innate response of rats to prefer darkness to light. The apparatus is a dark box connected with an illuminated elevated platform. Rats are placed on the platform and latency to enter the dark box is recorded. One trial is given on day 1 and three such trials on day 2. At the end of the third trial on day 2, the animals receive an electric footshock (0·25 mA) in the dark box for 1 sec. The next day latency to enter is recorded again in the first retention trial at 24 h after the single acquisition trial. At 48 h a second retention session is performed. LVP injected s.c. either 1 h before the first retention trial or immediately after the acquisition trial considerably increased avoidance latency. Avoidance latency was still augmented during the second retention trial at 48 h. Thus, the long-term preservation of an acquired response was also found in the passive avoidance situation (Ader and De Wied, 1972). A similar temporal relationship as in active avoidance behaviour was found for the retention of passive avoidance behaviour. Treatment at 6 h before the first retention trial was ineffective in increasing latency scores whereas injection at a 1 h time interval induced increased retention of the response. Thus the critical time period for the behavioural effect of vasopressin again was found to be approximately 1 h (Bohus et al., 1972). In general it can be stated that vasopressin is active when administered in association with behaviour which occurs 1 h prior to/or after injection (King and De Wied, 1974).

It was further investigated whether the long-term behavioural effect of LVP is specific for a particular response or whether generalization occurs to other adversely motivated responses (Bohus et al., 1972). Half of the animals were trained in the pole-jumping apparatus in the morning and subjected to the step through procedure 6 h later in the afternoon. The other half were trained first in the passive avoidance test in the morning and subjected to the pole-jumping avoidance test in the afternoon. Animals were injected on day 3 of the experiment with either saline or LVP 1 h prior to the morning session. Resistance to extinction was seen only in that situation where the training occurred in the morning 1 h after the administration of the peptides. No evidence of generalization or transfer of the effects of vasopressin from one behavioural situation to the other was found indicating that the effect on extinction is restricted to that behaviour which is occurring during the period of optimal vasopressin influence (Bohus et al., 1972).

4. Classical conditioning

In a series of experiments intended to dissociate classical and instrumental components underlying the behavioural effect, it appeared that classical conditioning alone was a sufficient behavioural substrate for the long-term effect of vasopressin on avoidance behaviour (King and De Wied, 1974), but instrumental conditioning was more effective. Thus, vasopressin administration to rats exposed to the CS and the US in the absence of an escape possibility significantly increased resistance to extinction of subsequent pole-jumping avoidance behaviour. However, a single correct response under the influence of vasopressin in the pole-jumping test is more effective in affecting resistance to extinction. The combination of the classical and instrumental components seems therefore optimal for the behavioural effect of vasopressin. These results are in agreement with findings on classically conditioned heart rate in free moving rats. The cardiac response in rats exposed to the sound of a buzzer (CS) followed by the US of shock appeared to be of a bradycardiac nature. Rapid extinction of this bradycardiac response takes place unless the animals are treated with LVP. It turns out that the influence of vasopressin on adaptive autonomic responses as heart rate appears only in situations where certain learning paradigms are involved such as in classical conditioning or in passive avoidance behaviour. The heart rate of non- or pseudo-conditioned rats is not affected by the peptide. The cardiac response in rats submitted to passive avoidance behaviour is of a bradycardiac nature and this bradycardia is further facilitated by DG-LVP. It is suggested that also in this situation vasopressin-like peptides affect specific memory functions (Bohus 1975).

5. Approach behaviour

Attempts to demonstrate behavioural effects of vasopressin analogues on other than fear motivated behaviour initially were not very successful. Garrud et al. (1974) failed to observe an effect of LVP or DG-LVP on extinction of a straight runway approach response for food in food-deprived rats. Although DG-LVP is practically devoid of antidiuretic activities, an interaction between the peptide, hunger drive and water metabolism cannot be excluded. However, the behaviour of food-deprived rats in a continual punishment situation which were trained to hold a lever down for 8 sec in order to obtain a food reward can be affected by vasopressin. When electric shock was introduced after training to a stable level contingent upon the completion of an 8 sec level hold at the same time as the food, treatment with lysine vasopressin prolonged the time needed to make the next response after each shock, and increased the efficiency with which the animals performed (Garrud, 1975). A straight runway may be too simple and therefore inadequate to study the influence of agents which may affect memory processes. The influence of vasopressin on approach behaviour was (therefore) studied in a maze. Male rats trained in a T maze to run for a receptive female chose the correct arm of the maze in a significantly higher percentage following DG-LVP treatment after each acquisition session. The effect again is of a long-term nature. Copulation reward appeared to be essential for this effect since unrewarded rats do not display more correct choices than placebo treated animals after cessation of the treatment (Bohus, 1976). DG-LVP also delays the disappearance of intromission and ejaculatory behaviour of male rats following castration. Thus, vasopressin analogues not only affect the maintenance of aversely motivated behaviour but also extinction of other behavioural patterns. Evidence for an effect on memory processes was further obtained when it appeared that vasopressin analogues antagonize retrograde amnesia. Lande *et al.* (1972) found that DG-LVP protects against puromycin induced memory loss in mice. Rigter *et al.* (1974) demonstrated that amnesia for a one trial passive avoidance response in rats as induced by CO_2 or by electroconvulsive shock is reversed by treatment with DG-LVP immediately after the learning trial. These authors suggested that the peptide promotes memory consolidation either by facilitating the consolidating process or by protecting memory consolidation from the adverse effects of the amnesic treatment. The possibility that vasopressin influences retrieval was also considered since DG-LVP exhibited anti-amnesic effects also if injected 1 h prior to the retention test.

6. Development of resistance to morphine analgesia

Recently, Krivoy *et al.* (1974) reported that DG-LVP facilitates the development of resistance to the analgesic action of morphine in mice. This might suggest a physiological role of vasopressin in the development of tolerance to narcotic analgesics.

Development of resistance to morphine analgesia may be regarded as a form of learning or memory (Cohen *et al.*, 1965). This view is corroborated by observations showing that protein synthesis inhibitors, which impair learning and memory, prevent the development of tolerance to narcotic analgesics also (Cox and Osman, 1970). Thus, similar mechanisms as in learning and memory processes may be involved in the development of tolerance. In addition, in homozygous diabetes insipidus animals which lack vasopressin (see below), in contrast to heterozygous litter mates, development of resistance to the analgesic action of morphine as measured on the hotplace is severely retarded (De Wied and Gispen, 1976). Their data indicate that lack of vasopressin interferes with the development of tolerance to morphine analgesia. Failure to develop resistance to morphine analgesia in diabetes insipidus rats can be amended by chronic treatment with either AVP or DG-LVP.

B. *Behavioural Profile of Rats Which Lack Vasopressin due to a Genetic Failure*

That vasopressin is physiologically involved in memory processes has recently been demonstrated in rats with hereditary hypothalamic diabetes insipidus. A homozygous variant of the Brattleboro strain lacks the ability to synthesize vasopressin due to a mutation on a single pair of autosomal loci (Valtin and Schroeder, 1964; Valtin, 1967). A radioimmunoassay of AVP, developed recently (van Wimersma Greidanus *et al.*, 1974; Dogterom *et al.*, in preparation) revealed that the pituitary vasopressin content in homozygous diabetes insipidus (HO-DI) rats is approximately 5% of that in heterozygous animals, which in turn is about 40% of the pituitary vasopressin content in homozygous normal Brattleboro rats (Table 2a). The small amount of vasopressin in pituitaries of diabetes insipidus rats is probably partly due to oxytocin which has some cross reactivity with the antiserum in the radioimmunoassay or to other, unknown, vasopressin-like peptides. The oxytocin content in the pituitaries of HO-DI rats is also lower than that of heterozygous (HE-DI) and of normal rats (Table 2b). This difference, however, is not dramatic and may be an accompanying phenomenon of the defect in the neurohypophysial system of the HO-DI animals in peptide synthesizing capacity. Moreover, it has been shown that these HO-DI Brattleboro rats have a total absence of arginine-8-vasoticin also (Rosenbloom and Fisher, 1975). The availability of rats with hereditary diabetes insipidus (DI) provided a model to study memory function in the absence of vasopressin. HO-DI rats are inferior in acquiring and maintaining active and passive avoidance behaviour (Bohus *et al.*, 1975). The behaviour deficits are most obvious in a step-through one trial passive avoidance test and least obvious in a multiple trial one way avoidance paradigm. Thus, the rate of acquisition of a shuttle-box avoidance response is slower in HO-DI rats as compared to that of heterozygous litter mates or Wistar strain animals. Extinction of the behaviour is very rapid in HO-DI and somewhat less rapid in HE-DI as compared to that of Wistar rats. The rate of acquisition of the pole-jumping response appeared to be the same in HO-DI and HE-DI rats but Wistar rats acquire the response much faster. Extinction is very rapid in HO-DI rats, somewhat slower in HE-DI animals and least rapid in the Wistar rats.

Memory function of HO-DI rats is completely impaired in a one trial passive avoidance situation when retention is tested 24 h or later after shock exposure. Arginine vasopressin (AVP) and DG-LVP given

Table 2a

Posterior pituitary vasopressin content in rats homozygous
or heterozygous for hereditary hypothalamic diabetes
insipidus as measured by radioimmunoassay

	Body weight (g)	Posterior pituitary weight (mg)	Vasopressin content (mU/whole posterior pituitary)	Vasopressin content (mU/mg posterior pituitary)
Homozygous DI (9)	243 ± 6	$1 \cdot 24 \pm 0 \cdot 07^a$	$8 \cdot 2 \pm 2 \cdot 0^b$	$6 \cdot 6 \pm 1 \cdot 6^b$
Heterozygous (9)	283 ± 7	$0 \cdot 84 \pm 0 \cdot 03$	163 ± 23^a	196 ± 27^a
Homozygous normal (6)	354 ± 9	$0 \cdot 90 \pm 0 \cdot 04$	425 ± 47	472 ± 51

[a] $p < 0 \cdot 05$.
[b] $p < 0 \cdot 02$.
( ) Number of animals per group.

Table 2b

Posterior pituitary oxytocin content in rats homozygous
or heterozygous for hereditary hypothalamic diabetes
insipidus as measured by radioimmunoassay

	Body weight (g)	Posterior pituitary weight (mg)	Oxytocin content (mU/whole posterior pituitary)	Oxytocin content (mU/mg posterior pituitary)
Homozygous DI (9)	254 ± 7	$1 \cdot 20 \pm 0 \cdot 07^a$	422 ± 60^a	352 ± 64^a
Heterozygous (9)	310 ± 6	$0 \cdot 87 \pm 0 \cdot 07$	696 ± 60	800 ± 64
Homozygous normal (6)	354 ± 9	$0 \cdot 90 \pm 0 \cdot 04$	610 ± 32	678 ± 42

[a] $p < 0 \cdot 05$.
( ) Number of animals per group.

immediately after the learning trial readily restore passive avoidance
behaviour in HO-DI rats (De Wied et al., 1975). This favours the
hypothesis that memory rather than learning processes are disturbed
in the absence of vasopressin. Indeed, as mentioned before, HO-DI
rats are able to acquire fear motivated responses in the shuttle-box or in

the pole-jumping test. Furthermore, full retention of passive avoidance behaviour is obtained in HO-DI rats when retention is tested shortly after the learning trial. The main disturbance is in the ability to maintain the behaviour. The passive avoidance response at 3 h after the learning trial is only partial, and completely absent at the 24 h retention test. These observations suggest that consolidation of memory is impaired in the absence of vasopressin. The pituitary–adrenal response also shows a marked relationship with passive avoidance behaviour in DI rats (Bohus et al., 1975). At the immediate retention test when full passive avoidance behaviour is displayed by HO-DI rats, an elevation of plasma corticosterone is found which is of the same magnitude as that of HE-DI rats. At the 3 h retention test a partial avoidance behaviour is associated with a reduced corticosterone response, while retention impairment is coupled with the absence of a significant increase in plasma corticosterone. These observations therefore indicate that the absence of vasopressin in HO-DI rats which results in an impairment of a psychological mechanism also results in an impairment of the accompanying endocrine response in an otherwise fear provoking environment. This might suggest that the behavioural effect of vasopressin is mediated by ACTH or other pituitary hormones. Vasopressin, however, effectively restores avoidance behaviour in hypophysectomized rats (Bohus et al., 1973; Lande et al., 1971).

Recent electrophysiological studies of the brain (Urban and De Wied, 1975) show that rhythmic slow activity (RSA) of HO-DI rats contains substantially lower hippocampal theta frequencies during paradoxical sleep (PS) than that of HE-DI animals. Differences are found in all spectral parameters and the averaged peak frequency of homozygous diabetes insipidus rats is approximately 1 Hz lower than that of heterozygous animals. Thus, PS fails to produce normal frequency of RSA in the absence of vasopressin, indicating a qualitatively different PS. Administration of DG-AVP enhances the generation of higher frequencies in HO-DI rats and almost completely restores the distribution of hippocampal theta frequencies. Deprivation of paradoxical sleep has been shown to interfere with the consolidation of learned responses (Leconte and Bloch, 1970; Stern, 1971; Fishbein, 1971). It might be therefore that the impaired memory of HO-DI rats is due to the low quality of PS found in these animals. In addition, Longo and Loizzo (1973) have reported that drugs which facilitate memory functions, increase theta frequency in the post-learning period suggesting that changes in the excitability in hippocampal theta activity may be related to memory consolidation.

Landfield *et al.* (1972) maintain that theta activity in the post-learning period may be a brain state which is optimal for memory storage. Hypophysectomized rats which also show learning deficits (De Wied, 1964) have shorter PS episodes and lack the normally present PS circadian rhythmicity (Valatx *et al.*, 1975). PS is also markedly disturbed in the chronic pontine cat without hypothalamus or pituitary gland (Jouvet, 1965). These deficits can be restored by treatment with various pituitary principles. Thus, these electrophysiological investigations in diabetes insipidus rats support the hypothesis that vasopressin is involved in the consolidation of memory processes.

Purified Lysine Vassopressin (LVP)

C. CNS Site of Action of Vasopressin in Relation to Avoidance Behaviour

The site of action for the behavioural effect of vasopressin was determined by intracerebral administration of the peptide and by means of lesion experiments. For these studies the pole-jumping avoidance test was used. Micro-injections of small amounts (0·1 µg) of LVP were placed in various limbic midbrain structures. Application of LVP in the posterior thalamic area, including the parafascicular nuclei, resulted in a preservation of the pole-jump avoidance response. Other brain areas, including ventromedial and antero-medial parts of the thalamus, posterior hypothalamus, substantia nigra, reticular formation, substantia grisea, putamen and the dorsal hippocampal complex appeared to be ineffective sites. Thus, the behavioural effect of vasopressin seemed to be located in the parafascicular area (van Wimersma Greidanus *et al.*, 1973, 1975b). However, ineffective micro-injections may not always represent non-sensitive structures of the brain, since a unilateral local micro-injection of a small amount of vasopressin into a restricted brain area may be unable to influence the activity of the functions of this area sufficiently to induce behavioural changes (van Wimersma Greidanus, 1975b). In addition, intraventricular administration also increased resistance to extinction (van Wimersma Greidanus *et al.*, 1973).

Rats bearing lesions in the parafascicular area were employed for further evaluation of the significance of these structures for the behavioural effect of vasopressin. Extensive lesions in the posterior thalamic area interfere with both acquisition and extinction of the pole-jumping avoidance response, whereas smaller lesions, restricted to the parafascicular area, interfere with the extinction processes only and induce facilitation of extinction (Bohus and De Wied, 1967a). The lesions reduced but did not prevent the behavioural effect of vasopressin in the pole-jumping test. Thus, although the parafascicular region is sensitive to the action of vasopressin, it does not seem to be essential in this respect. Such lesioned animals only require more vasopressin to increase resistance to extinction (van Wimersma Greidanus et al., 1974, 1975b).

To search for additional brain structures of the midbrain limbic system which would be sensitive to vasopressin, rats with extensive bilateral lesions either in the preoptic rostral septal area or in the dorsal hippocampal complex were used. These brain regions were chosen because marked behavioural changes have been reported in rats following ablation of the septum (Brady and Nauta, 1953; Fried, 1972) or in rats following dorsal hippocampectomy (Altman et al., 1973). Moreover, both brain regions are thought to be involved in learning processes (Albert and Mah, 1972; Altman et al., 1973). Extensive lesions in the rostral septum or in the dorsal hippocampus prevented vasopressin induced preservation of avoidance behaviour (van Wimersa Greidanus et al., 1975b), whereas the lesions themselves did not interfere with the rate of extinction of the avoidance response. Acquisition of the response was retarded in animals with extensive hippocampal lesions. Smaller lesions which caused partial damage of the dorsal hippocampal complex partly inhibited, but did not completely block the behavioural effect of vasopressin (van Wimersma Greidanus and De Wied, 1976). These results point to an important role of midbrain limbic structures in vasopressin induced effects on avoidance behaviour. In view of present knowledge on septal and hippocampal areas in relation to behaviour this is not unexpected. With a few exceptions, septal lesions have been shown to affect acquisition of a shuttle-box avoidance task (Deagle and Lubar, 1971; King, 1958) and of one way avoidance conditioning (Kenyon and Krieckhaus, 1965). Differences are described between the effects of septal lesions on behaviour of rats in one-way and two-way active avoidance situations (Dalby, 1970). The type of conditioning stimulus also appears to play an important role in the effect of septal lesions on avoidance behaviour (Dalby, 1970; Thomas and McClearly, 1974).

The hippocampal complex plays an essential role in behavioural performance (Douglas, 1967; Segal and Olds, 1972). Although the variability in lesion size has been an obstacle in comparing results from different laboratories, the literature agrees that hippocampal lesions affect behaviour. It should be mentioned that smaller lesions have sometimes different effects than larger lesions. The effect of hippocampectomy on one-way conditioning is not clear. Small lesions do not produce deficits (Liss, 1968), but large lesions do (Liss, 1968; Rich and Thompson, 1965). Retardation of acquisition as observed in our experiments is in agreement with observations by Nadel (1968), who suggested that the dorsal hippocampus may function in the modulation of responses to motivating stimuli. It is also suggested that in situations associated with high arousal, hippocampectomized subjects show a tendency of repeating previous responses due to either greater response perseveration or deficient response inhibition (Douglas, 1967; Kimble, 1968). This tendency is frequently observed in two-way active avoidance situations. In our one-way avoidance situation, however, no effect of dorsal hippocampectomy on extinction could be observed.

The present results suggest that vasopressin acts on midbrain–limbic circuits including septal and hippocampal structures to enhance the storage and/or retrieval of recently acquired information which is used when the animal is confronted again with the same environmental stimuli. In addition the theory that the hippocampus serves as a "gateway to memory" (Hirsch, 1974) fits the concept that this brain structure is a site of the memory consolidating action of vasopressin. In which way vasopressin acts on memory processes is not known. Long-term memory processes are generally considered to involve protein synthesis in the brain (Matthies, 1975). This behavioural effect of vasopressin may thus be a consequence of an influence of vasopressin on protein synthesis. Vasopressin effects on such peripheral target organs as the toad bladder and mammalian kidney involve activation of the adenylcyclase–3'5'-cyclic AMP system, which in turn initiates the activation of protein kinase and the phosphorylation of a specific protein. The behavioural effects of vasopressin could also be mediated by the adenylcyclase–cyclic AMP system. Increased synthesis of cyclic AMP as a consequence of an activation of adenyl cyclase may enhance the synthesis of proteins in specific brain regions which play a role in processes of learning and memory. Identification of the characteristics and of the localization of specific bindings sites and/or receptors for vasopressin in the brain are essential in this respect.

D. *The Role of the Cerebrospinal Fluid as a Route of Transport for the Behavioural Effect of Vasopressin*

Morphological and functional evidence has accumulated for the release of hypothalamic hormones from neural tissue into the liquor of the brain ventricular system. Recent studies indicate that neurosecretory axons run to the walls of the brain ventricular system (Sterba, 1974a; Vorherr *et al.*, 1968; Rodriguez, 1970). Morphological observations point to a connection between neurosecretory cells and the ependyma of the infundibular recess of the third ventricle. Axons originating in the supraoptic area, filled with neurosecretory substances have been shown to end in the infundibular recess (Wittkowski, 1968). In addition, vasopressin and/or vasotocin has been shown to be present in rabbit (Heller *et al.*, 1968) and human cerebrospinal fluid (Gupta, 1969; Pavel, 1970; Coculesco and Pavel, 1973). Rodriguez (1970) reviewed the relation between vasopressin in blood and in cerebrospinal fluid (CSF) and noted that blood levels of vasopressin are approximately twice as high as CSF levels (Heller *et al.*, 1968) and he calculated from these data that the amount of vasopressin released into the CSF is 200–400 times less than the amount released into the blood. To his opinion this may explain the fact that the number of neurosecretory fibres that reaches the third ventricle is relatively scarce in comparison with the number of those ending in capillaries to the neural lobe. We, however, found approximately 3–5 times higher vasopressin levels in the CSF than in peripheral blood (5 pg/ml CSF v. 1·5 pg/ml plasma) using a recently developed radioimmunoassay for vasopressin (Dogterom *et al.*, in preparation). However, the anaesthesia itself, which was used for collecting the CSF samples, may have caused a rise in the vasopressin levels in the CSF. It has been suggested that neurohumors are released directly into the CSF from liquor contacting terminals of neurones (Sterba, 1974a). With the use of electron microscopic and immunocytochemistry techniques Goldsmith and Zimmerman (1975) demonstrated that neuronal processes containing granules with neurophysin and with vasopressin were present close to portal capillary loops (see also p. 225) also protruding into the third ventricle along its ventral border. These results again point to a direct secretion of vasopressin from neurone terminals into portal blood and into the CSF as well (Goldsmith and Zimmerman, 1975; Zimmerman *et al.*, 1975). In which way the hormone is channelled from the CSF to the effector site is not clear. Maybe different pools of ependymal cells or some circumventricular organs act as mediators in this respect (Sterba, 1974b). Various possibilities for the function of vasopressin in the CSF has been suggested, such as a role in the feedback of its own secretion, in the homeostasis of ionic concentration in the brain etc. (Rodriguez, 1970). However, the cerebroventricular system may be the way of transport *par excellence* for vasopressin from its hypothalamic site of synthesis to the locus of action in the limbic midbrain system, in order to induce its behavioural effects. Indeed the fact that the intracerebroventricular administration of vasopressin analogues affects avoidance behaviour at much lower doses than after systemic injection support this hypothesis (De Wied, 1976). Since the CSF is a circulating medium bathing several brain regions the suggestion that it serves as a vehicle for intracerebral transport is not new (Milhorat, 1975). In 1910 it had been suggested by Cushing and Goetsch that posterior pituitary principles might be released into the third ventricle of the brain for distribution within the CNS. Moreover, a variety of hypothalamic peptides have been demonstrated to be distributed in many brain regions. Release of these peptides from peptidergic nerve terminals in extrahypothalamic limbic structures may be of biological importance in regulation of behaviour (Martin et al., 1976).

Recent studies revealed that the amounts of vasopressin required to stimulate ACTH release from the anterior pituitary, are approximately the same when administered intravenously or intracerebroventricularly, whereas the effect of vasopressin on blood pressure is initiated at lower doses following intravenous injection than after intracerebroventricular administration (van Wimersma Greidanus et al., in preparation). These data support the idea that the cerebroventricular fluid is the preferential route of transport for the behavioural influence of vasopressin, the portal vessel system for the hypophysiotropic action and the general circulation for the systemic effects of vasopressin.

E. *Intraventricular Administration of Vasopressin Antiserum Inhibits Retention of Passive Avoidance Behaviour*

Administration of vasopressin antiserum developed for the radioimmunoassay of this peptide hormone (van Wimersma Greidanus et al., 1974; Dogterom et al., in preparation), into one of the lateral ventricles of the brain, immediately after the learning trial induced an almost complete deficit in the one trial passive avoidance tasks when tested at 6, 8, 24 or 48 h after the learning trial. No interference with the behaviour was observed when the animals were tested for retention at 2 min, at 1 or 2 h after administration of the vasopressin antiserum. Treatments with oxytocin antiserum or with control rabbit serum, was ineffective in this respect (van Wimersma Greidanus et al., 1975a).

Intravenous injection (i.v.) of one hundred times as much vasopressin antiserum, which effectively removed the peptide from the circulation as indicated by the virtual absence of vasopressin in the urine and by the marked increase of the urine production, did not affect passive avoidance behaviour. These results indicate the importance of intraventricular release of vasopressin in relation to avoidance behaviour. In addition the observation that passive avoidance behaviour was normal in animals tested shortly after the administration of vasopressin antiserum indicates that memory consolidation rather than learning processes are influenced by vasopressin (van Wimersma Greidanus *et al.*, 1975a). Further proof for this assumption was obtained from experiments in which vasopressin antiserum was administered into the brain ventricular system during a multiple-trial learning procedure. The antiserum was administered each day, half an hour prior to the acquisition session of the pole-jumping avoidance response. Acquisition of rats treated with 1 µl vasopressin antiserum tended to be slower than that of animals treated with control serum, but both groups reached the learning criterion of 75% in the same period of time. During extinction, which was started at day 5, treatment was not continued. It appeared that extinction of the avoidance response was much faster in the group of animals which had been injected intraventricularly with vasopressin antiserum during acquisition (van Wimersma Greidanus *et al.*, 1975c). These findings reinforce the notion that learning can take place in the absence of vasopressin but the behaviour cannot be maintained, probably as the result of a disturbed memory consolidation.

V. Concluding Remarks

Recently the neurohypophysial hormone vasopressin has been demonstrated in the CSF and evidence has been obtained for direct secretion into the CSF (Heller and Saidi, 1974). Vasopressin seems to be transported to midbrain limbic structures which probably are the sites of the behavioural action of this neuropeptide. It is, however, also possible that a direct hypothalamic–limbic pathway exists which may be an integral subsystem of the main peptidergic neurosecretory system, as suggested by Sterba (1974b). In that case neuropeptides would influence limbic system structures directly by means of this subsystem. Recently evidence has been obtained by Pfaff (1975, personal communication) for a direct neuronal connection between anterior hypothalamic regions and limbic midbrain structures. Lately the existence of neurophysin-containing fibres to limbic system structures has been demonstrated (Kozlowski *et al.*, 1976). Martin *et al.* (1976) postulated that hypothalamic peptidergic neurones are part of a diffuse neural network that terminates in widespread areas of the brain which may be important in terms of neurobiologic regulation. One might state that the hypothalamic–neurohypophysial system serves the general circulation for peripheral effects of posterior pituitary hormones, the portal vessel system for anterior pituitary function and the cerebrospinal fluid for CNS activities.

Vasopressin, the mammalian antidiuretic principle induces re-absorption of water by increasing the permeability of the distal convoluted tubules and collecting ducts to water in the mammalian kidney. This effect of vasopressin is mediated by $3'5'$-cyclic AMP. The vasopressin secretion is mainly regulated by changes in plasma osmolality and in blood volume. Furthermore psychogenic stimuli increase vasopressin release.

Although posterior pituitary hormones may under certain conditions produce the discharge of TSH and LH (Martini and Morpurgo, 1955) and GH secretion from the anterior pituitary the most pronounced adenohypophysiotropic effect of vasopressin is in terms of ACTH release. Despite the fact that vasopressin stimulates the release of ACTH, and that several authors have proposed that vasopressin is the corticotrophin releasing factor, the physiological role of vasopressin in this respect remains to be elucidated.

Evidence is provided that vasopressin and analogues of this posterior pituitary principle facilitate the consolidation of new behaviour patterns. These peptides under certain conditions facilitate acquisition of active avoidance behaviour, increase resistance to extinction of active and passive avoidance behaviour and of sexually motivated approach behaviour. Vasopressin analogues antagonize retrograde amnesia also. Conversely, in the absence of vasopressin as found in hereditary diabetes insipidus rats severe memory disturbances are found. Intraventricular administration of minute amounts of vasopressin analogues facilitate memory consolidation, supporting the notion that the behavioural effect of these polypeptides is centrally mediated. Vasopressin antiserum which is assumed to neutralize vasopressin released into the CSF prevents memory consolidation. Studies on paradoxical sleep in diabetes insipidus rats revealed disturbances in hippocampal theta frequencies and enforce the hypothesis that memory processes are under the influence of vasopressin analogues. The development of resistance to the analgesic action of narcotic analgesics is facilitated by administration of vasopressin analogues and markedly retarded in diabetes insipidus rats. These and other results suggest that the memory consolidating effect of vasopressin analogues may be of a more general nature.

It is conceivable that the behavioural effects of vasopressin under

244   TJ. B. VAN WIMERSMA GREIDANUS AND D. DE WIED

physiological conditions result from an increased release of this or related peptides into the CSF in response to emotional stress which accompanies various types of behaviour, in the same ways as its release into the bloodstream is augmented in a similar behavioural situation (Thompson and De Wied, 1973). In this way, the neurohypophysial system is involved in the consolidation of memory processes which enables the organism to cope adequately with environmental changes.

References

Ader, R. and Wied, D. de (1972). *Psychon. Sci.* **29**, 46–48.
Ader, R., Weijnen, J. A. W. M. and Moleman, P. (1972). *Psychon. Sci.* **26**, 125–128.
Albert, D. J. and Mah, C. J. (1972). *Learning and Motivation* **3**, 369–388.
Altman, J., Brunner, R. L. and Bayer, S. A. (1973). *Behav. Biol.* **8**, 557–596.
Arimura, A., Sawano, S., Redding, T. W. and Schally, A. v. (1968). *Neuroendocrinology* **3**, 187–192.
Barnett, R. J. (1954). *Endocrinology* **55**, 484–501.
Berliner, R. W. and Bennett, C. M. (1967). *Amer. J. Med.* **42**, 777–789.
Bohus, B. (1975). *In* "Progr. Brain Res.", Vol. 42 (W. H. Gispen, Tj. B. van Wimersma Greidanus, B. Bohus and D. de Wied, eds). Elsevier Press, Amsterdam, pp. 275– 283.
Bohus, B. (1976). *Horm. Behav.* (in press).
Bohus, B. and Wied, D. de (1967a). *J. Comp. Physiol. Psychol.* **64**, 26–29.
Bohus, B., Ader, R. and Wied, D. de (1972). *Horm. Behav.* **3**, 191–197.
Bohus, B., Gispen, W. H. and Wied, D. de (1973). *Neuroendocrinology* **11**, 137–143.
Bohus, B., Wimersma Greidanus, Tj. B. van and Wied, D. de (1975). *Physiol. Behav.* **14**, 609–615.
Bonjour, J. P. and Malvin, R. L. (1970). *Amer. J. Physiol.* **218**, 1128–1132.
Boyar, R. M., Rosenfeld, R. S., Kapen, S., Finkelstein, J. W., Roffwarg, H. P., Weitzman, E. D. and Hellman, L. (1974). *J. Clin. Invest.* **54**, 609–618.
Brady, J. V. and Nauta, W. J. H. (1953). *J. Comp. Physiol. Psychol.* **46**, 339–346.
Buckingham, J. C. and Wimersma Greidanus, Tj. B. van (1977). *J. Endocrinol.* (in press).
Burlet, A. and Marchetti, J. (1975). *C.R. Soc. Biol. (Paris)* **169**, 148–151.
Chalmers, T. M. and Lewis, A. A. G. (1951). *Clin. Sci.* **10**, 127–135.
Clayton, G. W., Librik, L., Horan, A. and Sussman, L. (1965). *J. Clin. Endocrinol.* **25**, 1156–1162.
Coculescu, M. and Pavel, S. (1973). *J. Clin. Endocrinol.* **36**, 1031–1032.
Corson, S. A. and O'Leary Corson, E. (1967). *Fed. Proc.* **26**, 264.
Cohen, M., Keats, A. S., Krivoy, W. A. and Ungar, G. (1965). *Proc. Soc. Exp. Biol.* **119**, 381–384.
Cox, B. M. and Osman, O. H. (1970). *Brit. J. Pharmacol.* **38**, 157–170.
Cushing, H. and Goetsch, E. (1910). *Amer. J. Physiol.* **27**, 60–86.
Dalby, D. A. (1970). *J. Comp. Physiol. Psychol.* **73**, 278–283.
Deagle, J. H. and Lubar, J. F. (1971). *J. Comp. Physiol. Psychol.* **77**, 277–281.
Demin, N. N. (1974). "Advances in Neurochemistry" (E. M. Kreps *et al.*, eds). Nauka, Leningrad, pp. 29–39.

Doepfner, W., Stürmer, E. and Berde, B. (1963). *Endocrinology* **72**, 897–902.
Douglas, R. J. (1967). *Psychol. Bull.* **67**, 416–442.
Douglas, W. W. (1974). *In* "Handbook of Physiology" Section 7, Vol. 6, Part 1, (E. Knobil and W. H. Sawyer, eds). Amer. Physiol. Soc., pp. 191–224, Washington, D.C.
Dousa, T. P. (1973). *Life Sci.* **13**, 1033–1040.
Dunn, F. L., Breunan, Th. J., Nelson, A. E. and Robertson, G. L. (1973). *J. Clin. Invest.* **52**, 3212–3219.
Feinberg, I. and Earts, E. V. (1969). *Proc. Amer. Psychopath. Ass.* **58**, 334–343.
Fishbein, W. (1971). *Physiol. Behav.* **6**, 279–282.
Fried, P. A. (1972). *Psychol. Bull.* **78**, 292–310.
Garrud, P. (1975). *In* "Progr. in Brain Res." Vol. 42 (W. H. Gispen, Tj. B. van Wimersma Greidanus, B. Bohus and D. de Wied, eds). Elsevier Press, Amsterdam, pp. 173–186.
Garrud, P., Gray, J. A. and Wied, D. de (1974). *Physiol. Behav.* **12**, 109–119.
Glushenko, T. S. and Demin, N. N. (1971). *Dokladi Akad. Nauk SSSR* **197**, 1222–1225.
Goldsmith, P. C. and Zimmerman, A. E. (1975). *Endocrinology, Suppl. to* **96**, A–377.
Grantham, J. J. (1970). *Science* **168**, 1093–1095.
Grantham, J. J. (1971). *Fed. Proc.* **30**, 14–21.
Grantham, J. J. and Burg, M. B. (1966). *Amer. J. Physiol.* **211**, 255–259.
Guillemin, R. (1964). *Recent Progr. Hormone Res.* **20**, 89–130.
Gupta, K. K. (1969). *Lancet* **1**, 581.
Gwinup, G. (1965). *Metabolism* **14**, 1282–1286.
Harris, G. W. (1955). "Neural control of the pituitary gland". Edward Arnold, London.
Hays, R. M. and Franki, N. (1970). *J. Membrane Biol.* **2**, 263–276.
Hays, R. M., Franki, N. and Soberman, R. (1971). *J. Clin. Invest.* **50**, 1016–1018.
Hedge, G. A., Yates, M. B., Marcus, R. and Yates, F. E. (1966). *Endicronology* **79**, 328–340.
Heller, H. and Zaidi, S. M. A. (1974). *In* "Ependyma and neurohormonal regulation" (A. Mitro, ed.). Veda Publishing House, Bratislava, pp. 229–250.
Heller, H., Hasan, S. H. and Saifi, A. Q. (1968). *J. Endocrinol.* **41**, 273–280.
Hirsh, R. (1974). *Behav. Biol.* **12**, 421–444.
Hynie, S. and Sharp, G. W. G. (1971). *Biochim. Biophys. Acta* **230**, 40–51.
Jard, S. (1971). *J. Physiol. (Paris)* **63**, 99–146.
Jewell, P. A. and Verney, E. B. (1957). *Phil. Trans. B.* **240**, 197–224.
Jouvet, M. (1965). *In* "Aspects Anatomo-fonctionels de la Physiologie du Sommeil", CNRS, Paris, pp. 397–449.
Joy, M. R. and Prinz, P. N. (1969). *Physiol. Behav.* **4**, 809–814.
Kachadorian, W. A., Wade, J. B. and DiScala, V. A. (1975). *Science* **190**, 67–69.
Kelsall, A. R. (1949). *J. Physiol. (London)* **112**, 54–58.
Kenyon, J. and Krieckhaus, E. E. (1965). *Psychon. Sci.* **3**, 113–114.
Kimble, D. P. (1968). *Psychol. Bull.* **70**, 285–295.
King, F. A. (1958). *J. Nerv. Ment Dis.* **126**, 57–63.
King, A. R. and Wied, D. de (1974). *J. Comp. Physiol. Psychol.* **86**, 1008–1018.
Koefoed-Johnson, V. and Ussing, H. H. (1953). *Acta Physiol. Scand.* **28**, 60–76.
Kozlowski, G. P., Brownfield, M. S. and Hostetter, G. (1976). *In* "Evolutionary Aspects of Neuroendocrinology" (A. L. Polenor, W. Bargman and B. Scharrer, eds). Springer-Verlag, Berlin (in press).

Krivoy, W. A., Zimmerman, E. and Lande, S. (1974). *Proc. Nat. Acad. Sci. U.S.A.* **71**, 1852–1856.

Kurtzman, N. A. and Boonjarern, S. (1975). *Nephron* **15**, 167–185.

Lande, S., Witter, A. and Wied, D. de (1971). *J. Biol. Chem.* **246**, 2058–2062.

Lande, S., Flexner, J. B. and Flexner, L. B. (1972). *Proc. Nat. Acad. Sci. U.S.A.* **69**, 558–560.

Landfield, P. W., McGaugh, J. L. and Tusa, R. J. (1972). *Science* **175**, 87–89.

Leaf, A., Anderson, J. and Page, L. B. (1958). *J. Gen. Physiol.* **41**, 657–688.

Leconte, P. and Black, V. (1970). *C.R. Acad. Sci. (Paris) (Série D)* **271**, 226–229.

Liss, Ph. (1968). *J. Comp. Physiol. Psychol.* **66**, 193–197.

Longo, V. G. and Loizzo, A. (1973). *In* "Pharmacology and the Future of Man" (F. E. Bloom and G. H. Acheson, eds), Vol. 4. Karger, Basel, pp. 46–54.

Malvin, R. L. (1971). *Fed. Proc.* **30**, 1383–1386.

Martin, J. B., Renaud, L. P. and Brazeau, P. (1976). *Lancet* (in press).

Martini, L. and Morpurgo, C. (1955). *Nature (London)* **175**, 1127–1128.

Matthies, H. (1975). *Life Sci.* **15**, 2017–2031.

McCann, S. M. (1957). *Endocrinology* **60**, 664–676.

McCann, S. M. and Brobeck, J. R. (1954). *Proc. Soc. Exp. Biol.* **87**, 318–324.

McCann S. M., Antunes-Rodriguez, J., Naller, R. and Valtin, H. (1966). *Endocrinology* **79**, 1058–1064.

McDonald, R. U., Weise, V. K. and Patrick, R. W. (1956). *Proc. Soc. Exp. Biol.* **93**, 348–349.

Milhorat, Th. H. (1975). *In* "Brain–Endocrine Interaction II" (K. M. Knigge, D. E. Scott, H. Kobayashi and S. Ishii, eds). Karger, Basel, pp. 270–281.

Miller, N. E., DiCara, L. V. and Wolf, G. (1968). *Amer. J. Physiol.* **215**, 684–686.

Miller, L., Drew, W. G. and Schwartz, I. (1971). *Percept. Motor Skills* **33**, 118.

Miller, R. E., Yueh-Chien, H., Wiley, M. K. and Hewitt, R. (1974). *Neuroendocrinology* **14**, 233–250.

Mirsky, I. A., Stein, M. and Paulisch, G. (1954). *Endocrinology* **55**, 28–39.

Moore, W. W. (1971). *Fed. Proc.* **30**, 1387–1394.

Mulder, A. H., Geuze, J. J. and Wied, D. de (1970). *Endocrinology* **87**, 61–79.

Nadel, L. (1968). *Physiol. Behav.* **3**, 891–900.

Nash, F. D. (1971). *Fed. Proc.* **30**, 1376–1377.

O'Connor, W. J. and Verney, E. B. (1942). *Quart. J. Exp. Physiol.* **31**, 393–408.

Orloff, J. and Handler, J. S. (1967). *Amer. J. Med.* **42**, 757–768.

Orloff, J. and Handler, J. S. (1971). *Ann. N.Y. Acad. Sci.* **185**, 345–450.

Pavel, S. (1965). *Endocrinology* **77**, 812–817.

Pavel, S. (1970). *J. Clin. Endocrinol.* **31**, 369–371.

Pearlmutter, A. F., Rapino, E. and Saffran, M. (1974). *Neuroendocrinology* **15**, 106–119.

Pickering, B. T., Jones, C. W. and Burford, G. D. (1971). *In* "Neurohypophysial Hormones" (G. E. W. Wolstenholme and J. Birch, eds). Churchill Livingstone, Edinburgh and London, pp. 58–74.

Rich, I. and Thompson, R. (1965). *J. Comp. Physiol. Psychol.* **59**, 66–74.

Rigter, H., Riezen, H. van and Wied, D. de (1974). *Physiol. Behav.* **13**, 381–388.

Rodriguez, E. M. (1970). *In* "Aspects in neuroendocrinology" (W. Bargmann and B. Scharrer, eds). Springer-Verlag, Berlin, pp. 352–365.

Roosenbloom, A. A. and Fisher, D. A. (1975). *Neuroendocrinology* **17**, 354–361.

Rydin, H. and Verney, E. B. (1938). *Quart. J. Exp. Physiol.* **27**, 343–374.

Sacks, H., Fawcett, P., Takabatake, Y. and Portonova, R. (1969). *Recent Progr. Hormone Res.* **25**, 447–491.

Saffran, M., Schally, A. V. and Benfey, B. G. (1955). *Endocrinology* **57**, 439–444.

Saffran, M., Pearlmutter, A. F., Rapino, E. and Upton, G. V. (1972). *Biochem. Biophys. Res. Comm.* **49**, 748–751.

Sawyer, W. H. (1964). *Endocrinology* **75**, 981–990.

Sawyer, W. H. (1974). *In* "Handbook of Physiology", Section 7, Vol. 6, Part 1, (E. Knobil and W. H. Sawyer, eds). Amer. Physiol. Soc., Washington, D.C., pp. 443–468.

Sawyer, W. H. and Manning, M. (1973). *Annu. Rev. Pharmacol.* **13**, 5–17.

Schally, A. V., Saffran, M. and Zimmerman, B. (1958). *Biochem. J.* **70**, 97–103.

Segal, M. and Olds, J. (1972). *J. Neurophysiol.* **35**, 680–690.

Seif, S. M., Huellmantel, A. B., Stillman, M., Recht, L. and Robinson, A. G. (1975). *Endocrinology, Suppl. to Vol.* **96**, A–272.

Shapiro, C. M., Griesel, R. D., Bartel, P. R. and Jooste, T. L. (1975). *J. App. Physiol.* **39**(2), 187–190.

Share, L. (1961). *Endocrinology* **69**, 925–933.

Share, L. (1965). *Amer. J. Physiol.* **208**, 219–223.

Share, L. (1967). *Endocrinology* **81**, 1140–1146.

Smelik, P. G. (1960). *Acta Endocrinol. (Kbh.)* **33**, 437–443.

Smelik, P. G., Gaarenstroom, J. H., Konijnendijk, W. and Wied, D. de (1962). *Acta Physiol. Pharmacol. Neerl.* **11**, 20–33.

Smith, H. W. (1957). *Amer. J. Med.* **23**, 623–657.

Sobel, H., Levy, R. S., Marmorston, J., Schapiro, S. and Rosenfeld, S. (1955). *Proc. Soc. Exp. Biol.* **89**, 10–13.

Sterba, G. (1974a). *In* "Ependyma annneurohormonal regulation" (A. Mitro, ed.). Veda Publishing House, Bratislava, pp. 143–173.

Sterba, G. (1974b). *In* "Neurosecretion—The final neuroendocrine pathway" (F. Knowles and L. Vollrath, eds). Springer-Verlag, Berlin, pp. 38–47.

Stern, W. C. (1971). *Physiol. Behav.* **7**, 345–352.

Swaab, D. F., Pool, C. W. and Nijveldt, F. (1975). *J. Neural Transmission* **36**, 195–215.

Taylor, A., Mamelak, M., Reaven, E. and Maffly, R. (1973). *Science* **181**, 347–350.

Thompson, E. A. and Wied, D. de (1973). *Physiol. Behav.* **11**, 377–380.

Urban, I. and Wied, D. de (1975). *Brain Res.* **97**, 362–366.

Valatx, J. L., Chouvet, G. and Jouvet, M. (1975). *In* "Progress in Brain Research", Vol. 42 (W. H. Gispen, Tj. B. van Wimersma Greidanus, B. Bohus and D. de Wied, eds). Elsevier Press, Amsterdam, pp. 115–120.

Valtin, H. (1967). *Amer. J. Med.* **42**, 814–827.

Valtin, H. and Schroeder, H. A. (1964). *Amer. J. Physiol.* **206**, 425–430.

Vander, A. J. (1968). *Circulat. Res.* **23**, 605–609.

Verney, E. B. (1947). *Proc. Roy. Soc. B.* **135**, 25–106.

Vliegenthart, J. F. G. and Versteeg, D. H. G. (1965). *Proc. Kon. Ned. Akad. Wetensch.* **68**, 1–10.

Vliegenthart, J. F. G. and Versteeg, D. H. G. (1967). *J. Endocrinol.* **38**, 3–12.

Vorherr, H., Bradbury, M. W. B., Hoghoughi, M. and Kleeman, C. R. (1968). *Endocrinology* **83**, 246–250.

Wal, B. van der, Wiegman, T., Janssen, J. F., Delver, A. and Wied, D. de (1965). *Acta endocrinol. (Kbh.)* **48**, 81–90.

Wied, D. de (1961). *Endocrinology* **68**, 956–970.

Wied, D. de (1964). *Amer. J. Physiol.* **207**, 255–259.

Wied, D. de (1965). *Int. J. Neuropharmacol.* **4**, 157–167.

Wied, D. de (1968). *Neuroendocrinology* **3**, 129–135.

248   TJ. B. VAN WIMERSMA GREIDANUS AND D. DE WIED

Wied, D. de (1971). *Nature (London)* **232**, 58–60.
Wied, D. de (1976). *Life Sci.* **19**, 685–690.
Wied, D. de and Gispen, W. H. (1976). *Psychopharmacologia* **46**, 27–29.
Wied, D. de, Bohus, B., Ernst, A. M., Jong, W. de., Nieuwenhuizen, W., Pieper, E. E. M. and Yasamura, S. (1968). *In* "Memoirs of the Society for Endocrinology No. 17" (V. H. T. James and J. Landon, eds). Cambridge University Press, Cambridge, pp. 159–173.
Wied, D. de., Greven, H. M., Lande, S. and Witter, A. (1972). *Brit. J. Pharmacol.* **45**, 118–122.
Wied, D. de., Bohus, B. and Wimersma Greidanus, Tj. B. van (1974). *In* "Progr. Brain Res.", Vol. 41 (D. F. Swaab and J. P. Schadé, eds). Elsevier Press, Amsterdam, pp. 417–428.
Wied, D. de., Bohus, B. and Wimersma Greidanus, Tj. B. van (1975). *Brain Res.* **85**, 152–156.
Wied, D. de., Bohus, B., Urban, I., Wimersma Greidanus, Tj. B. van and Gispen, W. H. (1976). *In* "Chemistry, biophysics and biology of peptides" (R. Walter and J. Meienhofer, eds). Ann Arbor Science Publishers (in press).
Wiley, M. K., Pearlmutter, A. F. and Miller, R. E. (1974). *Neuroendocrinology* **14**, 257–270.
Wimersma Greidanus, Tj. B. van, Bohus, B. and Wied, D. de (1973). *In* "Progr. Endocrinol." Int. Congr. Ser. No. 273 (R. Scow, ed.). Excerpta Medica, Amsterdam, pp. 197–201.
Wimersma Greidanus, Tj. B. van, Bohus, B. and Wied, D. de (1974a). *Neuroendocrinology* **14**, 280–288.
Wimersma Greidanus, Tj. B. van, Buys, R. M., Hollemans, H. J. G. and Jong, W. de (1974b). *Experientia* **30**, 1217–1218.
Wimersma Greidanus, Tj. B. van, Dogterom, J. and Wied, D. de (1975a). *Life Sci.* **16**, 637–644.
Wimersma Greidanus, Tj. B. van, Bohus, B. and Wied, D. de (1975b). *In* "Anatomical Neuroendocrinology" (W. E. Stumpf and L. D. Grand, eds). Karger, Basel, pp. 284–289.
Wimersma Greidanus, Tj. B. van, Bohus, B. and Wied, D. de (1975c) *In* "Progr. Brain Res.", Vol. 42 (W. H. Gispen, Tj. B. van Wimersma Greidanus, B. Bohus and D. de Wied, eds). Elsevier Press, Amsterdam, pp. 133–141.
Wimersma Greidanus, Tj. B. van and Wied, D. de. (1976). *Pharmacol. Biochem. Behav.* (in press).
Wittkowski, W. (1968). *Z. Zellforsch.* **92**, 207–216.
Yates, F. E., Russell, S. M., Dallman, M. F., Hedge, G. A., McCann, S. M. and Dhariwal, A. P. S. (1971). *Endocrinology* **88**, 3–15.
Zimmerman, E. A. (1976). *In* "Frontiers in Neuroendocrinology", Vol. 4 (L. Martini and W. F. Ganong, eds). Raven Press, New York (in press).
Zimmerman, E. A., Hsu, K. C., Robinson, A. G., Carmel, P. W., Frantz, A. G. and Tannenbaum, M. (1973a). *Endocrinology* **92**, 931–940.
Zimmerman, E. A., Carmel, P. W., Husain, M. K., Ferin, M., Tannenbaum, M., Frantz, A. G. and Robinson, A. G. (1973b). *Science* **182**, 925–927.
Zimmerman, E. A., Kozlowski, G. P. and Scott, D. E. (1975). *In* "Brain–Endocrine Interaction" II (K. M. Knigge, D. E. Scott, H. Kobayahsi and S. Ishii, eds). Karger, Basel, pp. 123–134.

Chapter 8

Experience, Learning and Brain Metabolism

STEVEN P. R. ROSE and JEFF HAYWOOD

Brain Research Group, Open University,
Milton Keynes, England and Department of Biochemistry, University of
Leeds, Leeds, England

I. Specificity and Plasticity: Learning and Memory

There are three general features which any nervous system must possess if it is to carry out its functions effectively. The first may be defined as specificity: that is, during the development of the organism, the complex of sense organ → interneurone → effector pathways must necessarily become wired in such a way that the organism can respond in a predictable and reliable manner to predictable and reliable inputs. The details of this wiring must be fairly precisely specified by the organism's own internal programme of development, and be rather insensitive to fluctuating changes in the organism's environment, if it is to survive.

The second and third properties of the nervous system are the reverse of the first, and both are encompassed by the term plasticity. Thus a nervous system must be able to respond to short-term and transient changes in the environment by a modulation of its output so as to adapt it to changing circumstances. However, these modulations must be brief alterations in what we may, somewhat naively, refer to as the "normal ground state" of the system. Finally, the nervous system must be able to respond to long-term, repetitive or "significant" alterations in the environment by long-term or permanent changes in its output. Some of these long-term changes are rather general sequelae of environmental modification or experience, especially during development. For example, as discussed by Balázs (Chapter 3) undernutrition during periods of major brain growth in young mammals results in apparently irreversible changes in brain cell number, while changes in hormone level during development—thyroidectomy for instance—may affect cell number and wiring. Such insults result not merely in cellular defects but apparently irreversible behavioural sequelae as well (Dobbing and Smart, 1974).

More subtle environmental changes, for example between "enriched" and "impoverished" environments during development or even adulthood in the rat will result in long-term changes in cellular connectivity, as evidenced both biochemically, in the levels of certain supposed neurotransmitter enzyme systems, and morphologically, in terms of dendritic branching and synaptic structure (see below and Rosenzweig and Bennett, 1975; Greenough, 1975). These long-term environmental effects on brain and behaviour are examples of the plastic adaptation of the organism to experience, but must be distinguished from learning, that is the very precise and predictable modification of behaviour in response to particular experiences. In the sense we use the word here, learning is the set of processes whereby particular experiences have specific effects on behaviour. We assume that there is a continuity between the physiological, biochemical and morphological events in the brain which underlie both experience in the broad sense and learning in the narrow sense (Horn et al., 1973a; Rose et al., 1975; Rose, 1976a and b).

In this chapter, we are going to review evidence concerning both the biochemical sequelae of experience in the broad sense, and of learning and memory in the narrow sense. Before embarking upon such a review however, it will be useful to clarify some of the conceptual issues involved, so as to make it clear what sorts of biochemical evidence and systems we should be looking for. To start with why should one expect experience to leave a biochemical "trace"? Whilst no neurobiologist would question that some sort of change in brain properties must occur to encode experience and to alter the subsequent output of the organism, is it reasonable to expect that this change should be expressed in an altered biochemistry?

To confront this argument, consider the situation when kittens are reared in a visually restricted environment, where they see only vertical or horizontal black and white stripes, or darkness punctuated by light points, or a stationary universe illuminated only by stroboscopic flashes. When electrical recordings are made in the visual cortex of cats whose early environment has been thus restricted, the response properties of the neurones are found to be altered in a predictable way to "model" the environmental restriction (see Blakemore 1976, for review). The physiological properties of the cells have been altered so as to code for the modified environment. Should we expect their biochemistry to change too? The physiology of the neurones could not change without some underlying structural reorganization of cell connectivity having occurred, either by the growth or restriction of particular synapses, the realignment of the dendritic tree or the modification of the membrane properies of the cell. (Or indeed, a modification of the surrounding glia which thereby modulate neuronal properties. The possible role of the glia is perhaps somewhat cavalierly dismissed in most discussions of memory mechanisms.) Structural reorganization of the neurones has indeed been shown to occur in varying conditions of visual deprivation and stimulation. Changes may occur in dendritic structure as observed by Golgi staining (Valverde, 1967, 1971) synaptic dimensions, numbers of vesicles (Cragg, 1967; Vrensson and de Groot, 1974; 1975), or neuronal domains (de Vay, 1976).

At the very least, even if the metabolic states of a neurone before and after reorganization of its response properties are so similar as to be indistinguishable with current biochemical techniques, there must be a stage during reorganization when considerable metabolic mobilization occurs, and biochemical detection is possible. This is also true for memory and learning. Behavioural studies have revealed a great deal, in both human subjects and in animals, of the processes involved in memory consolidation. To simplify a voluminous literature, there are at least two separate processes involved in learning and memory formation (see e.g. McGaugh, 1966; McGaugh and Gold, 1975). During the first, known as short-term memory, the learned response or memory is very labile and easily disrupted by electrical, mechanical or chemical insult to the brain. This period lasts from minutes to hours. During the second period, which may last the remainder of the organism's lifetime, the memory trace appears to be extraordinarily stable, as there seems to be no way short of death or large scale ablation of the cerebral cortex, of permanently erasing the memory from the store (although it may be obliterated by other learned responses, such as learning the reverse of a prior habit). Such a labile consolidation period followed by considerable stability must again imply a structural reorganization of cellular properties into a new, essentially permanent configuration. There is anatomical, physiological and behavioural evidence (and some biochemical, too, based on the use of inhibitors— see below) that the process of learning, short-term memory and long-term memory are distinct, involving both different brain regions and different physiological mechanisms (for review see Rosenzweig and Bennett, 1975). This is not to argue that the properties of the nervous system can be "solved" exclusively at the molecular or cellular level, of course, but simply to insist that the biochemical changes which take place are one part of the hierarchical jigsaw we are trying to assemble. Nor is it to assume that because biochemical changes must in principle take place in response to experience, our present level of technology is of necessity adequate to detect them. We are always working with small differences in rates of production of molecules, in levels of metabolites and in enzyme activities, which are barely at the level of reliable detectability. Nor may we assume that, because we find biochemical changes associated with a particular experience, then these changes must be the necessary, sufficient and exclusive correlates of this experience. The implications of these questions are considered in the next two sections.

II. Behavioural Methods and Problems

It is relatively easy to alter the environment of an organism in a defined manner; it is much harder to predict precisely the response of any particular animal to that change. Most of the behavioural problems in this area arise from attempting to define more precisely that aspect of experience with which the changed biochemical parameter most directly correlates. Some approaches make use of relatively extreme environmental modification without attempts to dissect them out more distinctly. For example, visual deprivation, from birth or for relatively long periods during adulthood, followed by visual stimulation, is a functional stimulus to the animal, but one in which any observed biochemical sequelae may be the result of changed sensory input *per se*, altered motor, hormonal or circulatory activity, altered arousal states, disrupted circadian rhythms, or the learning of some aspect of the stimulus situation. Thus we have a "strong" stimulus situation likely to produce large biochemical effects the behavioural significance of which may be obscure.

A second favoured situation is that of environmental enrichment versus impoverishment, developed originally by Krech, Bennett and Rosenzweig in Berkeley (reviewed in Rosenzweig and Bennett, 1975). In this, animals, generally rats, are reared either in varying degrees of social and sensory isolation, or in communal cages with a large number of toys, opportunities for exploratory behaviour and to run mazes. Clearly the differences between the two groups are manifold—in particular there will be stress and hormonal differences—and to dissect out which, if any one, of these environmental and behavioural differences is associated with which observed morphological or biochemical difference would seem well nigh impossible.

We come next to the more specific learning tasks. Here, it might be argued that the likely biochemical effects would be smaller than in strong stimulus situations, but also that there would be fewer problems in controlling for effects external to the learning itself. Unfortunately this has not proved as straightforward as is sometimes believed. The commonest learning situations have been those in which the animal learns to avoid aversive situations or seek rewarding ones. Aversive stimuli are generally electric shocks and the animal has to learn that a light or a buzzer indicates that a shock is imminent, and to move to another compartment or to press a lever to avoid it. A jump-box, where a mouse jumps off an electrified grid to a shelf above the floor has been used by the Chapel Hill group (Glassman, 1969; Entingh *et al.*, 1975), and a shuttle-box, where a goldfish swims over a barrier which divides its tank, by Agranoff (e.g. Agranoff, 1971). Controls in such situations are often described as "yoked"—that is animals which see the light or hear the buzzer, but cannot escape the shock, and therefore cannot learn how to avoid their fate. Another "quiet control" group which remains in its home cages during the period of the experiment is sometimes introduced. However, "yoked" controls have a number of disadvantages (see e.g. Bateson, 1970; 1976); notably, that it may not be true that the yoked controls are learning "nothing". For example, they may be learning that there is "no" escape from the shock and hence arousal and stress will be different between the two groups. In addition, whilst one has a measure of the behaviour of the experimental animal—how many trials it takes to learn the escape route—there is no adequate measure for any aspect of the behaviour of the yoked control group.

An example of the learning of a rewarded discrimination comes from the experiments of Hydén (e.g. Hydén, 1973) in which rats with a natural preference for reaching for their food with a particular paw are forced instead to learn to reach for it with the non-preferred paw. Once an animal learns, that is reverses its preference, this behaviour remains stable for very long periods, and in such an experiment the two sides of the brain can be compared, the non-learning hemisphere serving as a control for the learning one. However any biochemical changes found during the acquisition of such a skill may not necessarily be correlates of learning; they may for example, be sequelae of the attention that the animal has to pay to the situation, or of the altered motor requirement involved. Other types of learning situation which have been used include the induction or reversal of the natural responses of the animal. These include such one-trial learning situations as the induction of "fear of the dark" in rodents which, given a choice between a dark and a lit compartment will normally choose the darkened one. However, if they are shocked when they try to enter the dark compartment they will thereafter shun it. The situation has been used by Ungar in his "transfer of learning experiments" (e.g. Ungar et al., 1972); Mark and his colleagues have used one-trial learning in the chick, in which the bird learns to discriminate between small differently coloured objects on the floor of its cage, and to avoid pecking at the class of objects which have been coated in an evil-tasting substance such as methylanthranilate (e.g. Watts and Mark, 1971).

Finally, our own work has utilized the imprinting situation, a "natural" learning process whereby the recently hatched chick learns to show a preference for a particular prominent moving object, which it subsequently follows as "mother" (Bateson, 1966, 1971). This natural learning can successfully be modelled under controlled conditions: hatching the chick in the dark, exposing it for defined periods to the object on which it is to be imprinted (generally a flashing light) and later testing the chick's approach behaviour when confronted with a choice between the light on which it was imprinted and an alternative of different colour and pattern (Bateson and Jaeckel, 1974; Bateson and Wainwright, 1972). In the imprinting situation, in addition to learning the chick is likely to be involved in motor activity, stress, arousal and sensory stimulation. Some of the behavioural controls which may discriminate between the biochemical correlates of these different aspects of the bird's behaviour in the learning situation are described below.

III. Biochemical Methods and Problems

There are two fundamentally different views of the way in which biochemical mechanisms operate in the processes of learning and memory, one involving quantitative and the other qualitative biochemical changes. The former is the majority view at present. Quantitative changes depend upon alterations in the relative proportion of substances already present in the brain, e.g. increased amounts or activities of certain enzymes or their metabolites. The coding and storage ability of the brain then depends upon changes in spatial parameters or neuronal interconnectivity modulated by rather general biochemical processes. Qualitative changes also result from the action of experiential events on metabolism, but in this case the response is the production of substances which are unique, i.e. code for, that experience alone. A consequence of this model would be that memory should be transferable between individuals by biochemical means, assuming they all use the same code. This is the rationale of experiments by Ungar and others (e.g. Ungar, 1970; 1971; Ungar et al., 1972). As we do not consider the case for biochemical mechanisms of this sort either experimentally or theoretically convincing, we do not discuss them here at all, and readers wishing to examine the evidence in their favour should consult the references cited above.

There are two main methods available to those interested in showing quantitative biochemical changes correlated with experience. Either look at enzymic and metabolic differences between experienced and naive animals, or else pharmacologically intervene in particular metabolic pathways and observe the behavioural consequences. These two approaches, which complement each other but have quite distinct features and problems, are termed "correlative" and "pharmacological" respectively, and are treated separately below.

Both approaches, of course, demand prior hypotheses concerning the nature of the biochemical changes likely to occurring; of all the possible metabolic systems or pharmacological interventions, which to study? For semi-accidental, historical rather than theoretical reasons, RNA and protein metabolism have been the most intensively studied (see Rose, 1970 for a discussion of the reasons why this has been the case); amongst enzyme systems, despite the fact that there is no conclusive evidence for any particular candidate as a transmitter in the cerebral cortex, closest attention has been paid to those enzymes involved in metabolism of substances known to be transmitters elsewhere in the CNS, such as acetylcholine, or believed to have a general membrane transport role, such as Na^+, K^+, ATPase (e.g.

Deutsch, 1971). By contrast, although the brain has a considerable lipid content, most of it integrated in membranes, especially the functionally important axonal membrane and its sheath, virtually no work has been done on the effects of experience on the lipid portion of lipoproteins. Only part of the reason for this lack is the difficulty of lipid and lipoprotein chemistry; the fact that proteins have played a more dominant role in biochemical research, and hence are more strongly favoured as candidates for cellular modification has also been important. This restricted approach can lead to misinterpretation. For instance changes in protein metabolism found as a result of experience may be interpreted as representing the end product of the metabolic chain, perhaps regarded as potential receptors or neurotransmitter enzymes, rather than as enzymes involved in lipoprotein metabolism. Further, observed changes may, unless the necessary controls to exclude such possibilities are performed, be artefacts; for instance an apparent elevation in the rate of protein synthesis may merely reflect enhanced uptake of radioactive precursor into the cell as a result of altered blood flow or changed levels of free-pool amino acids, or alterations in the rate of degradation of proteins (Rose *et al.*, 1975; Hambley *et al.*, 1976). Alternatively the changes may lie on a

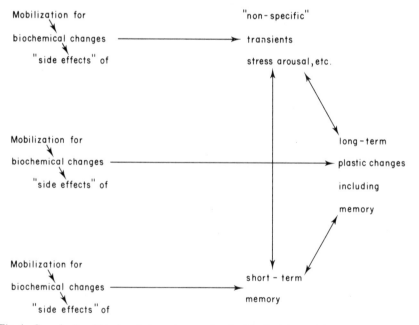

Fig. 1. Complexity of biochemical results associated with plasticity and learning.

biochemical sidepath to the "real" correlate—for instance, a genuine underlying biochemical correlate may be a process requiring ATP, and the level of ATP may be rate-limiting for protein synthesis. Hence protein synthesis will be modified indirectly when plastic responses to experience and learning occur. Finally, those changes that are detected may be biochemical correlates not of learning at all, but of a feature of the organism's behaviour which is a precondition for learning—an alteration in sensory input or arousal level, for example (Lat *et al.*, 1973; Bateson, 1976). These interactions among, and distinctions between, mobilization for, side effects of, and directly correlated biochemical changes associated with experience are shown in Fig. 1.

IV. Correlation Studies

A. *Background*

Correlation studies try to demonstrate that during or after learning there is a measurable change in some metabolic parameter of the brain of a learning as compared to a control animal. Ideally they also ought to show that the extent of the biochemical change correlates with the extent of the behavioural change, although such attempts have rarely been made. Another major methodological consideration is that of the time at which the biochemical observation is made in relation to the experience. Should it be during the early phase of learning, during the consolidation period, or during the subsequent recall period? There is ample evidence, which will be discussed below, to show that many biochemical changes are transient, occurring at the onset of the experience or at a particular period during consolidation. A time-course of change of all metabolites over the entire period of learning may be the only way to obtain a meaningful picture of the biochemical mechanisms concerned, but is likely to prove impractical except in particular cases. An example of the type of time-dependent effects that occur in the imprinting situation is given in Section IV.C.3.

There are three experimental approaches in common use:

1. measurements of changes in enzyme activities,
2. direct measurement of changes in absolute levels of substances such as RNA, protein and small metabolites, and
3. indirect measurements of levels of macromolecules or of rates of turnover by isotopic techniques.

The first approach is quite precise in its intentions: the enzyme under scrutiny is a defined entity, and changes in activity are potentially interpretable in terms of function. It does however suffer from the inevitable problem of relating *in vitro* enzyme specific activities to the *in vivo* situation.

The second is also clearly defined; one can specify a type of RNA, e.g. tRNA; or protein, e.g. S-100, to be measured; but it is rather little used except for small molecules. This is mainly because the changes in absolute levels of most macromolecules, at least averaged over relatively large regions of tissue, are likely to be so low that conventional assay techniques do not have sufficient sensitivity to detect them. However methods such as electron microscopy and histochemistry may prove of use in circumventing this question.

However, both the first two approaches are "needle in the hay-stack", relying on biochemical intuition as to which substances or enzymes may prove interesting. The third approach is by far the most used, and in many respects is the most fraught with problems of interpretation. The relationship between an administered precursor (e.g. amino acid or nucleotide), its macromolecular product and subsequent catabolic products is far from simple, whether the precursor is delivered via an intracranial or peripheral route (Oja, 1973; see also Dunn, 1975). Peripherally administered precursors must first enter the blood stream, be carried into the cerebral blood vessels and penetrate the capillary walls. Penetration is not by free diffusion; the brain has uptake and exclusion properties ("blood–brain barrier") and much of the precursor does not enter the cerebral tissue, but is lost in the rest of the body. Hence body blood flow characteristics will affect the distribution of the precursor and these are likely to be affected by prolonged or intense motor activity or fluctuating hormone levels during stress. Cerebral blood flow has itself been shown to vary with activity, for instance visual stimulation (Bondy *et al.*, 1974). For intracranially administered precursors both the trauma of injection, and the need for diffusion of the precursor throughout the brain from its initial area of high concentration, can influence the incorporation data obtained. Even when the precursor has reached the extracellular fluid there are still uptake problems related to the heterogeneity of the cell types present. A valid measure of the pool of precursor available for incorporation must refer to the subcellular compartment in which synthesis of the macromolecule occurs. In addition it must be remembered that the immediate precursor for protein synthesis is not the amino acid but the aminoacyl t-RNA. As the observed rate of incorporation of a radioactive precursor into its product macromolecule is dependent upon the ratio radioactive/total precursor in the immediate pool (specific radioactivity), fluctuations in this ratio will give different rates of incorporation even with a constant rate of macromolecular synthesis. Clearly in the initial stage of the experiment, just after injection, the ratio is rising from zero to a value which will remain steady for some period of time. Differences in this rate of increase will generate different summated incorporation rates. Moreover, as macromolecules are also being degraded, the precursor is being liberated, possibly to be quickly reutilized, and so the extent of incorporation at the end of the experiment is related to turnover, rather than synthetic rate. Clearly the longer the incorporation period, the greater these problems will become. In no case has it been possible to adequately define and measure all the variables, although degrees of approximation have been achieved. Instead, series of experiments have been performed in which different precursors have been used, and different aspects of the same metabolic sequence have been shown to vary in similar manner. Such studies tend to suggest that the interpretation in terms of changed synthesis is correct, even if any individual experiment itself cannot entirely rule out precursor-pool effects.

B. *Correlates of Broad Sense Plasticity*

1. *Enriched versus impoverished environments*

We consider two examples of experiments showing biochemical correlates of experience or environmental modification likely to involve learning but in which the behavioural sequelae of the experience have not been distinguished: the enriched/impoverished environment work of the Berkeley group of Bennett, Rosenzweig and their coworkers, and our own studies of dark rearing and light exposure.

The enriched/impoverished paradigm has been described above. Over the past 15 years there have been numerous reports of morphological and biochemical differences in the brains of rats exposed to the differing conditions, and a variety of factors such as onset of assignment to conditions, period per day of exposure to enrichment, and types of enrichment procedure, have been investigated. For example, recently it was shown that mere exposure to an enriched situation without the possibility of active participation in it is inadequate to produce the brain weight differences characteristic of enrichment (Ferchmin *et al.*, 1975). The morphological and biochemical differences which have been examined however are relatively few. There is a general growth of the posterior neocortex (Bennett *et al.*, 1964) accounted for both by an increased dendritic branching (Greenough, 1975), so that neuropil volume increases, and also an increased size of neuronal nuclei and perikarya (Diamond *et al.*, 1975). Such changes are generally of the order of 5–12%. There is an increase in the dimensions of the synaptic thickening, although recent reports suggest that this is not so marked as was at first believed (Møllgaard *et al.*, 1971; Greenough, 1975; Bennett, 1975). There is an enhanced incorporation of amino acids into protein in synaptosomal and nuclear fractions from the cerebral cortex and hippocampus (Levitan *et al.*, 1972) and some rather less well-defined changes in glucosamine incorporation (Ramirez *et al.*, 1974). There are also changes in the specific activity of certain enzymes, such as AChE (Rosenzweig *et al.*, 1972). However, in our view the value of further studies using this type of paradigm is likely to be limited by the very generality of the experiential situation and the experimental difficulties lying in the way of refining it further. What the studies have provided is convincing evidence of the existence and extent of experientially imposed biochemical and morphological modification of the brain; they do not enable us to go further in either elucidating the biochemical mechanisms or the exact nature of the experiential trigger(s) that may be involved.

2. Dark rearing and light exposure

A somewhat more precisely controlled experiential contrast is provided in the dark rearing/light exposure situation. Dark-reared, or light-deprived animals, may be compared with light-exposed litter mates, with "normals" or with animals deprived of sight by eyelid suturing or enucleation. Both the nature and extent of the light stimulus can be controlled and "visual" and "non-visual" regions of the brain compared. In some experiments, for example using light stimulation in birds, where the optic tract shows complete decussation (Chakrabarti *et al.*, 1974; Chakrabarti and Daginawala, 1975; Bondy *et al.*, 1974) one half of the brain can be used as a control for the other. Some recent experiments involving a visual discrimination task in rats (Křivánek *et al.*, 1975) have also been able to match control and trained halves of the brain. However, in general, experiments involving dark rearing and light exposure may only be regarded as measuring general sequelae of plasticity rather than learning *per se*.

Dark rearing and subsequent light exposure have been shown to result in measurable morphological changes in the visual pathways and also frontal cortex in several rodent species, studied either using Golgi methods or at the e.m. level. According to Valverde (1967, 1971) there is a reduction of dendritic spines on the apical dendrites of visual cortex pyramidal cells during dark rearing in mice, with a sprouting of spines taking place on light exposure. Cragg (1967, 1970) has shown changes in synaptic number and density in the visual cortex and lateral geniculate in dark-reared rats subsequently exposed to light, whilst Vrensson and de Groot (1974, 1975) have claimed that dark rearing for seven months in the rabbit results in a 40% deficit of synaptic vesicles, but no change in the number of synaptic zones. Subsequent light exposure did not reverse this deficit, which remained even after a year of normal visual experience.

Mareš et al. (1975) have followed DNA metabolism autoradiographically with ^{3}H-thymidine, and shown that in rats the normal decline in the rate of glial proliferation which occurs during development proceeds faster than during visual deprivation in the lateral geniculate and visual cortex. Dewar and his coworkers (Dewar and Reading, 1973; Dewar et al., 1973) found a lowered rate of incorporation of precursor into RNA in blind compared with sighted rats, and in dark-reared compared with light-exposed rats.

Our own studies* have been primarily concerned with protein metabolism. The initial observations (Rose, 1967a; Richardson and Rose, 1972) were that when incorporation of lysine into protein was compared in light-exposed (L) and dark-reared (D) animals, there was a transient elevation of incorporation into visual cortex protein between one and three hours after the onset of exposure of the L animals. With a one hour pulse of radioactivity, the elevation in incorporation was maximal, about 20% above control levels, after one hour of exposure to the light. However, within three hours the incorporation was back to control levels, and if exposure was prolonged thereafter, then depending on the conditions of illumination, there was a depression of up to 20% in incorporation in Ls compared with Ds which could last for up to four days. A similar transient elevation in incorporation, followed by a long lasting depression, occurred in the lateral geniculate and retina (where the effect was much larger than in the cortex). However, there was no elevation in the motor cortex, and there was no change in incorporation rate in the liver.

* Collaborators in this work include Dr A. Jones-Lecointe, Dr K. Richardson and Dr A. K. Sinha.

Thus there is an apparent transient elevation in protein synthetic rate along the visual pathway following the first exposure to light of dark-reared rats. In the further study of the biochemical significance of this effect we have concentrated on the visual cortex at the height of the elevation, one hour after the onset of light exposure. Biochemically, a key question is whether the apparent elevation in protein synthetic rate is real, or reflects merely changes in precursor pools, blood flow or turnover. If it is real, what is the molecular biological mechanism involved; are we observing a generalized elevation in synthesis of all cell proteins, or a particular response in a limited number? From the cell biological point of view we may then ask: are the new proteins cell-specific, and if so, what is their role in the cell's economy?

To approach this question, we labelled the proteins of one hour L and D animals as before and, following the labelling, separated the proteins from visual cortex and retina into soluble and insoluble fractions. Each group was then further subdivided, using polyacrylamide gel electrophoresis and a double-labelling procedure (Richardson and Rose, 1973a and b). Ten out of 41 retinal protein fractions, and six out of 41 visual cortex protein fractions, showed reliable elevations in incorporation of up to 2–300% in Ls compared with Ds; three retinal and one visual cortex protein fraction showed depressions of incorporation. Thus it does seem as if incorporation into only a limited number of proteins is affected by the light exposure of dark-reared animals.

However, while gel fractionation is a useful diagnostic technique, it is difficult to further subfractionate the gel bands which are of interest, partly because the gels are capable of receiving only very limited quantities of material, and the effects we are studying are themselves small. It therefore seemed preferable to try an alternative method of purification of the fractions in bulk.

This has involved subcellular fractionation of the visual cortex. Tissue from one hour L and D lysine-injected animals was homogenized either separately, or, in double-labelling experiments, after pooling, and subjected to a standard subcellular fractionation protocol (Jones-Lecointe et al., 1976). In the primary subcellular fractions, a difference between L and D appeared only in a ribosomal pellet (240%; p < 0·01). The subcellular fractionation also made possible an internal comparison between labelling in the motor and visual cortex of the same animal (Fig. 2). In the dark control animals the incorporation of precursor into visual cortex ribosomes was only some 74% of that into motor cortex, whilst in the light it was 185%. The elevated labelling of a ribosomal fraction which contains only 2·3% of the protein of the initial homogenate may reflect a change in the rate of production of ribosomes themselves, or represent label present in nascent protein bound to the ribosomes but awaiting release into the cell cytoplasm. So far we have not distinguished between these possibilities, though we consider the second to be the more probable, especially as subfractionation of the crude nuclear fraction did not

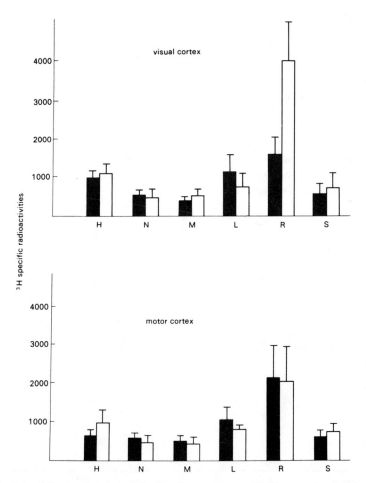

Fig. 2. Subcellular fractionation of visual and motor cortex of light-exposed and dark control rats. 100 µCi ^{3}H-lysine was injected i.p. into light-exposed and dark-reared rats. After 1 h incorporation in their respective conditions, animals were killed and total homogenate (H) and primary subcellular fractions: nuclei (N), mitochondria (M), lysosomes (L), ribosomes (R), and soluble cytoplasm (S) were prepared from visual and motor cortex. Results are means ± S.E.M. of 6 animals in each group. Black bars: dark controls, Open bars: light exposed. (Data derived from Jones-Lecointe et al., 1976.)

reveal any differential labelling between L and D, although this might have been expected if new ribosomal synthesis has occurred. On the other hand, although there was no overall change in the labelling of cytoplasmic protein, further subfractionation using gel filtration (A. Jones-Lecointe, unpublished results) suggests that there is an elevation of incorporation into three soluble protein fractions following light exposure.

A further approach to the cellular identification of the protein synthetic response is made possible by the existence of techniques for the bulk preparation of neuronal cell body and glial (neuropil) fractions from the cortex (Rose, 1967b, 1975). In cerebral cortex from normal animals, the rate of synthesis of protein is higher in neurones than in neuropil or glia, as has been known for some time on the basis of autoradiographic (Droz and Koenig, 1970) and electron microscopic (Palay and Chan-Palay, 1972) evidence. Recently this has been directly confirmed by measurement of the rate of incorporation of precursors into protein in neurones and neuropil both *in vivo* and *in vitro*. Depending on the precursor conditions, a one hour labelling period following intraperitoneal (i.p.) injection of amino acid results in about a 1·3- 1·6-fold higher incorporation rate into neurones than neuropil

Table 1

Incorporation of ^{3}H-lysine into protein in neurones and neuropil in normal, dark-reared and light-exposed rats

Brain region	Incorporation period, (h)	Neuronal/neuropil incorporation ratio in		
		Normal	Dark-reared	Light-exposed
Visual cortex	1	1·45 ± 0·18	0·67 ± 0·03	0·98 ± 0·09
	4	0·35 ± 0·04	0·75 ± 0·05	—
	24	0·44 ± 0·06	0·70 ± 0·05	—
Motor cortex	1	1·58 ± 0·09	1·35 ± 0·13	1·45 ± 0·07
	4	—	—	—
	24	—	—	—

Incorporation ratio is dpm/mg protein in neuronal fraction dpm/mg in neuropil fraction after i.p. injection of 250 µCi 4,5 ^{3}H-lysine in 1 ml 0·9% saline and after the incorporation period shown. Dissections were made and cells separated as described in the papers from which this table is compiled (Rose et al., 1973; Rose and Sinha, 1974b). Data are given as mean ±S.E.M. of n between 5 and 25. Differences between N and D in visual cortex are significant (p < 0·01) at all times; differences between D and L and L and N at 1 h are significant at p < 0·01 and <0·05 respectively. From Rose, 1976a.

(but see below). What would happen if we compared incorporation into neurones and neuropil from the visual cortex of one hour L and D animals?

Table 1 shows the results of such an experiment. Compared with normal animals, incorporation into visual cortex neuronal protein was depressed. When dark-reared animals were exposed to one hour of light there was no change in the rate of incorporation in the neuropil, but a significant elevation in the neuronal cell body fraction. The effect was region specific, and in the motor cortex of the dark-reared animals the incorporation ratio was at the normal control level. We conclude that a fraction of visual cortex neuronal protein synthesis is thus suppressed in dark rearing and is switched on when the animal is exposed to the light (Rose et al., 1973).

We can tell more about the nature of this suppressed fraction of neuronal protein synthesis from a study of the kinetics of incorporation of precursor into protein in normal animals (Rose and Sinha, 1974a). Although the rate of neuronal to neuropil incorporation is 1·3 to 1·6 following an hour of labelling in normal animals, if the labelling period is prolonged, within four hours there is a dramatic fall in the ratio to around 0·4 to 0·6. Thereafter it is stable for several days. This data indicates that, whilst the overall rate of synthesis and degradation of neuronal and glial proteins are roughly comparable, there is present in the neurone in the "normal" animal a rapidly synthesized protein fraction which, present in the cell body after short labelling periods, is transported out over a period of a few hours. The presence of this rapidly labelling and exported fraction can also be observed auto-radiographically (Droz and Koenig, 1970). Its fate is unclear, and over the four hour time period it does not accumulate in glial cell bodies or in synaptosomes. We have also observed, again in normal animals, that the rapidly labelling and exported fraction is apparently particulate, and probably at least in part glycoprotein in nature. Its synthesis is very sensitive to cycloheximide, a protein synthesis inhibitor, and its export from the neuronal cell body is blocked by the axonal flow inhibitor, colchicine. It therefore seems probable that this fraction is part of the axonally or dendritically transported neuronal material (Rose, 1976b; Rose and Sinha, 1976). Table 1 shows that when the period of incorporation is prolonged in dark-reared animals, the characteristic fall in neuronal/neuropil incorporation rate does not occur. The ratio is low, but stable (Rose and Sinha, 1974b). Thus we conclude that it is the synthesis of the rapidly labelling and exported glycoprotein which is switched off in the visual cortex of dark-reared animals, and which is apparently switched on in light exposure. Very recently we have been able to show that one component of this fraction, whose rate of incorporation is doubled on light exposure, is the microtubular protein tubulin (Rose *et al.*, 1976). Before turning to consider some biochemical correlates of more specific learning experiences, the available information on the biochemistry of dark rearing and visual stimulation should be completed by referring to evidence on changes in enzymic activity. There are data available for a number of lysosomal enzymes, the membrane enzyme Na$^+$, K$^+$ ATPase, and the enzymes of the acetylcholine (ACh) transmitter system (although there is no evidence that ACh is a transmitter in the visual pathways (Bigl *et al.*, 1975). Our own and some other results are summarized in Table 2, and indicate that the enzymic activity changes found in the D and L conditions compared with Normal, seem to fall

Table 2

Enzyme changes in visual system of normal, dark-reared and light-exposed animals

Enzyme	System	L/N	D/N	Interpretation	Reference
CAT[a]	Rat visual cortex	↑	Nil	Transient	1
CAT[a]	Chick forebrain roof	↑	—	Transient	2
AChE	Rat visual cortex	↑	Nil	Transient	1
BChE[b]	Chick forebrain roof	Nil	Nil	Nil	1
AChE	Chick forebrain roof	↑	—	Transient	2
AChE	Pigeon optic lobe	—	↓	Lasting	3
MAO[c]	Rat visual cortex	Nil	↑	Transient (?)	4
COMT[d]	Rat visual cortex	?	↓	Transient (?)	4
Na,K,ATPase	Rat cortex	↑	↓	Transient	5
Na,K,ATPase	Rat visual cortex	Nil	Nil	Nil	1
Na,K,ATPase	Pigeon optic lobe	—	↓	Lasting	6
Glutamate decarboxylase	Rat visual cortex	Nil	Nil	Nil	1
Glucosidase	Rat visual cortex	Nil	↓	Lasting	1
Galactosidase	Rat visual cortex	Nil	↓	Lasting	1
Glucosaminidase	Rat visual cortex	↑	Nil	Transient	1
Glucuronidase	Rat visual cortex	Nil	Nil	Nil	1
Galactosaminidase	Rat visual cortex	Nil	Nil	Nil	1
Acid phosphatase	Rat visual cortex	Nil	Nil	Nil	1
Acid phosphatase	Pigeon optic lobe	Nil	Nil	Nil	6

Directions of observed changes in enzyme specific activity (on a protein basis) compiled from the literature are indicated by the arrows; the interpretations are ours. References are 1. Sinha and Rose, 1976. 2. Haywood *et al.* (1975) (see also Table 4); 3. Chakrabarti *et al.* (1974); 4. Bigl *et al.* (1974); 5. Meisami and Timiras (1974); 6. Chakrabarti and Daginawala (1975). N: Normal; D: Dark-maintained; L: Light-exposed. [a] Choline acetyl transferase; [b] butylcholinesterase; [c] monoamine oxidase; [d] catecholamine-O-methyltransferase.

into two classes. In our experiments there are apparently lasting changes in the activities of some of the acid hydrolases, and more transient changes in the ACh enzymes. There are conflicting reports concerning Na^+, K^+ ATPase, perhaps reflecting treatment or species differences.

C. Correlates of Learning

There are a multitude of reports in the literature of experiments claiming to show a correlation between a specific biochemical response—generally an elevation of protein or RNA synthesis—and the learning of a specific skill. This chapter is not a comprehensive review and we shall not mention all these experiments. In our view many of them have not dealt rigorously with the problem of controls at the behavioural or biochemical level. The type of conclusion which can be drawn, and some of the experimental and interpretational problems encountered, will be indicated by referring in detail to three sets of experiments: those of the Chapel Hill group; Hydén, at Gotëborg and our own imprinting experiments. There is other work of relevance, mostly on RNA synthesis, including that of Shashoua (e.g. Shashoua, 1968, 1970), using a novel goldfish swimming response. Bowman and Strobel (1969) using maze learning in the rat, and Matthies and his colleagues (Popov et al., 1976) on enhancement of fucose incorporation during shock-motivated brightness discrimination in rats. We do not have space to consider these experiments in detail; however the biochemical conclusions (and problems) of such experiments point broadly in the same direction as those we do discuss.

1. The Chapel Hill experiments

Glassman and his coworkers at Chapel Hill have worked with mice in a jump-box (see Section II), comparing trained with yoked and quiet controls, and examined both RNA and protein metabolism during and after the acquisition of the new behaviour. As an RNA precursor they injected ^{3}H-uridine intracranially (i.c.) at the start of training and found that 15 minutes later there was increased incorporation into RNA, both nuclear (28%) and polysomal (40%), in the brain of trained versus yoked mice (Zemp et al., 1966; Adair et al., 1968b). Subsequent work showed that the response was restricted mainly to the dien-cephalon, and, by autoradiography, to the neurones of this region (Zemp et al., 1967; Kahan et al., 1970). To decide whether the metabolic effect was related primarily to learning, an experimental design was used in which already trained or prior-yoked animals were trained; only the prior-yokeds showed an incorporation increase. Prior-trained animals only showed the increase when the behaviour was extinguished (Adair *et al.*, 1968a; Coleman *et al.*, 1971b). Stress-related hormones are known to affect cerebral nucleic acid metabolism (Jakoubek *et al.*, 1972) so the experiments were repeated using hypophysectomized animals. The absence of such hormones as ACTH did not markedly affect the uridine incorporation (Coleman *et al.*, 1971a) (see also de Wied, Chapter 5). Some of these experiments have been supported by other groups. For instance Uphouse found an increased polysome to monosome ratio in trained versus yoked animals, and also increased polysome labelling by precursor (Uphouse *et al.*, 1972). Matthies showed, using shock-motivated light discrimination, that whereas total ribosome content in hippocampus increased in both trained and active-control animals, only trained animals had an increased number of membrane-bound ribosomes (Wenzel *et al.*, 1975).

Some of the problems that Glassman's group faced are good examples of the difficulties in the use of radioactive precursors mentioned earlier. They generally calculated their data as the ratio of incorporated radioactivity to that in uridine monophosphate (UMP), in an attempt to correct for pool radioactivity variations, even though uridine triphosphate (UTP), not UMP, is the immediate precursor of RNA, and the relationship between these two may not be constant. (The group were aware of this flaw but found UTP radioactivity too difficult to determine.) Also their method of calculating UMP radioactivity was incorrect, as they later showed (Entingh *et al.*, 1974) and when the earlier data was revised the increased incorporation into nuclear RNA was found to be non-existent. There was still a polysomal effect, but much reduced. This example emphasizes the need for extreme caution in the use of pool-corrected radioactivities, and the need to present uncorrected as well as corrected data (see also below).

Entingh also switched from an intracranial to a subcutaneous route of precursor administration, probably to avoid the hazards of the former. Not only are misplaced injections and trauma (detectable in the experimental but not the yoked animal) probable sources of error resulting from the use of intracranial injections but also the metabolism of the precursor is quite different from that given peripherally (Marchisio and Bondy, 1974; Schotman *et al.*, 1974; Damstra *et al.*, 1975).

In a very interesting set of experiments Glassman's group have looked at the effects of recall on prior-trained animals (Machlus *et al.*,

1974a, b). Using radioactive pyrophosphate they showed that there was greater labelling of non-histone nuclear proteins in the basal forebrain of trained than yoked or quiet animals, and that this could be detected at an absolute level as phosphoserine without the use of radioactive precursors. When the precursor was given to prior-trained and prior-yoked animals and these merely placed in the training apparatus, only the prior-trained showed an increased incorporation. Thus the reminding effect did not seem to be related to stress.

Glassman et al. have also looked at the effects of training and related factors on amino acid incorporation into protein (Rees et al., 1974). They exposed animals to one of several conditions: a training schedule, handling, buzzers or shocks and measured ^{3}H-lysine incorporation into protein in brain and liver. While with uridine as precursor the effects of training decreased with time, the converse was found to be true for lysine, which supports to some degree a model of a temporal sequence in which altered RNA metabolism is followed by altered protein metabolism. They measured both incorporated and free-pool (lysine) radioactivities and also calculated their ratio, the relative radioactivity. Training, 30 handlings or 30 buzzers (and to a lesser degree 20 shocks) increased the relative radioactivity in brain with respect to controls but when the incorporated and free radioactivities were considered separately a complex pattern emerged. Handling increased incorporated radioactivity (26%) but had no effect on pool, and buzzers increased both. However the resultant relative radioactivities were the same. In the liver there was a massively increased relative radioactivity following all treatments, without there being any effect on pool. Hence the use of relative radioactivities in this way serves to mask quite different responses of the organism to different stimuli, and any realistic theory of metabolic response to experience must cope with this problem. Although such effects are difficult to explain, their presence is rather satisfying; the possibility that, when an animal is subjected to obviously significant stimuli such as electric shocks, it responds only with a single type of biochemical response, limited to the brain, would run counter to the obvious facts of physiological and behavioural sensitivity to such massive insults.

In their most recent work Glassman's group have extended their study of protein metabolism, this time by using three different amino acids; leucine, lysine and methionine (Hershkowitz et al., 1975). They changed from an avoidance to an appetitive task (milk reward) to avoid the noxious aspects of the shock-avoidance learning. Training was shown to increase the catabolism of leucine to non-amino acid products and decrease the labelling of protein in the brain. This was found to be even more extreme for ^{3}H-methionine, where 90% of the isotope was found in ^{3}H$_2$O within 20 minutes following the injection, while ^{35}S-methionine seemed to lose ^{35}S into some other substance. Lysine appeared to be the most stable amino acid and the brains of trained animals compared with controls contained more radioactivity in the nuclear protein fraction after 20 minutes labelling and in the nuclear, microsomal and cytoplasmic proteins after 60 minutes labelling. To obtain a more uniform labelling effect a radioactive protein hydrolysate was used and with this the cytoplasmic fraction showed the greatest increase. These results clearly indicate the diversity of effects that training can have on different substances in terms of both metabolism and uptake, and the dangers of extrapolating from one precursor to others.

2. The Hydén experiments

Hydén's work in this field stretches back over more than two decades, and some of his earlier experiments are well known and will not be reviewed in detail. In summary they depended on analyses of RNA content and base ratio composition in some of the large neurones and surrounding neuropil of the Deiters' nucleus region, which has a functional role in relationship to vestibular responses. The claim was that in learning animals, though not passively stimulated ones, there is an increase in total RNA and a shift in its composition towards a more DNA-like type, indicative of the production of mRNA (e.g. Hydén and Egyházi, 1962). The problem in these experiments was both the relative lack of specificity of the learning task, and the interpretation of the biochemical data as representing a shift to mRNA synthesis, which was of necessity somewhat inferential.

More recently, experiments involving learning to reach for food with a non-preferred paw have been used (see Section II). This behaviour change enables the animal to be used as its own control. Because of the operational asymmetry of the task the contralateral hemisphere is the learning and the ipsilateral the control. Thus to some extent hormonal and other whole-body variations are compensated for. Hydén found both an increased RNA content in neurones from the sensori–motor cortex and also a large shift in base ratio towards an adenine and uracil-rich type (Hydén and Egyházi, 1964). Again he postulated this to represent increased mRNA production, and the largely nuclear response in these neurones seemed to fit with the large ratio of nuclear to cytoplasmic volume. However the elevation in RNA content was between 40 and 50% of total content, which is greater than that given by spinal motor neurones after ACTH treatment or intense motor activity. (These neurones in fact produce RNA with a high guanine and cytosine content, supposedly ribosomal.) As well as the doubt this casts on Hydén's interpretation, the choice of brain region for analysis may be queried on the grounds that the motor cortex may well respond to the novel use of the non-preferred paw in the absence of learning (Bateson, 1970, 1976), while the fact that the task involves a high degree of vigilance both during training and testing means that there may well have been altered RNA metabolism during both parts of the experiment. This type of effect has only been tackled to any degree by Glassman (Section IV.C.1). Later studies have used the transfer-of-handedness paradigm to look at protein metabolism by ^{3}H-leucine incorporation into several brain regions both during and after the acquisition of the new behaviour (Hydén, 1973a). The pattern that emerged was that during training there was a shift of leucine incorporation from limbic to cortical regions, followed during over-training by a similar or lowered incorporation in these regions, to that found during early training. The one exception to this was a maintained high incorporation in the thalamus. However the data had some curious aspects. Hydén analysed his results in terms of "corrected specific radioactivities" which were the ratio of the specific radioactivity in a given brain region of a trained animal to that in the control. In all cases the ratio was less than 1·0, i.e. there was less incorporation in trained than control. In the cortex the ratio was 0·3 at the start of training, 0·5 during increasing learning, and back at 0·3 with overtraining. The ratio in the limbic system fell from almost 1·0 initially to 0·25 throughout the training period, which lasted several days. No clear reason for the occurrence of this low ratio was given, but it could not have been due to overall activity levels because the animals were matched on this measure. Such gross effects may be true components of the responses to the training situation, but may also reflect the inadequacy of the controls. Either way the pattern of incorporation changes shown are of interest and give an indication of the involvement of different parts of the brain in learning and related processes in a way that examination of the biochemical sequelae of brief experiences cannot. Subsequent experiments using the transfer-of-handedness paradigm have been concerned with the hippocampus, which may be involved in acquisition (but see Nadel and O'Keefe, 1974 for a view of the hippocampus as a space-mapping region).

Hydén and his colleagues looked at the changes in the content of the S-100 protein of neurones in a discrete region (CA3) of hippocampus during training, and found an increased content of both this protein and Ca^{2+}. Using polyacrylamide gels, a new protein band was found close to S-100 during training. This was interpreted as being S-100 with a different conformation, possibly due to interaction with calcium ions (Hydén and Lange, 1968, 1970; Hydén, 1973a). The increased Ca^{2+} levels were not accompanied by increased Na^+ or K^+, suggesting that there was no tissue swelling. However the source of the extra calcium is not clear. Nor indeed need this effect be related to long-term memory, for such ion effects would seem to be more likely to be involved in short-term phenomena. Both the level of S-100 and its specific radioactivity increased, which suggests that de novo synthesis had occurred, although it is not clear that this was the only protein fraction which changed, as a tactical decision seems to have been made to study only S-100 and related proteins, rather than scan the entire range of PAGE fractions.

That S-100 protein plays some role in learning is further suggested by the action of S-100 antibody, which, in an active form, prevented the acquisition of the new skill (Hydén, 1973a). However such an inhibitory action of the antibody might not necessarily only relate to a specific process such as the prevention of learning, but may be a sequel of a more general action (see discussion of metabolic inhibitors, Section V). So far only S-100 and 14-3-2 proteins have been examined, so the specificity of these responses is still an open question. The roles of S-100 and 14-3-2 have not yet been demonstrated unequivocally, although S-100 is suggested to be involved with a filamentous web below the nerve cell membrane which Hydén believes he has been able to demonstrate on the basis of electron microscopic studies of dissected and fragmented synapses (Hydén, 1973c; 1976). S-100 has also been suggested to be related to synaptic structure by Walters and Matus (1975). 14-3-2 protein is a soluble protein of unknown properties.

3. Imprinting

The merits of the chick imprinting system as a model for learning have been mentioned (Section II); the significance of imprinting to the young bird and the fact that it occurs early in life, suggest that it may involve metabolic effects of a magnitude greater than in other learning situations in adult animals.

Our strategy in the imprinting experiments* has been first to define a relatively large anatomical region in which biochemical changes

* Collaborators in this work include: Dr P. P. G. Bateson, Sub Department of Animal Behaviour, Madingley, Cambridge; Professor G. Horn, Department of Anatomy, University of Bristol; Mr J. Hambley and Dr A. K. Sinha of the Brain Research Group.

occur during learning; second to attempt to show that such changes are specific correlates of the learning; and third (the stage we are now entering) to focus down more precisely on the exact sequence of biochemical events and their more exact anatomical localization (Rose, 1976a). In these experiments, dark-hatched chicks are exposed to an imprinting stimulus (a coloured flashing light) or maintained in the dark and after appropriate periods of exposure and rest are tested for their preference for the familiar object, a variety of other behavioural measures being made concurrently (Bateson and Wainwright, 1972; Bateson and Jaeckel, 1974). Incorporation of precursors is measured into several different brain regions—the midbrain, containing the optic tectum and most of the thalamic nuclei; the base of the forebrain, containing predominantly neo, ecto-and palaeostriatum; the posterior forebrain roof containing hippocampus, and the anterior forebrain roof containing hyperstriatum.

The early experiments (summarized in Bateson et al., 1972; reviewed in Horn et al., 1973a) showed that there is increased incorporation of ^{3}H-uracil into RNA and ^{3}H-lysine into protein in the forebrain roof of chicks which have been exposed to the imprinting stimulus for 78 and 150 minutes respectively, but not in birds exposed either to diffuse overhead illumination or kept in darkness. Longer exposure results in RNA incorporation changes which are not region specific.

To partially control for the effects of visual stimulation alone, in more recent experiments birds were exposed to the stimulus, injected with ^{14}C-lysine and then returned to darkness, so that both they and the control dark group were in identical conditions during the incorporation period (Hambley et al., 1976). Birds exposed for 60 minutes to the stimulus had greater lysine incorporation into protein in the anterior forebrain roof during the subsequent 20 minutes in the dark than did the birds which had been maintained in the dark throughout. This effect was specific to the anterior forebrain roof, although there was a generalized increase in free radioactive precursor in all regions. Following a shorter (30 minutes) or a longer (120 minutes) time of exposure there was no difference between the groups. The difference in radioactivity acutely posed the problem of precursor pool specific radioactivities, and as a partial answer we showed that there was no difference in total tissue lysine specific radioactivity between exposed and dark maintained birds. An amino acid which is taken into the tissue but not incorporated into protein (2-aminoisobutyrate) also showed a generalized increase in uptake in the exposed birds. These effects are summarized in Table 3.

Table 3

Changes in uptake and incorporation rates of precursors in chick brain during and after exposure to an imprinting stimulus

System	Stimulus onset (offset) to killing (min)	Incorpora- tion time (min)	Brain region	(I/D) × 100
³H-Uracil into RNA	76 150	150 150	Roof All regions	120 ~125
³H-Lysine into protein	150	90	Roof	117
¹⁴C-Lysine into protein	80(20)	20	Anterior roof	125
¹⁴C-Lysine into pool	80(20)	20	All regions	~121
¹⁴C-2 Amino- isobutyrate into pool	80(20)	20	All regions	~122

Incorporation, as dpm/mg protein, either in acid insoluble (RNA and protein) or acid soluble (pool) fractions from the studied brain regions from day-old chicks, is expressed as that into (Imprinted/Dark controls) × 100. Only differences which are significant at $p < 0.05$ or better are shown; n is 15 or more for each condition. No significant differences occur at other times or regions. In the ³H-precursor experiments incorporation took place during exposure; in the ¹⁴C-precursor experiments it took place immediately following exposure. ¹⁴C-2 amino-isobutyrate is a non-metabolizable amino acid used as a marker for uptake (and hence probably blood flow) changes. Data are calculated from Bateson et al. (1972) and Haywood et al. (1976). (From Rose, 1976a.)

The observed changes in incorporation into the anterior forebrain roof are preceded by an increased activity of the enzyme RNA polymerase in cell nuclei isolated from the forebrain roof of birds exposed to 30 minutes of imprinting stimulus, but not to shorter (15 minute) or longer (45 minute) periods of exposure (Haywood et al., 1970; 1975). Hence there appears to be a temporal sequence of metabolic events following stimulus onset which are compatible with an activation of a transcription–translation sequence. In addition, it seems that at least two processes, one rather general and affecting all brain regions, and the second more specific and limited to the anterior forebrain roof, are occurring. The existence of a biochemical sequence of this nature, including a transient change in an enzyme activity which is not explicable as a simple precursor artefact, is encouraging, although we have yet to demonstrate that the changes in incorporation of precursor into protein are limited to certain specific protein fractions. This essentially represents the key conclusion to the first phase of our strategic approach.

Both transient effects prior to RNA polymerase elevation and those involved in short-term memory processes are likely to involve membrane and synaptic events. On general biochemical grounds, we anticipated that one likely early component of the metabolic events associated with imprinting would be cyclic AMP. After 15 minutes exposure the level of cyclic AMP was lower in forebrain roof of exposed than dark birds, and higher in their midbrain (Hambley *et al.*, 1972). An increase in cAMP content in forebrain roof did not occur until 60 minutes exposure, and was accompanied by higher adenyl cyclase activity. This suggests that cAMP, if involved in the activation of RNA polymerase, was not restricted to this role, but might for instance, be involved in other transport phenomena or synaptic modulation.

Another obvious marker for synaptic events is the level of transmitter metabolism, and we have compared the activities of AChE and CAT following exposure to the imprinting stimulus with that in dark maintained chicks (Haywood *et al.*, 1975). After 60 minutes exposure the activity of CAT was raised in the midbrain of exposed birds but after a further 60 minutes in the dark fell to the control level and remained unchanged for at least 24 hours. In contrast, AChE activity did not alter until one hour after the end of exposure. There was then an increase in the forebrain roof of exposed birds. By six hour post-exposure there was a generalized increase in AChE activity in the brains of exposed birds and after 12 hours a depression of activity in their midbrain. At 24 hours after exposure there was no difference between the groups. It is at present unclear whether these transient AChE and CAT changes reflect the phase of reorganization of connectivity or are less specific consequences of the training experience. Nor do we know whether the change represents an absolute increase or decline in the number of enzyme molecules present, or is a post-translational effect. The enzyme and metabolite changes are summarized in Table 4.

The second phase of our strategy was to try to identify which aspects of the observed biochemical changes correlated most closely with the learning. One problem of working with learning and biochemistry together is that the technical requirements of the one tend to restrict the experimental manipulation of the other. The only way round this is to design some experiments to give maximum behavioural data using simple biochemical manipulations, and the others to give the converse.

Table 4

Changes in metabolite levels and enzyme activities in chick
brain after exposure to an imprinting stimulus

System	Stimulus onset (offset) to killing (min)	Brain region	(I/D) × 100	Reference
cAMP	15	Roof	35	1
	15	Midbrain	160	1
RNA polymerase	30	Roof	134	2
Adenyl	30	Midbrain	78	3
cyclase	60	Roof	150	3
Choline acetyltransferase	60	Midbrain	110	4
Acetylcholinesterase	120(60)	Roof	111	4
	420(360)	Roof	113	4
	420(360)	Base	112	4
	420(360)	Midbrain	110	4
	780(720)	Midbrain	87	4

Enzyme activities were determined in brain regions from day-old chicks at varying times after exposure to imprinting stimulus. Maximum length of stimulus exposure, 60 min. Data are expressed as (activity in Imprinted/Dark control) × 100, and only significant elevations or depressions are shown (p < 0.05 or better; n is 12 or more for each condition. Data are calculated from 1. Hambley et al. (1972); 2. Haywood et al. (1970); 3. Hambley and Rose (1973); 4. Haywood et al. (1975). (From Rose, 1976a.)

Hence all the behavioural control experiments we have conducted have used a single biochemical measure, the incorporation of ^{3}H- or ^{14}C-uracil into RNA.

The first (Horn et al., 1973b) utilized the fact of the complete decussation of the optic tract, which makes possible a "split-brain" preparation (Fig. 3). In these experiments, the supraoptic commissures of 12 chicks were divided shortly after hatching, and after recovery from the operation, one eye of each chick was covered with a patch. The animal was exposed to the stimulus for one hour, then tested first with the trained eye and then with the untrained eye. No transfer of learning took place; there were no differences in pool between trained and untrained sides of the brain (tending to rule out asymmetric blood flow); but incorporation into RNA in the forebrain roof (but no other region) in the trained side was significantly elevated by comparison with the control side. Hence it is unlikely that the

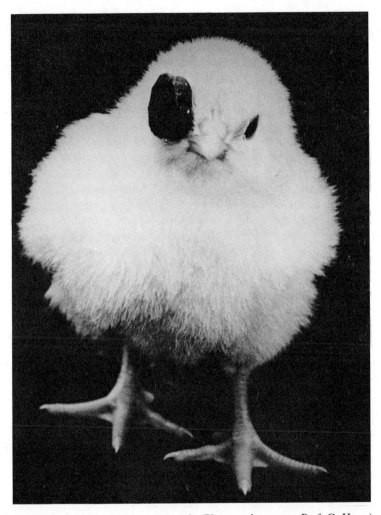

Fig. 3. A split-brain chick wearing an eyepatch. (Photograph courtesy Prof. G. Horn.)

changed incorporation resulted from general hormonal response to stress, non-visual sensory input or differences in motor activity.

In the next experiment, we attempted to rule out sensory stimulation as a cause of the differences in RNA incorporation (Bateson *et al.*, 1973). To do this, we divided the learning period into two sessions, on two successive days. On the first, birds were exposed to the stimulus, in the absence of precursor, for varying periods of time. Thus by the next session some birds still had a considerable amount to learn about the stimulus, while others had learned a great deal of what there was to know. On the second session all the birds were exposed for the same period and thus received similar amounts of sensory stimulation, and during this session incorporation was measured. Incorporation was higher in the anterior forebrain roof in the birds which had been exposed for the shorter periods on the first day. That is, the more the birds had to learn about the stimulus, the more precursor they incorporated into RNA in the anterior forebrain roof. Birds which were not exposed to the stimulus on the second day showed identical incorporation on this day irrespective of their previous treatment. This tended to rule out sensory stimulation itself as the cause of the incorporation effect, and also, as the activity of the birds did not differ on day 2 between the groups exposed for varying periods on day 1, the results run counter to any simple "vigilance" interpretation. There remains the possibility that light *per se* acts as a trigger, setting in train a process of cellular differentiation which requires a given amount of exposure to complete. This possibility, which might be implied by some experiments by Rogers *et al.* (1974) on the effects of cycloheximide in the chick (see Section IV.C), can still not be ruled out on the basis of our experiment.

In the latest of this series of experiments (Bateson *et al.*, 1975) we used only trained birds. There is great variability between birds from the same hatch in their behaviour towards the imprinting stimulus; some respond very early in the exposure period and others much later; some develop a weak and others a strong preference for the familiar stimulus. There is also great variability in biochemistry between individual birds. By training all birds identically and looking at the correlations between incorporation and a large number of behavioural responses, we were able to show that, when effects due to motor activity, etc. had been accounted for, there remained only one significant correlation, namely between the incorporation into RNA in the anterior forebrain roof and the bird's preference for the familiar as opposed to a novel stimulus. To put it simply, the more the birds learned, the more uracil they incorporated into RNA. No other behavioural measure amongst those we made could be related to an elevation in incorporation into macromolecules, although there were some changes in pool uptake which were not region specific and may be related to motor activity.

These behavioural controls are not, of course, exhaustive. For example, it could be argued that both the birds propensity to learn and to incorporate uracil into RNA are consequences of a quite separate prior effect—for example ontogenetic differences in "attention" or "motivation" or any other of the possible behavioural subsystems that may be postulated as components of a given animal's response in a particular situation. And, of course, the fact that one of our biochemical measures is only correlated with learning does not logically allow the inference that the same is true for the others, either the protein incorporation or the enzyme changes. Indeed, the balance of probability suggests that some of the biochemical changes may indeed be correlates of more general phenomena. One may also ask whether it is even possible to have an episode of "learning" without other attendant, but distinct, behavioural processes occurring, or to distinguish a unique biochemical event which codes for "pure" learning. Such reductionism may be inappropriate (see Section VI).

V. Pharmacological Studies

A. *Background*

The pharmacological approach is the inverse of the correlative approach. In it, substances with a hopefully defined biochemical effect are introduced into the animal and their effects on learning, retention or recall are assayed. If the biochemical effect is on one system only, and if the behavioural effect can really be shown to be highly specific (and localized in a particular tissue region), then it should be possible to draw valid conclusions concerning the role of the biochemical process in the behaviour.

However, a consideration of the interactions of Fig. 1 makes it clear that, even granted biochemical specificity, there are many potential sites of action of a pharmacological agent which may have effects on long- or short-term memory or their behavioural antecedents, without proving that the biochemical system is necessarily, exclusively and sufficiently related to the behaviour. For instance, an agent which acts on the kidneys may result in a depletion of brain amino acids, hence lowering protein synthesis and impairing long-term memory fixation, but we may not therefore conclude that the kidneys are the site of memory.

In general the agents that have been used are inhibitors, and most, though not all, attention has focussed on agents which affect RNA and protein metabolism. An example of a pharmacological approach which does not utilize inhibitors is that of the injection of large amounts of orotic acid, which has been shown to alter the rate of discrimination learning (Matthies *et al.*, 1971). Such effects may not be directly on learning. A great deal of pharmacological work has shown that there exist agents (such as the amphetamines or certain peptides for example) which increase attention, arousal level, or exploratory behaviour and therefore can result in more rapid learning. (See Section II and Chapter 7). This work will not be discussed here.

From all the drug studies, a number of clear indications have emerged. First, there appears to be a critical element in the timing of drug administration, which varies with the drug, the animal, the task and the type of behavioural process (e.g. learning; recall) inhibited. This is apparently the reason why some of the very early inhibitor studies gave negative results (e.g. Flexner et al., 1962; Barondes and Cohen, 1967a, b). Second, inhibition of protein synthesis seems to be more consistent in its amnesic effects (that is, inhibition of retention but not learning) than does inhibition of RNA synthesis, perhaps because the latter cannot prevent synthesis of protein on already present mRNA. Third, the degree of amnesia is an inverse function of drug dose and strength of training, and for any given training procedure the degree of amnesia is strictly related to the size of the dose. Fourth, not all the amnesic effects found are related to impairment of retention; some, like those of puromycin, seem to be producing a loss of ability to recall. (This is an interesting area, which has been little studied.) The effects of inhibitors on learning and memory have been fully reviewed by Flood and Jarvik (1975).

B. Inhibition of RNA Synthesis

8-Azaguanine, which is incorporated into RNA, and produces a non-functional molecule, does not seem to have any specific action on memory, but instead produces depressed activity (Chamberlain et al., 1963; Jewett et al., 1965). Actinomycin D, which inhibits DNA-dependent RNA polymerase, gave amnesic effects in some cases (Agranoff et al., 1967) but not others (Cohen and Barondes, 1966). These investigators used goldfish and mice respectively, which may not respond to the drug in the same manner. Moreover the effect of actinomycin D seems to be dependent on the extent of training, for the more rigorous the criteria of learning, the less was the amnesic effect (Squire and Barondes, 1970). It has been shown that actinomycin D does not have a "blanket effect" on all RNA synthesis, but that at low doses, as probably used in these studies, only ribosomal RNA synthesis is impaired (Schluederberg et al., 1971). The amnesic effects do not seem to relate to degree of inhibition of RNA synthesis, for reduction of RNA synthesis by 15% was sufficient to produce amnesia when a low training criterion was applied, whereas even 80% inhibition was not sufficient to impair memory if a rigorous criterion was adopted. Thus it has not been convincingly shown on the basis of inhibitor studies that there is an obligatory involvement of RNA synthesis in memory formation.

C. Inhibition of Protein Synthesis

Inhibition of protein synthesis on the other hand has given less equivocal results. Puromycin prevents protein synthesis by causing premature release of the nascent polypeptide chain from the ribosome in the form of peptidyl-puromycin. The time of injection is important, for animals injected before or after learning developed deficits in retention (Flexner et al., 1965; Agranoff et al., 1965; Barondes and Cohen, 1967a). However, subsequent injections of saline proved effective in counteracting the amnesic effects (Flexner and Flexner, 1967, 1969) which suggested that the action of puromycin was perhaps not as specific as originally supposed. Other agents were also found to counter puromycin-induced amnesia, such as ACTH and adrenergic drugs. (Flexner et al., 1971; Flexner and Flexner, 1971). Subsequently it was shown that the radioactive peptidyl-puromycin remained in the brain for long periods of time and could be found in mitochondria, nuclei and synaptosomes (Gambetti et al., 1972). Puromycin also apparently causes mitochondrial swelling. That long-term amnesic effects of puromycin may well be due to the animal's inability to recall information, is suggested by the protective action of cycloheximide against a puromycin-induced amnesia. Although cycloheximide is an amnesic agent in its own right (see below), it prevents the formation of peptidyl-puromycins (Flexner and Flexner, 1966). This was not a general phenomenon in that no such effect was seen in goldfish (Lim et al., 1970); perhaps here the puromycin derivatives were not toxic.

Because of these apparently diverse actions of puromycin, unrelated to protein synthesis inhibition per se, it has generally been abandoned as an inhibitor in learning studies, and the emphasis has shifted to cycloheximide and acetoxycycloheximide, which have so far not been shown to have such side effects. They act by preventing the transfer of amino acids from tRNA to the polypeptide, but do not produce long-lived products (Siegel and Sisler, 1963). In fact they stabilize the mRNA from degradation and after their removal protein synthesis continues at the same or a higher rate than previously (Trakatellis et *al.*, 1965; J. Hambley and J. Haywood, unpublished data). They act very rapidly and precursor incorporation in brain falls by 90% or more within 10–20 minutes of injection (even at a peripheral site).

The amnesic effects found are a function of injection time and training strength; administration just before or immediately after training is most effective (Cohen and Barondes, 1968a, b; Geller *et al.*, 1970) and the more intensive the training programme, the later did the amnesic effects occur. This correlates with the postulated action of cycloheximide on long- rather than short-term memory. Such treatments as electro-convulsive shock (ECS) disrupt retention for a short time after testing whereas with cycloheximide short-term retention is normal but deficits occur at a later time (Andry and Luttges, 1972; Mark and Watts, 1971; Watts and Mark, 1971a).

Most recently a very clear demonstration has been made that the degree of retention is related to the extent of inhibition of protein synthesis and its proximity to the time of training (Flood *et al.*, 1975). Using anisomycin as an inhibitor they showed that if protein synthesis was allowed to occur for short periods after training then the degree of retention correlated with the extent of synthesis, and that the nearer this period was to the end of training the greater retention. Related to this is the demonstration by Squire and Becker (1975) that anisomycin also impairs habituation, a short-term plastic response of the nervous system which many behaviourists regard as analogous to learning. Such experiments elegantly demonstrate the kinds of results needed to validate the inhibitor approach.

The criticisms of inhibitor studies are twofold. One is behavioural in nature and can be answered provided very careful measurements are made of the behaviour of the experimental and control animals. It is by no means sufficient in these experiments to state that "the animals did not appear to be sick", for significant differences in activity and responsiveness could be present which were not easily detectable by eye. To prove this, training programmes are needed which give data on as many aspects of the animal's behaviour as possible. For instance cycloheximide increased and then decreased the activity of rats (Squire *et al.*, 1970) and increased distress calls by chicks in the testing apparatus (P. P. G. Bateson, J. Haywood, J. Hambley and S. P. R. Rose, unpublished results). Only by such measurements can one be sure that the only variable affected is that of learning or retention.

The other criticism is more difficult to resolve. Protein synthesis is an integral and important function of living cells, and the faster the rate of protein synthesis, e.g. in growing cells, the more drastic will be the results of inhibiting it. Indeed this is why the inhibitors were originally developed as antibiotics. Thus long periods of protein synthesis inhibition could cause a generalized, but low level, impairment of cellular function. A possible indication of this may be found in the evidence that memory sometimes reappeared after a period of amnesia (e.g. Squire and Barondes, 1972) or could be easily evoked by a "reminder" (Quartermain et al., 1970).

Relevant here may be the inhibitor experiments of Mark and his colleagues. They have shown that cycloheximide causes amnesia for recall of a one-trial aversive learning response involving visual discrimination in chicks (see Section II) when retested a day after training. However, in later experiments they administered cycloheximide to young chicks in four conditions; in the dark; in auditory isolation; in the light; exposed to auditory stimuli. Weeks later, chicks in which protein synthesis had been inhibited whilst they were in the light or exposed to sound, proved to have impairments in learning visual or auditory skills respectively. Those which had been given cycloheximide in the absence of sensory stimuli however, were unimpaired in their learning (Rogers et al., 1974). This suggests that the inhibition of protein synthesis permanently impairs some cellular differentiation which is essential for later modification of the brain in response to environmental (sensory) stimuli. This impairment is more profound than merely a transient blockage of learning.

Thus the effects of inhibitors on memory may be one of several impairments, but it is the only one rigorously tested. In addition these drugs may have biochemical effects other than those studied, which are usually limited solely to protein synthesis. Cycloheximide has been reported to cause decreased tyrosine hydroxylase activity in vitro, and thus lowered noradrenaline levels (Flexner et al., 1973; Flexner and Goodman, 1975) although Squire et al. (1974) did not find such an effect to be responsible for the amnesia. However, the point was made that there may be other chemical changes caused by an inhibitor which could lead to decreased learning ability or retention.

D. *Other Inhibitory Effects*

While the evidence from the inhibitor studies that protein synthesis is necessary for the retention of long-term memory is quite strong, there are limitations to the amount of light this throws on biochemical mechanisms. This is partly because of the rather general effect on a fundamental cellular property that their use represents. In the last few years there has, therefore, been a tendency to seek for alternative inhibitors with rather more limited effects. One example is colchicine, which inhibits both cell division (which is unlikely to be relevant in the brain over the time period of the experiments) and axonal flow. In an interesting series of experiments, Cronley-Dillon and Perry (1975) have shown that in the goldfish, intracranial administration of colchicine prevents retention of a shuttle-box avoidance task without, apparently, any other behavioural deficit. This experiment represents in one sense the converse of our results with protein synthesis during sensory stimulation (Section IV.B.2) and may cast some light on the cellular role of the proteins involved in consolidation. Related to this approach may be the immunological one of using antisera to specific protein fractions. Thus the offspring of rats, injected intraperitoneally with antisera to synaptic membrane proteins, are claimed to show a permanently impaired learning and retention (Karpiak and Rapport, 1975).

An even more powerful role of the inhibitors has been in unravelling the temporal sequence of events in consolidation (e.g. McGaugh, 1966; Booth, 1967; Flood and Jarvik, 1975). This use is well illustrated in experiments using several different inhibitors in the chick by Mark (Watts and Mark, 1971b). Thus as well as showing that the time of injection of the cycloheximide is critical to whether retention loss occurs, these experiments have also used inhibitors of membrane transport, such as ouabain. In the presence of ouabain the chick behaves as if it cannot learn over the period of the training, but when tested subsequently shows full retention. Ouabain and cycloheximide together block both learning and retention. This suggests a dis-association of the learning and memory processes into biochemically and behaviourally distinct segments, one a short-term process involving ionic or other membrane effects, the other, longer term, requiring an unimpaired protein synthetic machinery.

VI. Conclusions

As we emphasized at the beginning of this chapter, we have not attempted to provide a comprehensive review of all the considerable number of research reports that in recent years have claimed to describe biochemical correlates of plasticity and learning. One whole area of research activity, into the so-called transfer of learning by injection of brain extracts, has been omitted, and we have been quite selective in our discussion of the correlative and pharmacological approaches. What we have attempted to do in this selection is to critically discuss certain types of research findings at sufficient length to make clear both the strengths and weaknesses of the available approaches.

Despite the criticisms that can be levelled at any individual experiment, when they are taken together, we believe that they add up to a convincing demonstration that when the consolidation of learning takes place, an organized sequence of transient metabolic events occurs in a limited cellular (probably neuronal) ensemble. This sequence has a specific temporal order, and although to our knowledge our own studies are the only ones that have actually attempted to define this time sequence, we may assume that learning commences with the activation of certain cells in a specified brain region by the arrival of a novel constellation of synaptic inputs. This results, within these cells, in an activation of the nuclear mRNA synthetic machinery, such that, within 30 minutes of the onset of the stimulus, there is an enhanced RNA polymerase activity, followed within one hour by an elevated production of certain specific proteins. Whilst the cellular role of these proteins is still not clear, at least some may be axonally (dendritically) transported and be involved in synaptic modulation at either pre- or postsynaptic sides of the junction. This process may take several hours, and proceeds independently (possibly also anatomically independently) of the processes involve in short-term learning and memory. These too may involve synaptic events, but if so are modulated by transient changes in ionic balance and/or transmitter activity levels. In the normal course of events, as these transient changes decline, the long-term change builds up in magnitude, so that eventually there is a "cross-over" when short-term memory ceases to be effective and long-term memory becomes dominant. Implicit in this model is the assumption that changes in the rates of protein synthesis, although themselves transient, result in long-lasting structural alterations responsible for the modulation of synaptic connectivity so as to produce a permanent trace or record in the brain. These processes are summarized in Fig. 4. This figure does not suggest a significance to the oscillatory changes we have observed in both protein incorporation and enzyme activity, as we remain uncertain as to their exact physiological or biochemical significance, although there are several obvious potential explanations.

This model implies that we consider the synthesis of specific neuronal proteins as a necessary condition for long-term memory to occur. We have not argued, and do not think that the evidence yet allows us to argue, that such syntheses are either exclusive or sufficient conditions for learning and memory. For example, until we know what

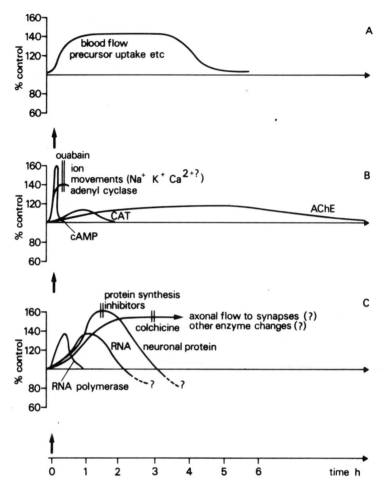

Fig. 4. Hypothetical scheme for biochemical events associated with learning. A. General, non-region-specific changes attendant on learning (postulated). B. Cell specific changes associated with short-term learning and memory showing some changes known to occur and the effects of inhibitors. C. Cell specific changes associated with long-term learning and memory, showing some changes known to occur in various systems and the effects of inhibitors. ↑ Onset of learning experience.

the cellular role(s) of the protein(s) is (are), we cannot be sure that they are not part of a much larger metabolic response whose end product is, for instance, the production of larger amounts of transmitters or membrane lipids. Indeed, that such changes also occur in learning and memory seems more probable than not. That is, we do not yet know which cellular processes (other, possibly, than enhanced DNA synthesis and cell division) do *not* occur during learning and memory. In addition, none of the data we have reviewed, it seems to us, can rule out the possibility that protein synthesis, etc. underlie not memory *per se* but some—as yet unspecified—behavioural process prior to and essential for memory to occur. While some of the inhibitor studies, such as those of Mark, make this less likely, they cannot exclude it entirely. This point has been emphasized by Bateson (1976) (see Fig. 1). If such processes are essential for learning, it may be that a reductionist attempt to define "the" cellular and metabolic locus of learning is always doomed to failure, and the most that can be hoped for is the type of correlative relationship between biochemistry and behaviour that is discussed above.

Two further points should be emphasized. The first is that to argue, as we have done, that specific biochemical sequences underlie learning, is not to imply that these are the *only* changes that occur when an animal learns. That is, in normal learning, many processes as well as memory formation are involved, some of which have been referred to already in this chapter. These include motor and sensory activity, arousal, stress, etc. Clearly, all of these generate brain-state changes which have transient biochemical correlates, and we have in passing commented on evidence for changed rates of cerebral blood flow and precursor uptake. There are likely to be many others, ranging from changes in energy metabolism to changes in transmitter levels; changes specific to learning are superimposed upon this continuous fluctuation. This is why we regard the normal biochemistry of the brain as dynamically "state-dependent" rather than constant.

The second point is that we have not argued for any biochemical specificity for the changes underlying learning. We do not regard them as likely to be unique to the particular piece of learning involved (as the transfer experiments would imply) but rather, special cases of the same general processes of plasticity with which we began the chapter, limited not by biochemical specificity but by the number and addresses of the particular cells whose connectivity is modulated (this point is discussed further in Rose *et al.*, 1975; Rose, 1976a and b).

The implications of this point are substantial, for they mean that there are strong theoretical limitations on what the biochemical approach to learning and plasticity will ever be able to achieve. These limitations are that we are never going to be able, on the basis of a particular biochemical structure, even at a given cellular locus, to predict that this is the engram for a particular item the animal has learned, be it the direction to turn in a maze, the taste of sugar, or the opening bars of Beethoven's Fifth Symphony. That is, what the biochemistry can at best profvide is a description of learning, its explanation in molecular terms, but not its prediction or control.

Acknowledgements

The work and ideas discussed in this chapter have benefited from discussion with many colleagues, and we would like in particular to mention Dr P. P. G. Bateson (University of Cambridge), Professor Gabriel Horn (University of Bristol), Mr J. W. Hambley (now at the Australian National University), Dr K. Richardson (now at The National Children's Bureau, London), Dr A. K. Sinha and Dr A. Jones-Lecointe of the Brain Research Group at the Open University. Experimental work was in part supported by grants to SPR from the Medical Research Council and Science Research Council.

References

Adair, L. B., Wilson, J. E. and Glassman, E. (1968a). *Proc. Nat. Acad. Sci. U.S.A.* **61**, 917–922.
Adair, L. B., Wilson, J. E., Zemp, J. W. and Glassman, E. (1968b). *Proc. Nat. Acad. Sci. U.S.A.* **61**, 606–613.
Agranoff, B. W. (1971). *In* "Animal Memory" (W. K. Honig and P. H. James, eds). Academic Press, New York and London, pp. 243–258.
Agranoff, B. W., Davis, R. E. and Brink, J. J. (1965). *Proc. Nat. Acad. Sci. U.S.A.* **54**, 788–793.
Agranoff, B. W., Davis, R. E., Casola, L. and Lim, R. (1967). *Science* **158**, 1600–1601.
Andry, D. K. and Luttges, M. W. (1972). *Science* **178**, 518–520.
Barondes, S. H. and Cohen, H. D. (1967a). *Brain Res.* **4**, 44–51.
Barondes, S. H. and Cohen, H. D. (1967b). *Proc. Nat. Acad. Sci. U.S.A.* **58**, 157–164.
Bateson, P. P. G. (1966). *Biol. Rev.* **41**, 177–220.
Bateson, P. P. G. (1970). *In* "Short-term changes in Neural Activity and Behaviour" (G. Horn and R. A. Hinde, eds). Cambridge University Press, Cambridge, pp. 553–564.
Bateson, P. P. G. (1971). *In* "The Ontogeny of Vertebrate Behaviour" (H. Moltz, ed.). Academic Press, New York and London, pp. 369–387.
Bateson, P. P. G. (1976). *In* "Perspectives in Experimental Biology" (P. Spencer-Davies, ed.), Vol. 1. Pergamon Press, Oxford, pp. 411–415.
Bateson, P. P. G. and Jaeckel, J. B. (1974). *Anim. Behav.* **22**, 899–906.
Bateson, P. P. G. and Wainwright, A. A. P. (1972). *Behaviour* **42**, 279–290.
Bateson, P. P. G., Horn, G. and Rose, S. P. R. (1972). *Brain Res.* **39**, 449–465.
Bateson, P. P. G., Rose, S. P. R. and Horn, G. (1973). *Science* **181**, 576–578.
Bateson, P. P. G., Horn, G. and Rose, S. P. R. (1975). *Brain Res.* **84**, 207–220.
Bennett, E. L. (1975). *In* "Neural approaches to learning and memory" (M. R. Rosenzweig and E. Bennett, eds). M.I.T. Press, Cambridge, Massachusetts.
Bennett, E. L., Diamond, M. C., Krech, D. and Rosenzweig, M. R. (1964). *Science* **146**, 610–619.
Bigl, V., Biesold, D. and Weisz, K. (1974). *J. Neurochem.* **22**, 505–509.
Bigl, V., Schober, W. and Lüth, H. J. (1975). *Abstr. Symp. Visual System Reinhardsbrunn*.

Blakemore, C. (1976). *Phil. Trans. Roy. Soc.* (in press).
Bondy, S. C., Lehman, R. A. W. and Purdy, J. L. (1974). *Nature* **248**, 440–441.
Booth, D. A. (1967). *Psychol. Bull.* **68**, 149–177.
Bowman, R. E. and Strobel, D. A. (1969). *J. Comp. Physiol. Psychol.* **67**, 448–458.
Chakrabarti, T. and Daginawala, H. F. (1975). *J. Neurochem.* **24**, 983–998.
Chakrabarti, T., Dias, P. D., Roychowdury, D. and Daginawala, H. F. (1974). *J. Neurochem.* **22**, 865–867.
Chamberlain, T. J., Rothschild, G. H. and Gerard, R. W. (1963). *Proc. Nat. Acad. Sci. U.S.A.* **49**, 918–924.
Cohen, H. D. and Barondes, S. H. (1966). *J. Neurochem.* **13**, 207–211.
Cohen, H. D. and Barondes, S. H. (1968a). *Behav. Biol.* **1**, 337–340.
Cohen, H. D. and Barondes, S. H. (1968b). *Nature* **218**, 271–273.
Coleman, M. S., Wilson, J. E. and Glassman, E. (1971a). *Nature* **229**, 54–55.
Coleman, M. S., Pfingst, B., Wilson, J. E. and Glassman, E. (1971b). *Brain Res.* **26**, 349–350.
Cragg, B. G. (1967). *Nature* **215**, 251–253.
Cragg, B. G. (1970). *Brain Res.* **18**, 297–307.
Cronley-Dillon, J. R. and Perry, G. W. (1975). *J. Physiol.* **252**, 27–28P.
Damstra, T., Entingh, D., Wilson, J. E. and Glassman, E. (1975). *Behav. Biol.* **13**, 121–126.
Deutsch, J. A. (1971). *Science* **174**, 788–794.
de Vay, S. (1976). *Phil. Trans. Roy. Soc.* (in press).
Dewar, A. J. and Reading, H. W. (1973). *Exp. Neurol.* **40**, 216–231.
Dewar, A. J., Reading, H. W. and Winterburn, (1973). *Exp. Neurol.* **41**, 133–149.
Diamond, M. C., Johnson, R. E., Ingham, C., Rosenzweig, M. R. and Bennett, E. L. (1975). *Behav. Biol.* **15**, 107–111.
Dobbing, J. and Smart, J. L. (1974). *Brit. Med. Bull.* **30**, 164–168.
Droz, B. and Koenig, H. L. (1970). *In* "Protein Metabolism of the nervous system" (A. Lajtha, ed.). Plenum Press, New York, pp. 93–108.
Dunn, A. (1975). *Brain Res.* **99**, 405–409.
Entingh, D., Damstra-Entingh, T., Dunn, A., Wilson, J. E. and Glassman, E. (1974). *Brain Res.* **70**, 131–138.
Entingh, D., Dunn, A., Glassman, E., Wilson, J. E., Hogan, E. and Damstra, T. (1975). *In* "Handbook of Psychobiology" (M. Gazzaniga and C. Blakemore, eds). Academic Press, New York and London, pp. 201–238.
Ferchmin, P. A., Bennett, E. L. and Rosenzweig, M. R. (1975). *J. Comp. Physiol. Psychol.* **88**, 360–367.
Flexner, J. B. and Flexner, L. B. (1967). *Proc. Nat. Acad. Sci. U.S.A.* **57**, 1651–1654.
Flexner, J. B. and Flexner, L. B. (1969). *Proc. Nat. Acad. Sci. U.S.A.* **62**, 729–732.
Flexner, L. B. and Flexner, J. B. (1966). *Proc. Nat. Acad. Sci. U.S.A.* **55**, 369–374.
Flexner, J. B. and Flexner, L. B. (1971). *Proc. Nat. Acad. Sci. U.S.A.* **68**, 2519–2521.
Flexner, L. B. and Goodman, R. H. (1975). *Proc. Nat. Acad. Sci. U.S.A.* **72**, 4660–4663.
Flexner, J. B., Flexner, L. B., Stellar, E., de la Haba, G. and Roberts, R. B. (1962). *J. Neurochem.* **9**, 595–605.
Flexner, L. B., Flexner, J. B., de la Haba, G. and Roberts, R. B. (1965). *J. Neurochem.* **12**, 505–514.
Flexner, L. B., Gambetti, P., Flexner, J. B. and Roberts, R. B. (1971). *Proc. Nat. Acad. Sci. U.S.A.* **68**, 26–28.
Flexner, L. B., Serota, R. G. and Goodman, R. H. (1973). *Proc. Nat. Acad. Sci. U.S.A.* **70**, 354–356.
Flood, J. F. and Jarvik, M. E. (1975). *In* "Neural approaches to learning and memory" (M. R. Rosenzweig and E. Bennett, eds). M.I.T. Press, Cambridge, Massachusetts.
Flood, J. F., Bennett, E. L., Orme, A. E. and Ronsenzweig, M. R. (1975). *Physiol. and Behav.* **15**, 97–102.
Gambetti, P., Hirt, L., Stieber, A. and Shafer, B. (1972). *Exp. Neurol.* **34**, 223–228.

Geller, A., Robustelli, F. and Jarvik, M. E. (1970). *Psychopharmacol.* **16**, 281–289.
Glassman, E. (1969). *Ann. Rev. Biochem.* **38**, 605–646.
Greenough, W. (1975). *In* "Neural approaches to learning and memory" (M. R. Ronsezweig and E. Bennett, eds). M.I.T. Press, Cambridge, Massachusetts.
Hambley, J. W. and Rose, S. P. R. (1973). *Abst. ISN meeting, Tokyo.*
Hambley, J. W., Rose, S. P. R. and Bateson, P. P. G. (1972). *Biochem. J.* **127**, 90P.
Hambley, J. W., Haywood, J., Rose, S. P. R. and Bateson, P. P. G. (1976). *J. Neurobiol.* (in press).
Haywood, J., Hambley, J. W. and Rose, S. P. R. (1975a). *Brain Res.* **92**, 219–225.
Haywood, J., Hambley, J. W., Rose, S. P. R. and Bateson, P. P. G. (1974). *Trans. Biochem. Soc.* **2**, 241–243.
Haywood, J., Rose, S. P. R. and Bateson, P. P. G. (1970). *Nature* **228**, 373–374.
Haywood, J., Rose, S. P. R. and Bateson, P. P. G. (1975b). *Brain Res.* **92**, 223–235.
Hershkowitz, M., Wilson, J. E. and Glassman, E. (1975). *J. Neurochem.* **25**, 687–694.
Horn, G., Rose, S. P. R. and Bateson, P. P. G. (1973a). *Science* **181**, 506–514.
Horn, G., Bateson, P. P. G. and Rose, S. P. R. (1973). *Brain Res.* **56**, 227–237.
Hydén, H. (1973a). *In* "Macromolecules and Behaviour" (G. B. Ansell and P. B. Bradley, eds). Macmillan, London.
Hydén, H. (1973b). *In* "Macromolecules and Behaviour" (G. B. Ansell and P. B. Bradley, eds). Macmillan, London.
Hydén, H. (1973c). *Abstr. 4th Meeting of Int. Soc. Neurochem, Tokyo.*
Hydén, H. (1976). *In* "Perspectives in Brain Research" (M. Corner and R. Swaab, eds). Elsevier Press, Amsterdam (in press).
Hydén, H. and Egyházi, E. (1962). *Proc. Nat. Acad. Sci. U.S.A.* **48**, 1366–1373.
Hydén, H. and Egyházi, E. (1964). *Proc. Nat. Acad. Sci. U.S.A.* **52**, 1030–1035.
Hydén, H. and Lange, P. W. (1968). *Science* **159**, 1370–1373.
Hydén, H. and Lange, P. W. (1970). *Exp. Cell Res.* **62**, 125–132.
Jakoubek, B., Buresova, M., Hakej, I., Etrychova, A., Pavlik, A. and Dedicova, A. (1972). *Brain Res.* **43**, 417–428.
Jewett, R. E., Pirch, J. H. and Norton, S. (1965). *Nature* **207**, 277–278.
Jones-Lecointe, A., Rose, S. P. R. and Sinha, A. K. (1976). *J. Neurochem.* **26**, 929–933.
Kahan, B., Krigman, M. R., Wilson, J. E. and Glassman, E. (1970). *Proc. Nat. Acad. Sci. U.S.A.* **65**, 300–303.
Karpiak, S. E. and Rapport, M. M. (1975). *Brain Res.* **92**, 405–413.
Krivanek, J. (1975). *Experientia* **31**, 1042–1043.
Lat, J., Pavlik, A. and Jakoubek, B. (1973). *Physiol. Behav.* **11**, 131–137.
Levitan, I. B., Mushynski, W. E. and Ramirez, G. (1972). *Brain Res.* **41**, 498–502.
Lim, R., Brink, J. J. and Agranoff, B. W. (1970). *J. Neurochem.* **17**, 1637–1647.
Luttges, M., Johnson, T., Buck, C., Holland, J. and McGaugh, J. L. (1966). *Science* **151**, 834–837.
Machlus, B., Entingh, D., Wilson, J. E. and Glassman, E. (1974a). *Behav. Biol.* **10**, 43–62.
Machlus, B., Wilson, J. E. and Glassman, E. (1974b). *Behav. Biol.* **10**, 63–73.
McGaugh, J. L. (1966). *Science* **153**, 1351–1358.
McGaugh, J. L. and Gold, P. (1975). *In* "Neural approaches to learning and memory" (M. R. Rosenzweig and E. L. Bennett, eds). M.I.T. Press, Cambridge, Massachusetts.
Marchisio, P. and Bondy, S. C. (1974). *Experientia* **30**, 335–336.
Mareš, V., Brückner, G., Biesold, D. and Narovec, T. (1975). *Abst Symp. Visual System, Reinhardsbrunn.*
Mark, R. F. and Watts, M. E. (1971). *Proc. Roy. Soc. Ser. B.* **178**, 439–454.

Matthies, H., Fähse, C. and Lietz, W. (1971). *Psychopharmacol.* **20**, 10–15.

Meisami, E. and Timiras, P. V. (1974). *J. Neurochem.* **22**, 725–729.

Møllgaard, K., Diamond, M. C., Bennett, E. L., Rosenzweig, M. R. and Lindner, B. (1971). *Int. J. Neurosci.* **2**, 113–128.

Nadel, L. and O'Keefe, J. (1974). *In* "Essays on the Nervous System" (R. Bellairs and E. G. Gray, eds). Clarendon Press, Oxford, pp. 368–390.

Oja, S. S. (1973). *Int. J. Neurosci.* **5**, 31–33.

Palay, S. and Chan-Palay, V. (1972). *In* "Metabolic Compartmentation in the Brain" (R. Balázs and J. E. Cremer, eds). Macmillan, London, pp. 287–304.

Popov, N. Rüthrich, H. L., Pohle, W., Schulzeck, S. and Matthies, H. (1976). *Brain Res.* **101**, 295–304.

Quartermain, D., McEwen, B. S. and Azmitia, E. C. (1970). *Science* **169**, 683–686.

Ramirez, G., Karlsson, B. and Perrin, C. L. (1974). *Brain Res.* **79**, 296–300.

Rees, H. D., Brogan, L. L., Entingh, D. J., Dunn, A. J. and Shinkman, P. G. (1974). *Brain Res.* **68**, 143–156.

Richardson, K. and Rose, S. P. R. (1972). *Brain Res.* **44**, 299–303.

Richardson, K. and Rose, S. P. R. (1973a). *J. Neurochem.* **21**, 521–530.

Richardson, K. and Rose, S. P. R. (1973b). *J. Neurochem.* **21**, 531–537.

Rogers, L. J., Drennan, H. D. and Mark, R. F. (1974). *Brain Res.* **79**, 213–233.

Rose, S. P. R. (1967a). *Nature* **215**, 253–255.

Rose, S. P. R. (1967b). *Biochem. J.* **102**, 33–43.

Rose, S. P. R. (1970). *In* "Short term changes in neural activity and behaviour" (R. Hinde and G. Horn, eds). University Press, Cambridge, pp. 517–551.

Rose, S. P. R. (1975). *Int. J. Neurosci. Res.* **1**, 19–30.

Rose, S. P. R. (1976a). *Phil. Trans. Roy. Soc.* (in press).

Rose, S. P. R. (1976b). "The Conscious Brain" 2nd edn Penguin, Harmondsworth.

Rose, S. P. R. and Sinha, A. K. (1974a). *J. Neurochem.* **23**, 1065–1076.

Rose, S. P. R. and Sinha, A. K. (1974b). *Life Sci.* **15**, 223–230.

Rose, S. P. R., Sinha, A. K. (1976). *J. Neurochem.* **27**, 963–967.

Rose, S. P. R., Sinha, A. K. and Broomhead, S. (1973). *J. Neurochem.* **21**, 539–546.

Rose, S. P. R., Hambley, J. and Haywood, J. (1975). *In* "Neural approaches to learning and memory" (M. R. Rosenzweig and E. L. Bennett, eds). M.I.T. Press, Cambridge, Massachusetts.

Rose, S. P. R., Sinha, A. K. and Jones-Lecointe, A. (1976). *FEBS lett.* **65**, 135–139.

Rosenzweig, M. R. and Bennett, E. L. (eds) (1975). "Neural approaches to learning and memory". M.I.T. Press, Cambridge, Massachusetts.

Rosenzweig, M. R., Bennett, E. L. and Diamond, M. C. (1972). *In* "Macromolecules and Behaviour" 2nd edn (J. Gaito, ed). Appleton-Century Crofts, New York, pp. 205– 227.

Schluederberg, A., Hendel, R. C. and Chavanich, S. (1971). *Science* **172**, 577–579.

Schotman, P., Gipon, L. and Gispen, W. H. (1974). *Brain Res.* **70**, 377–380.

Shashoua, V. E. (1968). *Nature* **217**, 238–240.

Shashova, V. E. (1970). *Proc. Nat. Acad. Sci. U.S.A.* **65**, 160–167.

Siegel, M. R. and Sisler, H. D. (1963). *Nature* **200**, 675–676.

Sinha, A. K. and Rose, S. P. R. (1976). *J. Neurochem.* **27**, 921–927.

Squire, L. R. and Barondes, S. H. (1970). *Nature* **225**, 649–650.

Squire, L. R. and Barondes, S. H. (1972). *Proc. Nat. Acad. Sci. U.S.A.* **69**, 1416–1420.

Squire, L. R. and Becker, C. K. (1975). *Brain Res.* **97**, 367–372.

Squire, L. R., Geller, A. and Jarvik, M. E. (1970). *Commun. Behav. Biol.* **5**, 249–254.

Squire, L. R., Kuczenski, R. and Barondes, S. H. (1974). *Brain Res.* **82**, 241–248.

Traketellis, A. C., Montjar, M. and Axelrod, A. E. (1965). *Biochemistry* **4**, 2065–2071.

Ungar, G. (1970). *In* "Protein Metabolism in the Nervous System" (Lajtha, A. ed.). Plenum Press, New York, pp. 571–585.

Ungar, G. (1971). *In* "Chemistry of Acquired Information" (A. Schwarz, ed.). Appleton-Century Crofts, New York, pp. 479–514.

Ungar, G., Desiderio, D. M. and Parr, W. (1972). *Nature* **238**, 198–202.

Uphouse, L., MacInnes, J. W. and Schlesinger, K. (1972). *Physiol. Behav.* **9**, 315–318.

Valverde, F. (1967). *Exp. Brain Res.* **3**, 337–352.

Valverde, F. (1971). *Brain Res.* **33**, 1–11.

Vrensson, G. and de Groot, D. (1974). *Brain Res.* **78**, 263–278.

Vrensson, G. and de Groot, D. (1975). *Brain Res.* **93**, 15–24.

Walters, B. B. and Matus, A. I. (1975). *Nature* **257**, 496–498.

Watts, M. E. and Mark, R. F. (1971a). *Proc. Roy. Soc. Ser. B* **178**, 455–464.

Watts, M. E. and Mark, R. F. (1971b). *Brain Res.* **25**, 420–423.

Wenzel, J., David, H., Marx, I. and Matthies, H. (1975). *Brain Res.* **84**, 99–109.

Zemp, J. W., Wilson, J. E., Schlesinger, K., Boggan, W. O. and Glassman, E. (1966). *Proc. Nat. Acad. Sci. U.S.A.* **55**, 1423–1431.

Zemp, J. W., Wilson, J. E. and Glassman, E. (1967). *Proc. Nat. Acad. Sci. U.S.A.* **58**, 1120–1125.

Chapter 9

The Biochemistry of Sleep

ANTONIO GIUDITTA

International Institute of Genetics and Biophysics, via G. Marconi 10, Naples, Italy

I. Introduction

As in the case of other complex neural functions the contribution that molecular studies may give to the understanding of the function of sleep is evaluated differently according to the general attitude taken with regard to biological epistemology. For the believer in reductionism explanation follows solely or ultimately from knowledge of molecular events, and this view would make him willing to attribute the utmost importance to biochemical investigations of the sleep states. On the other hand, and this happens to be the minority view among scientists, other people prefer to emphasize the relevance of all levels of organization in the understanding of biological functions and in particular of neural activities. This attitude does not underestimate the need for a full elucidation of the molecular events occurring during sleep. It merely stresses the additional need to consider also supramolecular processes involving the cell, the tissue and the whole system. The behaviour of the brain and of the organism in the transition between the states of wakefulness and sleep is likely to be modified at all levels of organization and it will remain for the future scholar to assess their relative order of importance in the explanation of the functions of sleep. But even if we assume that the relevant processes are taking place above the molecular level, knowledge of the biochemical events would still be essential to prove the issue in our present condition of ignorance and to establish whether molecular reactions follow similar or different patterns in the switching of cerebral states. The problem is also operational, requiring the use of cellular and subcellular techniques to pinpoint differences which would otherwise average out in the heterogeneity of neural structures. In other words, it is conceivable that overall biochemical processes in brain may be basically similar in sleep and in wakefulness and that only their spatial distribution within the tissue is changed.

An obvious but important distinction should separate the biochemical processes occurring during sleep in the brain from those present in the remaining organs of the body. Sleep is a condition involving the whole organism and might significantly influence the biochemical operations of non-nervous tissues and organs. The hormonal changes which take place during the sleep–wakefulness cycle emphasize this point since they are presumably addressed to more cell types than the neural elements. Conceivably, in the brain itself sleep may bring about metabolic changes similar to those induced in other organs, in addition to more specific and telling effects. While tissue-specificity should definitely be established, there seems to be no compelling reason to disregard the brain changes occurring also in other organs and to consider them as irrelevant to the understanding of the neural functions of sleep. A metabolic event might actually assume different and specific meanings according to the type of cell and tissue in which it takes place.

This article was aimed at bringing together the available information on the biochemical behaviour of the brain during sleep from the point of view of the function subserved by this state. No attempt has been made to cover the voluminous literature dealing with the involvement of cerebral neurotransmitters in sleep. This task would have required an article in itself, and an extensive review has appeared recently (Jouvet, 1972). In addition, neurotransmitters are at the borderline with the neurophysiological and neuropharmacological approach (Steriade and Hobson, 1976) and at this stage of the game they are more likely to provide information on the mechanism of sleep rather than on its function.

II. The Sleep States

It is by now common knowledge that the period of sleep in higher vertebrates is structured in several phases or states, which differ on a number of parameters. On the basis of electroencephalographic (EEG) criteria the state which differs most from wakefulness (W) is the slow wave or synchronized sleep (SS), the first one to be described (Berger, 1929), characterized in man by the occurrence of high voltage oscillations of low frequency (<2 Hz) and of less frequent spindles (10–12 Hz) and K complexes (fast wave followed by slow oscillation). SS has been further distinguished in four states, the first one of which is characterized by mixed frequency low amplitude waves, and represents the first state entered from W. By some authors it is not considered part of SS. In state 2 the background of mixed frequency becomes slower and slow waves, spindles and K complexes appear. In states 3 and 4 slow waves increase in amount and the distinction becomes somewhat arbitrary (state 3, 20–50% slow waves; state 4, >50%). A different state is reached when the EEG pattern resumes a low amplitude mixed frequency similar to state 1 (emergent state 1) in association with a number of phasic events the most widely known of which are the rapid eye movements (REM). These occur singly but more usually in clusters on both eyes and are accompanied by the presence of rapid waves recorded from the pons, geniculate bodies and occipital cortex (ponto–geniculate–occipital or PGO waves). Since the EEG and other parameters are more similar to wakefulness than sleep, this state has received the name of paradoxical sleep (PS). During this state phasic movements can occur in many parts of the body, like limbs, fingers, vibrissae, facial muscles etc. Another important feature of this state is the lack of tone in antigravitary muscles (e.g. neck muscles). Muscle tone becomes lower but does not disappear during SS. An automatic procedure to deprive animals selectively of PS is based on this property. Animals are placed on small platforms surrounded by water in which they fall and awake whenever PS occurs. The tone of antigravitary muscles which persists during SS is sufficient to keep them on the platform. Autonomic functions like heart frequency, blood pressure and respiration which are less intense and quite regular during SS become activated and irregular during PS. Major psychic events during PS are the dreams which occur chiefly during this state, as shown by awaking subjects from various states of sleep. Thought-like activity prevails instead during SS (Recht-schaffen, 1973).

During the course of a sleep period, the first state to be entered is 1, followed by states 2, 3 and 4. There follows a return to 3 and 2 and finally entrance into PS. After the PS episode (lasting up to 20 min in man) a new cycle starts again and terminates with another PS episode. Duration of this cycle in adult humans is about 90 min. Stages 3 and 4 predominate during the initial half of the sleep period while PS prevails during the latter half.

Ontogenetic studies of sleep have revealed that the absolute amount of PS is higher in young animals and may reach 100% total time in foetuses before term. In newborn babies which sleep two-thirds of the time, 50% of the sleep time is PS. The remaining sleep does not develop into full SS until the first months of life. It would seem that the first type of sleep to appear in ontogenesis, even before the animal is exposed to the external environment, is PS. A mature SS appears later, after exposure to the external stimulation.

The phylogenetic picture is more complex. PS occurs chiefly in homeotherms, birds and mammals, but also in some reptilian species. In birds PS episodes are very short. An undeniable correlation exists between complexity of the brain (and of incoming information input) and amount of PS across species. Clear correlations exist furthermore across mammalian species between several sleep parameters and physiological variables like body weight, life span and gestational time which are known to be interrelated. Duration of the sleep period is directly related to the body weight of the species, and therefore inversely related to metabolic rate (Zepelin and Rechtschaffen, 1974).

Of special importance for the biochemical understanding of the sleep phenomena are the hormonal changes which accompany the occurrence of sleep. It has long been known that the blood level of ACTH and corticosteroids undergo a circadian fluctuation with a maximum in the early morning. This rhythm can be dissociated from the sleep–wakefulness rhythm (Rubin et al., 1974). On the other hand, the level of growth hormone (GH) increases during the first sleep cycle in association with stages 3 and 4 from which it cannot be dissociated by displacement of the sleep period to the original wakefulness time (Takahashi et al., 1968; Sassin et al., 1969a). Mechanisms triggering GH release in man may require short periods of stage 3 or may even be associated to stage 2 sleep since deprivation of stages 3 and 4 was not consistently accompanied by inhibition of GH secretion (Sassin et al., 1969b). In view of the anabolic function of this hormone (Korner,

1965; Tata, 1968) SS is considered a period of enhanced synthesis of protein and nucleic acids in the brain and in other organs of the body (Oswald, 1969). GH appears furthermore to participate in the induction of PS since a significant increase in PS time occurs after intraperironeal (i.p.) injection of the hormone in rats (Drucker-Colin et al., 1975) and cats (Stern et al., 1975). Several other hormones have been reported to vary during sleep periods (Rubin et al., 1974; Rubin, 1975). An increase during the latter part of the night occurs for testosterone (Evans et al., 1971) and prolactin (Sassin et al., 1972; Rubin et al., 1975), while blood levels of follicle stimulating hormone (FSH) and luteinizing hormone (LH) do not differ substantially between sleep and wakefulness (Rubin et al., 1972). An enhanced secretion of LH and of testosterone during sleep occurs however at the time of puberty (Boyar et al., 1974).

Several sleep parameters are genetically determined. Spindles (10–12 Hz) are present in CBA mice but absent in the C57BR strain. Other differences regard the duration of total sleep which is longer in CBA, the duration of PS which is longer in C57BR and the difference in sleep time between day and night which is considerably greater in the latter strain (Valatz et al., 1972). Interstrain hybrids are more similar to CBA mice with regard to sleep parameters, but lack the retinal degeneration of the parent strain. Back-crosses between first generation hybrids and C57BR mice show segregation of EEG spindling (Valatz and Bugat, 1974). Duration of SS and PS appears to be determined independently. Interstrain differences occur also in the distribution of REMs. In comparison with Balb mice the C57BR strain has a lower REM frequency and more REM clusters per PS episode but each cluster has a shorter duration (Cespuglio et al., 1975).

By recording the activity of single neurones impaled with microelectrodes in freely moving animals it has been ascertained that in general the average frequency of neuronal discharge tends to decrease during SS and to return to or even surpass W values during PS (Evarts, 1964; Evarts, 1967; Noda and Ross Adey, 1970; Desiraju, 1972; Steriade et al., 1974). In addition, the temporal pattern of discharge observed during W may become drastically different during sleep. For instance, in pyramidal tract neurones the relatively uniform spiking present during W is superseded by clusters of spikes followed by long silent periods during SS. The latter pattern becomes even more pronounced during PS (Evarts, 1967). On the other hand, the pattern of discharge in association cortex remains tonic with no bursts of spikes during sleep (Desiraju, 1972). With regard to the hypothetical relative rest of small (inhibitory) neurones during sleep, it is of interest that their frequency of firing has been found to remain at levels comparable or even higher than those prevailing during W (Steriade *et al.*, 1974). A reduced function of these neurones during sleep was presumed to be required for recovering from wakefulness activities.

The elevated neuronal activity which occurs in PS is accompanied by a marked increase in cerebral blood flow (CBF). In cats deprived of sleep for one to two days on a rotating treadmill the concentration of ^{14}C-antipyrine given intravenously (i.v.) at a constant rate for one minute increased in all the 25 brain regions examined with comparison to values obtained during W in non-deprived animals. The most pronounced changes were observed in brain stem and diencephalic structures. Among cortical sites CBF increased most in hippocampus and association areas and least in sensory-motor cortex (Fig. 1). By considering the size of each region the overall increase was calculated to reach 80% (Reivich *et al.*, 1968). While sleep deprivation, exercise and stress might have partly influenced CBF rates, the increase in CBF values during PS has been consistently verified with independent methods of analysis. In man, cortical blood flow during PS was found to increase up to 50% with relation to SS values using a thermal clearance technique (Seylaz *et al.*, 1971) and about 23% using curves of ^{133}Xe clearance (Townsend *et al.*, 1973). The moderate increase reported in the latter investigation should be considered to reflect more an average value in view of the relatively long time (10 min) required for analysis and of the correlation of CBF values with density of phasic events occurring during PS.

Somewhat more contradictory are the data relative to CBF during SS. In the study of Reivich *et al.* (1968), only 10 out of 25 brain regions showed an increased blood flow during SS. The increase reached 20–30% in the cerebellar and association cortex but remained insignificant in other cortical regions. The overall increase reached 15%. A similar increase (10–15%) with regard to W was found in human cortical blood flow using a thermal clearance technique, but the effect was not consistently observed (Seylaz *et al.*, 1971). On the other hand, human cortical blood flow was found to decrease about 10% during SS using the method of ^{133}Xe clearance (Townsend *et al.*, 1973). As W is not a homogeneous state, these discrepancies might be attributed in part to the different states of W taken as reference. It may be concluded, on the whole, that during SS CBF, and in particular cortical blood flow, remains essentially similar to the value prevailing during quiet W. This is somewhat surprising in view of the general trend towards a reduction in neuronal activity which occurs during SS. Although this lack of correlation has been taken to indicate vasomotor control of CBF

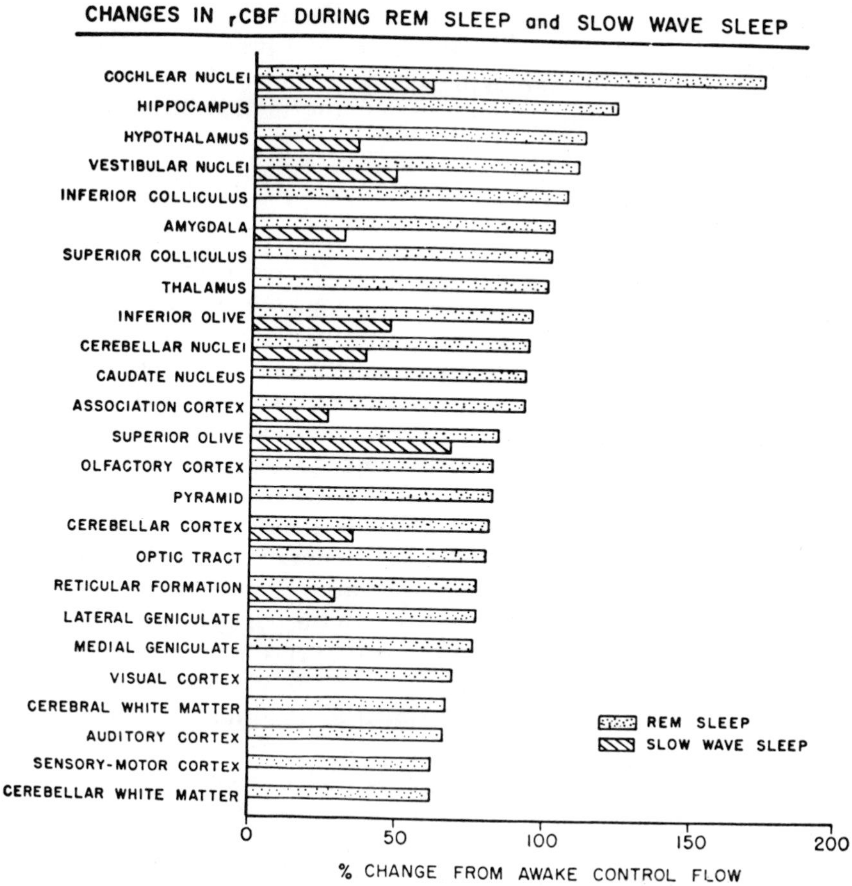

CHANGES IN rCBF DURING REM SLEEP and SLOW WAVE SLEEP

Fig. 1. Blood flow in various cerebral regions (rCBF) of the cat during REM sleep and slow wave sleep. Determinations were carried out with autoradiographic techniques after intravenous injection of ^{14}C-antipyrine at constant rate for one minute. (From Reivich et al., 1968.)

(Seylaz et al., 1971) neuronal activity actually monitors only part of the overall cerebral metabolism, which is also due to glial elements. Overall cerebral O_2 uptake measured by arterio-venous difference in sleeping men was not found to be substantially different from relaxed W although there was a slight tendency towards a decrease (Mangold et al., 1955). The possibility of regional variations was pointed out by the finding that in the dog the passage from W to SS was accompanied by a moderate but significant decrease in the rate of cortical O_2 uptake. In man, the cerebral blood volume was also shown to vary to a different extent in various cortical regions, with a general increase during PS in comparison with SS. The variation was more pronounced in frontal and parietal regions. Cerebral blood volume reflects CBF and may be taken as an index of functional activity (Ingvar, 1975).

III. Possible Functions of Sleep

In the adult mammal sleep is generally considered a period of recovery of mental abilities. This broad conclusion is based on the outcome of experiments of total and selective sleep deprivation, on observations relating brain functions with sleep parameters and on the refreshing effects experienced after a period of sleep. According to other views, sleep should be considered an instinct, endowed with appetitive and consummatory phases (Claparède, 1905; Moruzzi, 1969; Mancia, 1975) and addressed to maintain some central parameters within homeostatic limits (Moruzzi, 1972) or simply to prevent other behavioural responses and thus save energy and avoid negative environmental conditions such as predators (Webb, 1974). Although the recognition of the instinctive nature of sleep may help to categorize it with other responses of organisms and to classify sleep mechanisms under a new perspective, it does not seem to provide significant clues as to the role subserved by this functional state. Similarly, as the sleep–wakefulness cycle originated most probably from the rest–activity cycle of the most primitive organisms, to consider sleep merely as a state of non-responding would unnecessarily limit its role to that presumably prevailing in less evolved species.

More specific hypotheses have concerned the role of PS (for review, see Hennevin and Leconte, 1971). This type of sleep has been alternatively regarded as a recurrent "sentinel" state which facilitates monitoring of potentially dangerous environmental conditions (Snyder, 1966), as a period of enhanced neuronal activity required for the maturation and maintenance of brain circuitry (Roffwarg et al., 1966) or of oculomotor pathways (Berger, 1969), or as a condition involved in memory functions (Greenberg and Pearlman, 1974).

In the general framework of the recovery hypothesis it is clear that this process cannot be related to the maintenance of neuronal activity in the same way as the restoration of ionic unbalance across the cell membrane. It is well known that several nerve centres (e.g. respiratory centre) and non-nervous organs such as the heart maintain their activity throughout the life span of an organism without resorting to a special period of recovery. In more general terms it may be concluded that processes such as those related to the generation, conduction and transmission of impulses are not likely to require a long-lasting recovery period such as sleep. Optimal conditions for impulse trade are indeed continuously regenerated in individual neurones. This is actually borne out by the recognition that the overall rate of discharge of single brain neurones during SS remains comparable to that of wakefulness and may actually increase during PS (Evarts, 1967; Steriade et al., 1974). By the same token, it does not seem likely that sleep is required to convert biopolymers from a metastable to a stable state in order to counteract the inverse process presumed to take place during wakefulness (Kleinschmidt, 1974), unless it is further assumed that these changes are related to activities other than impulse flow. Recovery must therefore involve more complex operations resulting from the coordinated interplay of populations of nerve cells which may well be distributed over the whole brain. These operations are likely to be different from those prevailing during wakefulness, although it is conceivable that they might also occur in awake animals at an insufficient pace. The nature of these operations is still not clear, but a pertinent conceptual framework is being progressively laid down, mainly as result of deprivation experiments and with regard to the paradoxical phase of sleep.

Deprivation of total sleep brings about alterations in the subjective state, severe decrements in performance and an increased tendency to sleep. According to the lapse hypothesis periods of lowered reactive capacity which occur periodically in normal subjects increase in frequency and duration with the degree of sleep loss (Williams et al., 1959; 1966). The encoding of items in short-term memory appears impaired during these periods (Polzella, 1975).

When sleep is restricted to a few hours stages 3 and 4 remain essentially unchanged while all other stages decrease. PS and stage 2 decrease most markedly. In the following recovery night there is a lengthening of sleep duration which is chiefly accounted for by PS and stage 2 (Webb and Agnew, 1965; 1975). This finding appears in line with the structure of sleep observed in short and long sleepers and, in particular, with the relative predominance of stage 4 in short sleepers and with the increased duration of stage 2 and PS in long sleepers (Webb and Agnew, 1970).

After a period of total sleep loss recovery sleep is longer than normal but considerably less than the total sleep loss. The increase (rebound) concerns primarily SS and eventually PS. According to Jouvet (1972) SS is proportional to the log of the duration of the preceding W period while PS is proportional to the duration of the preceding W period

(1/10 approximately). Upon selective deprivation of PS or of stages 3 and 4 a pressure develops to reenter the deprived state, as shown by the marked increase in number of awakenings necessary to keep the subject out of it. This pressure is also evident in the selective increase in duration of the deprived state on recovery nights (Dement, 1960; Agnew et al., 1967). Differential effects have been reported to accompany PS and stages 3 and 4 deprivation with regard to mood which becomes irritable, anxious and hyperinstinctive in the former case and somewhat depressed and lethargic in the latter (Agnew et al., 1967). These differences have not been reproduced in other studies.

The state of PS has been correlated to memory functions by a number of observations. Indirect evidence on this point was based initially on the inverse relationship of amount of PS and mental retardation (Feinberg, 1968), on the increased PS time of recuperating aphasic but not stationary patients (Greenberg and Dewan, 1969), on the increased PS time of subjects wearing inverted prisms which imposed reorganization of spatial relationships. Recently more straightforward evidence has been obtained in animal studies which have shown enhancement of PS time following acquisition of a variety of tasks (Lucero, 1970; Fishbein et al., 1974; Hennevin et al., 1974; Smith et al., 1974) and failure in retention when acquisition was followed by selective PS deprivation (Leconte et al., 1974). While contradictory findings have also been reported, the most plausible conclusion appears to be that PS is required in memory functions triggered by acquisition of complex and emotion-laden inputs (Grieser et al., 1972), but not in the acquisition of simple and neutral tasks, and in general not of tasks commensurate to the behavioural repertoire of the species (Greenberg and Pearlman, 1974). In other words, only novel information inducing a behavioural response for which the organism is not prepared (Seligman, 1970; Bolles, 1970) should be expected to require PS in order to be properly memorized. This challenging situation does involve a strong emotional participation.

PS deprivation has been reported to maintain the memory trace in a labile state for days, as evidenced by its susceptibility to the amnesic effects of electroconvulsive shock (ECS) (Fishbein et al., 1971) which otherwise becomes ineffective with a sharp temporal gradient after acquisition (Mcgaugh, 1966). In addition, PS deprivation lowers the threshold to ECS (Cohen and Dement, 1965) and decreases the duration of the tonic phase of convulsions (Handwerker and Fishbein, 1975). On the other hand, ECS appears to act as a PS substitute since it decreases PS time without subsequent rebound (Cohen and Dement, 1966 and 1967). The adverse effect of PS deprivation on memory retention appears to be potentiated in man by administration of doxycycline, a tetracycline antibiotic endowed with the capacity to inhibit protein synthesis (Allen, 1975).

On the psychoanalytic level ego defence mechanisms are believed to be activated during PS (Hartman, 1973) mainly on the basis of personality changes produced by PS deprivation (Greenberg et al., 1970; Cartwright and Ratzel, 1972) and of surfacing of psychic contents of strong emotional tone. In general accord with this view is the relationship between duration of PS and type of personality in short and long sleepers and in variable sleepers (Hartman et al., 1973 and 1973a). Ego defence mechanisms are likely to be related to the memory functions occurring during PS and in a similar way imply an integration of novel percepts with past experience of similar modality. This process should not be considered a mere addition of new bits of information, but primarily a reorganization of preexisting memory clusters and a reprogramming of perceptual, decisional and output rules (Bryson and Schacher, 1969). From this point of view the concept of recovery is no longer sufficient to account for sleep functions and should be integrated by the concept of reprogramming (Dewan, 1970). An additional important feature of the recovery hypothesis, initially suggested by Jackson (1932) regards the shedding of irrelevant information from brain storage circuitry. The failure of PS deprivation to inhibit memory storage of a certain category of perceptual inputs (Pearlman, 1971; Pearlman, 1973; Joy and Prinz, 1969; Miller et al., 1971) indicates that the primary process of laying down the memory trace is not selectively occurring during PS. This is also borne out by the absence of PS in the majority of animal species (Tauber, 1974) which are nonetheless capable of long-term storage. What is more likely to occur during PS is the ordering of memories in organized patterns presumably aiming at a more efficient retrieval of individual sets or, conversely, in the case of memories with ego-destructive potentials, to their substantial protection from retrieval processes. It is also likely that ordering of memories implies formation of bonds or associations with memories of similar nature, according to rules which may be understandable at the psychological level but whose neuro-physiological codes are almost completely unknown (Bakan, 1975).

However penetrant these formulations may turn out to be, they concern only the role of PS and appear actually to be based on the concept of two different sleep phases with little if any mutual relationship. In a similar perspective the period of SS has been related to restoration following physical exercise (Baekeland and Lasky, 1966; Hobson, 1968; Matsumoto et al., 1968, Horne and Porter, 1975), to starvation (MacFadyen *et al.*, 1973) and, more generally, to anabolic processes of undefined nature and localization (Oswald, 1969; Hartman, 1973), mainly on the basis of the associated GH release in blood (Takahashi *et al.*, 1968).

While it is likely that each phase of sleep and in particular PS and SS subserve different functional roles, sleep as a whole should be considered an integrated mode of activity of the brain in the spiralling continuum of the sleep–wakefulness cycle. Some experimental support for this view may be derived from the observation that rearing rats in an enriched environment increases their total sleep time but does not change the percentage of PS (Tagney, 1973). In man, although a retention deficit for complex items has been reported to occur after selective PS deprivation (Emson and Clarke, 1970), other investigations have failed to differentiate the effects of PS and stage 4 deprivation on a number of performance and memory functions (Johnson, 1973) even after potentiation of the presumed deficits by a subsequent period of total sleep deprivation (Johnson *et al.*, 1974). In addition, the decrement in performance and mood capacities induced by loss of total sleep disappeared at equal rates regardless of the selective deprivation of PS or stage 4 sleep imposed during recovery (Lubin *et al.*, 1974). Retention may actually improve after a period of sleep with prevailing SS in comparison with a period of sleep of the same duration with prevalent PS (Fowler *et al.*, 1973). The latter finding is one of the very few (Latash *et al.*, 1975) which appears to suggest a memory function for SS. A correlation between amount of SS and intensity of visual stimulation has been reported in human subjects (Horne and Walmsley, 1975). From this point of view, the sequential occurrence of SS before PS (Jouvet, 1967), the prior SS rebound in experiments of sleep deprivation (Agnew *et al.*, 1967; Kales *et al.*, 1970; Berger and Oswald, 1962; Williams *et al.*, 1964; Dement and Greenberg, 1966; Webb and Agnew, 1965), the absence of PS in phylogenetically less developed species (Tauber, 1974) appear to indicate that some of the initial steps in information processing occur during SS and are required for the further processing that takes place during PS. The nature of these operations is unknown but might also be related to the ordering of memories. A similar interpretation of the relationship between SS and PS has been presented on the basis of some experimental evidence (Latash *et al.*, 1975).

IV. Sleep-inducing Factors

The possibility that sleep might be induced by injection of humoral factors accumulating during wakefulness was first considered in the classic work of Legendre and Pieron (1910, 1913). Adult dogs were deprived of sleep for several days (150–293 h) by sensory stimulation and by preventing them from laying down during the day and by walking them at night. Histological examination of the brain indicated that under these conditions chromatolytic changes and other severe alterations of the neuronal cytoplasm and nucleus were consistently occurring in the frontal cortex. These changes were roughly proportional to the duration of the period of sleep loss and were fully reversed when the dog was allowed to sleep. As physical exercise did not produce similar alterations, they were attributed to a specific effect of prolonged wakefulness.

In the first series of experiments aimed at the humoral transmission of sleep, blood or serum withdrawn from sleep-deprived and control dogs was injected in large amounts in the circulation of recipient animals. Although similar brain alterations were specifically induced by blood or serum of sleep-deprived animals, a state resembling sleep was also produced by blood or serum derived from control dogs. In order to reduce these unspecific effects, in the following series of experiments brain extracts, serum and cerebrospinal fluid (CSF) obtained from sleep-deprived and control dogs were injected into the fourth ventricle of recipient animals. Using this procedure results were more consistent and a state of sleep lasting several hours was specifically induced when the donor was a sleep-deprived animal. Several attempts were subsequently made to define the properties of the sleep factor or hypnotoxin, as it was called for the pathological alterations which it caused in brain. As a result of these studies the factor was found to be inactivated by heat and by treatment with oxygen, to be non-dialysable and to be precipitated with ethanol. In current terminology, it appeared to behave as a macromolecule.

Despite the provocative nature of these findings the experiments left much to be desired on methodological grounds since they involved the withdrawal and injection of large volumes of CSF (4–8 ml) without anaesthesia and inflicted severe stress to both donor and recipient animals.

A replication of the Legendre and Pieron experiment was reported several years later by Schnedorf and Ivy (1939) using essentially similar techniques. Dogs were deprived of sleep by keeping them in a standing position for 7–16 days and 8 ml of their CSF were injected into the cisterna magna of recipient animals after the previous withdrawal of a corresponding volume of CSF. Nine out of 20 dogs which received CSF from sleep-deprived donors showed the occurrence of a sleep-like state, while only four of the 24 animals which had received normal CSF, their own CSF or a saline solution were similarly but less intensely affected. However, the experimental results suffered from the concomitance of side effects such as increases in body temperature and in CSF pressure which appeared to stem from the withdrawal and reinjection of CSF.

The problem of the humoral transmission of sleep has been recently reconsidered in several laboratories using substantially improved techniques and different assay systems. The most impressive results have been obtained by infusing CSF from sleep-deprived goats into the ventricles of chronically implanted cats and rats (Pappenheimer et al., 1967) and by administration to rabbits of a blood dialysate obtained from rabbits induced to sleep by thalamic stimulation (Monnier and Hösli, 1966).

In Pappenheimer's laboratory goats were deprived of sleep for three days by an automatic device which provided electric shock and acoustic alarm to relaxing animals. Goats were chronically implanted with a cisternal tube permitting withdrawal of CSF at a rate of 0·1 ml/min for several hours while the animal remained free to move and apparently unstressed. CSF from sleep-deprived and normal goats was injected at the rate of 3·3 µl/min for 30 min (0·1 ml total volume) in the lateral ventricle of unrestrained rats which were chronically implanted with a guide tube.

The infusion was made in the afternoon before the nocturnal period of activity which was monitored by photocell recording. In comparison with baseline values obtained before the injection, sleep-deprived but not normal or artificial CSF induced a significant decrease in locomotor activity which lasted several hours. The state of sleep was assessed also behaviourally and found to be readily reverted to wakefulness upon stimulation (Pappenheimer et al., 1967). It was thus established that sleep could be transmitted by a humoral factor present in the CSF after moderate sleep-deprivation, using unstressful methods of CSF withdrawal and infusion. Furthermore, transmission of sleep appeared to occur across species since the sleep factor obtained from goats proved effective in cats and rats. These results were confirmed in later experiments (Fencl et al., 1971) which showed, in addition, that the sleep factor induced a parallel increase in slow wave EEG activity. The concentration of sleep factor in the CSF of donor goats became significant after one day of deprivation and reached a maximum after two days (Fig. 2). This gradual accumulation supported the hypothesis that the factor may be actually regulating the sleep–wakefulness cycle. Since infusions made over the dorsal cortex failed to elicit sleep, it appeared reasonable to assume that the compound was acting at a periventricular site. No evidence is available on the site of synthesis and release of the sleep factor. Induction of sleep was not obtained with several known compounds including serotonin, butyrolactone, 4-OH-butyrate, glutamate, ε-amino-butyrate and cAMP.

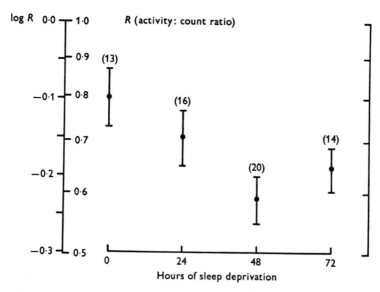

Fig. 2. Concentration of sleep-promoting factor in the cerebrospinal fluid (CSF) of a goat as function of the length of sleep deprivation. On the ordinate, nocturnal activity of rats infused with 0·1 ml CSF (means ±S.E.M.; in parenthesis number of infusions). R is defined as the activity counts in 6 h following infusion divided the activity counts in 6 h on the preceding night. (From Fencl et al., 1971.)

From experiments of molecular sieving carried out with calibrated membranes and Sephadex columns the sleep factor was estimated to be a peptide with molecular weight between 350 and 700, whose activity was completely lost upon incubation with pronase. Injection of 0·1 nmol (estimated by Fluorescamine fluorescence) into rats reduced their subsequent locomotor activity 30%. The factor was also active in rabbits which doubled the percentage of slow wave sleep for at least four hours after injection of 0·3 nmol (Pappenheimer et al., 1974).

During the course of these studies it became apparent that the CSF of normal and sleep-deprived goats contained an additional factor which was capable of inducing an immediate and long lasting excitatory behaviour in rats. Locomotor activity was markedly increased for several days but remained well coordinated. At variance with the sleep factor, the excitatory compound may be presumed to act on cortical tissue since its infusion over the dorsal cortex elicited the excitatory behaviour. Two excitatory peptides have been isolated from goat and human CSF by means of molecular sieving and paper electrophoresis. They have a similar amino acid composition (Asp, Glu, Lys, Ser, Gly, Ala and possibly Thr) but differ in the number of glutamic acid residues which are two or three in one peptide and nine or ten in the other one. Both peptides may be linked to carbohydrate (Pappenheimer et al., 1974).

The presence of "waking" factors had been previously noted in cross-circulation experiments carried out with "encéphale isolé" preparations from cats (Purpura, 1956) and in transfer experiments in rabbits (Monnier and Hösli, 1964).

In the experiments of humoral transfer of sleep carried out in Monnier's laboratory donor rabbits were subjected to extracorporeal countercurrent dialysis of the venous blood coming from the brain while hypnogenic centres present in the ventro-medial intralaminary thalamus were stimulated at low frequency. This procedure elicited a significant increase in the amount of slow wave activity in the EEG pattern with comparison to a previous unstimulated period and to sham-operated animals. In previous experiments of cross-circulation it had been shown that under these conditions sleep could be induced in the recipient rabbit (Monnier et al., 1963). In the initial experiments 20 ml of dialysate obtained from sleeping or control rabbits were injected intravenously in recipient animals (Monnier and Hösli, 1964) while in later work transfer was achieved by slow infusion of 0·05 ml of dialysate in the mesodiencephalic ventricle of mildly restrained or freely moving rabbits (Monnier and Hatt, 1971; Schoenenberger et al., 1972). Recipient rabbits were prepared the day before the experiment and were implanted in the morning under local anaesthesia. Upon infusion with the dialysate from sleeping animals a significant increase in slow wave activity was observed in the EEG record starting 10–15 min after the onset of the infusion. Normal EEG patterns were recovered within 15 min after the infusion was terminated (Fig. 3). In close correlation with the EEG effect the locomotor activity was markedly inhibited and the rabbit showed an evident sleep behaviour, while blood pressure, CSF pressure and respiration

A

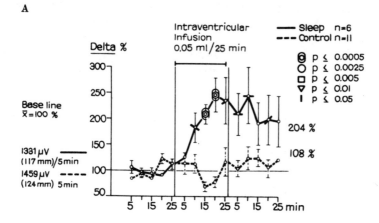

B

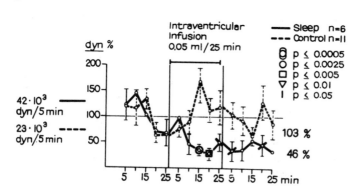

Fig. 3. Hypnogenic activity of the desalted fraction of a primary sleep dialysate obtained from the cerebral venous blood of rabbits subjected to stimulation of the thalamic sleep centre. A. Electroencephalographic test showing an increased delta activity symptomatic of orthodox sleep, during and after intraventricular infusion to recipient rabbits. B. Kinesigraphic behaviour test; decreased motor activity concurrent with delta sleep. (From Monnier *et al.*, 1973, with acknowledgements.)

remained unchanged. Only the heart rate was slightly reduced as in normal sleep. All these effects were not produced by infusion of a dialysate from a sham-operated rabbit (Monnier *et al.*, 1973). The activity of the sleep factor was sensitive to heat treatment and to acid and alkaline conditions (Monnier *et al.*, 1972; Monnier and Schoenenberger, 1972). Using gel filtration, thin layer chromatography and high voltage electrophoresis the sleep factor has been purified and shown to be a peptide with molecular weight around 800 yielding nine amino acids upon acid hydrolysis (Ser, Glu, 3 Gly, 2 Ala, Arg, Trp). Its active dose was calculated to be $3 \cdot 3 \times 10^{-9}$ mol.kg^{-1} (Schoenenberger and Monnier, 1975).

While this peptide was being successfully isolated from the blood of rabbits induced to sleep by thalamic stimulation, attempts to reproduce the same phenomenon using a blood dialysate from sleep-deprived rabbits met with failure (Ringle and Herndon, 1968). In this experiment rabbits were kept in a rotating cylinder for three days and stimulated periodically with light and buzzer. Plasma obtained from cardiac puncture was extensively dialysed, lyophilized and injected i.v. into rats, rabbits and mice. No significant effect was noted in the EEG of rats and rabbits recorded for 45 min after the injection nor in the locomotor activity of mice. In a second experiment CSF taken from sleep-deprived rabbits after electrocuting was slowly infused into the lateral ventricle of rats. Again, no significant effect was noted on locomotor activity, behaviour and EEG pattern in comparison with animals receiving control CSF (Ringle and Herndon, 1969). Although these data may be taken to suggest the absence of a sleep factor in sleep-deprived rabbits, a number of different reasons might explain the negative results, including electrocution of the rabbits before CSF withdrawal, or withdrawal of the blood from the heart instead of the cerebral venous system, as in Monnier's experiments. In any case, it remains well established that a sleep factor is present in sleep-deprived animals (Pappenheimer et al., 1974), even if the relationship of this compound with Monnier's peptide has not yet been elucidated.

A sleep promoting factor has been detected in the brain stem of rats deprived of sleep for one day by electric shock stimulation (Nagasaki et al., 1974). The tissue homogenate was dialysed against water and the lyophilized dialysate was injected i.p. into recipient rats where it produced a significant increase in the amount of EEG slow waves and a decrease in locomotor activity. Extracts from the brain stem of control rats had no effect.

Another sleep-inducing material has been obtained by means of a push–pull cannula from the mesencephalic reticular formation (MRF) of sleep-deprived cats. The perfusate obtained from sleeping animals, but not from awake cats, induced behavioural and EEG signs of normal sleep lasting 20–60 min upon its infusion in the MRF of recipient cats (Drucker-Colín et al., 1970). In later experiments it was confirmed that sleep perfusates from the cat MRF specifically increased the duration of SS and decreased its latency in recipient animals, without affecting PS (Drucker-Colín, 1973).

With regard to the possible humoral transmission of PS, experiments with rats have shown a significant synchrony of occurrence of PS in members of parabiotic pairs but not in rats joined through the skin and lacking a cross circulation (Matsumoto *et al.*, 1972). This finding might suggest the presence of humoral factors regulating the occurrence of PS. One such factor might indeed be GH whose administration has recently been reported to increase the duration of PS in cats (Stern *et al.*, 1975) and rats (Drucker-Colin *et al.*, 1975).

V. Intermediary Metabolism

Several studies have indicated that the lactate concentration decreases in the brain during SS while phosphocreatine and ATP increase slightly. These changes may be interpreted in terms of a reduced utilization of energy with a concomitant reduced utilization of glucose through the glycolytic pathway. The first report (Richter and Dawson, 1948) concerned young rats induced to sleep by a strong light, and killed by immersion in liquid nitrogen after 30 min. The brain of these animals was found to contain 35% less lactate than the brain of rats in a state varying from "dozing" to "resisting handling". Sleep was monitored by behavioural observation. Similar findings were later confirmed with young rats and extended to adult rats and hamsters (Cooks, 1967). In this experiment sleep was spontaneous for at least 30 min and the animals were killed by dipping into liquid nitrogen. Monitoring of sleep was again based on observation. In rats weighing 50 g the brain concentration of lactate decreased 15% during sleep, while in rats weighing 150 g the decrease reached 28%. The largest reduction (36%) was observed in adult hamsters of 100 g body weight. A decrease in brain lactate during sleep was also reported in older rats (250–300 g), but only if the animals had been previously exposed to the experimental situation. The reverse effect occurred with non-habituated animals (Reich *et al.*, 1972). Rats were implanted with cortical and muscle electrodes at least three weeks before the experiment. One group of animals had no previous experience of the experimental situation, while the rats of a second group were left in the experimental cage for at least two hours on four or more consecutive days before the experiment. On the experimental day, single rats were placed in the cage in the morning and were left undisturbed and free to move and take food and water. In the afternoon, after the occurrence of a period of sleep lasting more than 20 min, they were killed by immersion into liquid nitrogen. The following day a second rat matched by weight and date of implantation was killed at the same time and after the same period of wakefulness plus one hour of previous wakefulness. Mild auditory stimulation was used to keep the animal in a waking state. Sleep and wakefulness were monitored by EEG and EMG recording as well as by behavioural observation. In the group of habituated rats brain lactate was 21% lower and pyruvate 33% lower during sleep, while non-significant trends towards an increase were present in creatine phosphate, AMP and ATP. The animals of this group were calm and slept readily as soon as they entered the cage. On the other hand, the non habituated rats were restless and did not sleep during the first 1–2 h, although no difference could be detected in their EEG patterns during sleep in comparison with the habituated animals. In the group of non-habituated rats the concentration of brain lactate increased 64% during sleep. Pyruvate was 54% higher, but the difference was not significant. An opposite trend was found for creatine phosphate and ATP which decreased 15% and 11% respectively. The total content of adenine nucleotides and the lactate to pyruvate ratio remained unchanged in both experimental groups. This observation indicated that regulatory mechanisms were operating in the glycolytic pathway above the level of lactate dehydrogenase. The increase in brain lactate in non habituated rats may be related to the similar increase present in rat brain after stressful handling (Richter and Dawson, 1948). As no effect was noted in waking brains, it appeared as a physiological debt created by tension and anxiety was paid during sleep.

A decreased lactate concentration in the brain of sleeping rats was also found following a period of physical exercise (Van den Noort and Brine, 1970). Pairs of rats weighing 150 g were placed in a rotating drum and revolved for four hours. At this time one rat was decapitated while the other one was previously allowed one hour rest in a quiet, illuminated cage (sleeping). Heads were immediately frozen in liquid nitrogen. A significant loss of weight, 7 g, occurred during the period of sleep deprivation which was not restored during the recovery hour. In sleeping rats blood lactate was 40% lower, probably because of the intervening period of arrest of muscular activity. In brain there was a fall in lactate (10%), ADP (10%) and AMP (21%) and a concomitant increase in glucose (28%), fructose diphosphate (16%), ATP (10%) and creatine phosphate (20%) concentration. No change occurred in the content of total adenine nucleotides, glucose-6-phosphate, triose phosphate, phosphoenolpyruvate and pyruvate. In a second experiment rats were treated as above but their heads were kept at room temperature for 30 sec before freezing. Under these anoxic conditions the metabolic rate of brain remains closely related to that previously occurring *in vivo* (King *et al.*, 1967). From the rate of utilization of glucose and labile phosphates the metabolic rate of rat brain was found to be essentially the same in sleep-deprived and in sleeping animals. Nonetheless during the anoxic interval brains of sleeping rats accumulated less AMP and utilized more glucose. In all these experiments the behavioural state was not monitored by EEG techniques and actually no comment was provided as to how the state of sleep was assessed. EEG procedures were applied, however, in a smaller group of rats which were implanted with cortical electrodes five days before the experiment and recorded while freely moving. The observed changes in brain metabolites were less pronounced but essentially similar to those obtained with the unmonitored animals. As all the rats were kept in a rotating drum for four hours before analysis, it may be surmised that the levels of brain substrates might have been influenced by the previous period of physical exercise and associated stress. Brain lactate concentrations were actually higher than those reported in other studies, both in waking and in sleeping animals.

At variance with these results which supported the notion of an effect of sleep on the rate of brain glycolysis and energy utilization, in one report brain lactate levels were found to remain unchanged during sleep (Shimizu *et al.*, 1966). Young rats weighing 30–45 g were implanted with cortical and muscle electrodes 3–5 days before the experiment and were allowed to sleep spontaneously for 20 min, regardless of the type of sleep, before being dropped into liquid nitrogen. Under these conditions the cerebral concentration of lactate in the group of rats killed during SS and in those killed during PS was found to be undistinguishable from that of awake controls (Table 1).

Depriving animals of PS increases brain levels of lactate, pyruvate and malate, but does not modify the concentration of some nucleotides and of several other metabolites of the glycolytic and tricarboxylic acid cycle pathways (Mendelson *et al.*, 1974). Adult rats weighing 200 g were deprived of PS for four days by the platform technique. Control animals were kept in single cages while two other conditions were used to control stress. The rats of the first group were kept on larger platforms which allowed normal values of PS while those of the second group were kept in single cages and immersed in water at 19° for one hour each day. EEG recordings established that PS deprived rats had about half as much PS as control animals. Rats kept on larger platforms had initially the same degree of PS deprivation experienced by the PS deprived group but recovered a normal amount of PS by the end of the experimental period. PS time remained normal in the group of rats stressed in cold water. At the end of the fourth day a

Table 1

Concentrations of lactate and pyruvate in rat brain during sleep

Source of data	Weight of rat (g)	EEG monitor	Sleep Induction	Duration	Method of killing	Control	Lactate[a]	Ratio and[b] significance	Pyruvate[a]	Ratio and[b] significance
Richter and Dawson (1948)	30–40	No	Strong sunlight	30 min	Liq. air	Rest	S 1·36 (6) W 2·09 (10)	0·65 p < 0·01		
Cocks (1967)	Adult	No	Natural	30 min	Liq. N₂	Rest	S 2·25·(25) W 3·14 (30)	0·72 p < 0·005		
Shimizu et al. (1966)	30–45	Yes	Natural	20 min	Liq. N₂	Rest	S 2·78 (22) W 2·67 (7)	1·04 NS		
Van den Noort and Brine (1970)	150	No	4 h exercise	60 min	Decap. into liq. N₂	4 h exercise	S 4·51 (13) W 5·01 (13)	0·90 p < 0·05	0·21 (14) 0·25 (14)	0·84 NS
		Yes	4 h exercise	60 min	Decap. into liq. N₂	4 h exercise	S 4·08 (5) W 4·64 (6)	0·88 NS		
Present study	250–300	Yes	Natural	20 min	Liq. N₂	Rest	A[c] S 4·02 (7) W 2·62 (7) B[c] S 2·28 (7) W 3·00 (7)	1·64 p < 0·05 0·79 p < 0·05	0·24 (7) 0·19 (7) 0·15 (7) 0·22 (7)	1·54 NS 0·67 p < 0·01

[a] The values represent the means (in µmol/g wet wt.) with the number of reported animals given in brackets.

[b] Ratios of S/W, with probabilities, P, of ratios differing from 1·0 indicated.

[c] A, B, unacclimatized and acclimatized groups of animals, respectively, reported in the present study.

From Reich et al., 1972. Decap., decapitation; Liq. N₂, liquid nitrogen; S, sleeping; W, walking; NS, not significant (p < 0·05).

sample of brain tissue was taken in less than a second using a "brain blower" (Veech *et al.*, 1972). In comparison with cage controls, an increase was present in the brain concentration of lactate (29%), pyruvate (22%) and malate (18%) in PS deprived animals. The two stress control groups had intermediate values. No significant change was present in the levels of glucose, glucose-6-phosphate, citrate, isocitrate, α-ketoglutarate, adenine nucleotides and creatine phosphate. The pyruvate to lactate ratio remained equally unchanged. These results suggested that the rate of glycolysis increased in the brain of PS deprived animals. The increase was in part reflecting the stress associated to this condition.

PS deprivation has also been reported to selectively decrease the K^+ concentration in brain and in plasma (Heiner *et al.*, 1968). In rats deprived of PS for ten days by the platform method the content of K^+ ions decreased approximately 20% in the telencephalon and in the rest of the brain, while the concentration of Na^+, Ca^{2+} and Mg^{2+} ions remained unchanged. A comparable selective reduction in K^+ concentration was present in plasma. Since no stress control group was analysed it remains possible that the effect might be due in part to the stress produced by the prolonged PS deprivation. A similar comment applies to the results of a comparable experiment dealing with ammonia production in brain, which also lacked a stress control group (Haulică *et al.*, 1970). After six days of PS deprivation by the platform method the ammonia concentration in rat brain increased 3·5-fold in concomitance with a marked increase in the activity of glutaminase (53%) and AMP deaminase (159%) and with a decrease in the content of nucleic acids. These results were interpreted as indicating an accelerated catabolism of proteins and nucleic acids.

The influence of sleep and of sleep deprivation on the content and biosynthesis of cerebral amino acids has been investigated by several workers. For some of the amino acids this topic is at the borderline between intermediary metabolism and chemical transmission.

A significant increase in the content of γ-aminobutyric (GABA) and aspartic acids was reported to occur in the brain of sleeping rats (Godin and Mandel, 1965). Animals of approximately 100 g were induced to sleep by a strong light and left undisturbed for 20 min during which waking periods lasting up to 1·5 min were tolerated. Awake animals were treated similarly but were killed before sleep induction. A different group of rats was sleep-deprived for one day by being forced to walk on a rolling floor by electric shocks. At the end of this period rats were allowed to sleep spontaneously (without light) or kept awake for 30 min before immersion into liquid nitrogen. The state of sleep was monitored behaviourally. Analyses were carried out on a sample containing cerebral hemispheres, cerebellum and bulb. In comparison with awake controls, the content of aspartic acid was 29% higher in rats induced to sleep by the strong light and in those sleeping spontaneously after deprivation. No significant change was present in deprived rats killed during wakefulness. In the case of GABA the increase was smaller (15–19%) and it was present also in the latter group of animals. No significant change was noted in the concentration of glutamate, glutamine, glycine, alanine and lysine in any of the experimental groups.

PS deprivation in adult cats has similarly been reported to modify the content of GABA and aspartate depending on the cerebral structure examined (Mičič et al., 1967). Unfortunately, in this experiment the duration of the deprivation period and the conditions of the control cats were not stated. Sacrifice was accomplished by decapitation and heads were quickly frozen in liquid air. An increase in the content of GABA was found in the reticular formation (39%), thalamus (26%) and frontal cortex (15%) and a decrease in the colliculi (29%) and caudate nucleus (22%). The concentration of aspartate increased in the thalamus (29%), frontal cortex (18%) and reticular formation (16%) and decreased in the caudate nucleus (26%). The only significant change for glutamate was an increase in the thalamus (15·3%).

These results were essentially confirmed in a second experiment (Karadžić et al., 1971) in which adult cats were deprived of PS for five days. In order to monitor possible stress effects a group of animals was PS deprived for three days with allowance of eight hours sleep per day. Besides aspartate and GABA, PS deprivation significantly modified the concentrations of threonine, arginine, glycine, lysine and cysteine in several brain regions but did not affect the content of glutamate, tyrosine, histidine and serine.

An increased synthesis of brain glutamine is associated with deprivation of total sleep (Mark et al., 1969). Rats weighing about 100 g were kept for two days on pedestals surrounded by water (PS deprivation) or were forced to walk on moving belts with electric shocks (total sleep deprivation). Feeding periods of 30 min were allowed three times a day to experimental and control animals. After subcutaneous injection of uniformly labelled ^{14}C-glucose they were returned to their respective conditions and sacrificed by immersion into liquid nitrogen at 15, 30, 45 and 60 min. The decrease in the specific activity of brain glucose observed with time in control rats was not modified by total or PS deprivation. On the other hand, the specific radioactivity of brain glutamine relative to that of glucose or of glutamate was consistently higher at all times in animals deprived of total sleep. After 30 min the effect was most marked in the pons and medulla oblongata and least evident in the telencephalon. Similar increases in the relative (to glucose) specific activity of glutamate, aspartate and GABA were present after 15 min but not at later times in rats deprived of PS or total sleep. While the latter effect was tentatively attributed to synthesis of amino acids from a pool of glucose with a higher specific activity, the increased labelling of glutamine suggested a faster turnover, possibly in relation to an increased production of ammonia (Haulica et al., 1970).

A further indication that the metabolism of amino acids in brain may be affected by sleep was provided by the report that the activity of cortical aspartate transaminase increased 15–20% in the transition from a desynchronized to a synchronized EEG pattern. The experiments were carried out in unanaesthesized cats immobilized by muscle paralysis or by bulbo-spinal resection and artificially ventilated (Steriade et al., 1969).

PSdeprivation decreases the glycogen content of different brain structures to a different extent (Karadžić and Mršulja, 1969). Adult rats were deprived of PS for three days by the platform method. Stress controls were kept on larger platforms. Some of the PSdeprived rats were allowed to sleep for three, six or nine hours. After decapitation heads were plunged into liquid air. With comparison with normal and stress controls, PSdeprived rats showed a substantial decrease in glycogen concentration in the hippocampus, caudate nucleus and caudal brain stem, but not in the frontal and occipital cortex. After three hours of sleep the decrease was more marked in all areas and became significant also for the two cortical regions. Six or nine hours of sleep restored normal glycogen values. The effect occurred largely in the fraction of bound glycogen. If a fall in the concentration of glycogen is taken to indicate a mobilization of energy reserves to cope with enhanced cellular activity it appears that while hippocampus and subcortical regions may be sufficiently active during periods of PS deprivation, cortical regions become more active during periods of rebound sleep containing a higher proportion of PS.

A comparable fluctuation of brain glycogen has been found to follow a circadian rhythm in the teleost Serranus scriba, with minimum values attained in the evening hours during which the fish is most active (Mršulja and Rakić, 1974).

Some evidence that the oxidation of cerebral substrates may follow a different pattern during synchronized sleep was obtained by analysis of the output of radioactive CO_2 in perfused cat brain metabolizing ^{14}C-glucose. During periods of EEG synchronization produced by pretrigeminal midbrain transection (cerveau isolé) the specific activity of CO_2 decreased significantly in comparison with periods of de-synchronized EEG activity. The effect appeared to be specific since it was not reproduced when cortical synchronization was achieved by stimulation of the thalamic hypnogenic centre or by administration of barbiturates. A decrease in the specific activity of CO_2 had previously been observed in the same preparation after convulsive activity elicited by metrazol or ECS and appeared to reflect an increased oxidation of unlabelled substrates (Magnes *et al.*, 1967).

VI. Macromolecules

A. *The Phosphoprotein Story*

A substantial increase in the uptake of ^{32}P-phosphate has been reported to take place during sleep in a phosphoprotein fraction extracted from brain (Reich *et al.*, 1967). After 90 min of wakefulness maintained by mild stimulation the radioactive precursor was injected into the tail vein of 20-day-old littermate rats which were allowed to fall asleep spontaneously or were kept awake by gentle handling. Sleep was monitored by behavioural observation. Thirty minutes later the rats were decapitated and the brains were subjected to a sequential extraction procedure which yielded a lipid fraction, a hot TCA-extract and an alkali digest. The only differential effect was present in the hot TCA-extract whose specific radioactivity was 2·5-fold higher after sleep than after wakefulness. No change occurred in blood and in the hot TCA-extract obtained from liver. The observed increase in incorporation of ^{32}P-phosphate could not be attributed to differences in muscular activity between sleeping and waking rats since the specific activity of the hot TCA-extract remained essentially the same in resting and exercised animals. In addition, the effect appeared not to depend on differences in the availability of labelled phosphate since the increase in specific radioactivity was limited to only one of the phosphate-containing fractions. By chromatographic analysis of the hot TCA-extract the effect was traced to the presence of inorganic phosphate which had been hydrolyzed from a more complex molecule by the acid treatment. Incubation with alkaline phosphatase and alkaline hydrolysis of the tissue residue before extraction with hot TCA failed to solubilize a labelled compound with a higher specific radioactivity during sleep. These properties suggested that the phosphate compound affected by sleep was likely to be a phospho-protein.

Using improved procedures a similar increase in the incorporation of ^{32}P-phosphate into sleeping rat brain was later reported to occur also in adult animals (Reich *et al.*, 1973). Rats weighing 250–300 g were chronically implanted with a ventricular cannula and with cortical and muscle electrodes. On the day of the experiment in the morning one animal of a pair matched for weight and date of implantation was placed in the experimental cage and connected to an EEG recorder and to a push–pull pump. The rat was free to move and to have food and drink. Three hours later, at the beginning of a sleep period, the radioactive precursor was injected intraventricularly during a period of 10 minutes at a rate of 3 µl/min. The infusion did not appear to disturb the animal and did not modify electrical activities of brain and muscle. At the end of the injection the rat was allowed to complete a sleep period lasting 20 min regardless of the total time of incorporation which on the average remained slightly less than one hour. The experiment was terminated by plunging the rat into liquid nitrogen through a trapdoor placed in the cage floor. The following day the second animal of the pair was treated similarly, except that during the period of incorporation as well as for one hour previously it was kept awake by mild auditory stimulation. Incorporation time corresponded to that of the sleeping mate.

Two groups of animals were studied. Those of the first group were exposed to the experimental environment for the first time on the day of the experiment, while those of the second group were brought to the experimental cage and connected to the EEG cable for two hours or more on at least four consecutive days before the experiment. On the experimental day the animals of the first group were more restless and disturbed than the habituated rats, although normal sleep periods with similar EEG patterns were present in both groups at the time of precursor administration. In the group of animals not previously exposed to the experimental environment sleep induced a significant increase in the specific radioactivity of the hot TCA-extract which was less pronounced (1·8-fold) than the one observed with younger rats (Reich *et al.*, 1967). An increase was present also in the specific radioactivity of the alkali digest which remained, however, at the borderline of significance. Both these effects were not present in the group of animals previously accustomed to the experimental situation. This observation emphasizes the relevance of previous waking ex-periences on brain metabolism during sleep and the need to define these conditions in any biochemical study. In addition, it indicates that different chemical processes may take place in brain while EEG patterns remain essentially the same.

The substance responsible for the sleep effect was soluble in ionic detergents, such as sodium dodecyl sulphate (SDS) and deoxycholate. Prolonged digestion with pronase released a ^{32}P-containing dialysable material consisting largely of phosphopeptides.

Final proof that the increased uptake of ^{32}P-phosphate in the sleeping brain is due to a phosphoprotein has been recently provided by extensive purification of the active material and by its identification as the enzyme glucose-6-phosphatase (Anchors and Karnovsky, 1975). Using pairs of sleeping and waking rats respectively injected with ^{32}P- and ^{33}P-phosphate the relevant component was monitored throughout the purification procedure by the excess labelling associated with the sleeping extract. The phosphoprotein was solubilized with sodium deoxycholate from a myelin-free particulate fraction previously washed with Triton X-100. After gel filtration on Sephadex G-100 and chromatography on DEAE-Sephadex the purified protein was shown to yield a single band on SDS gel electrophoresis (mol.wt 28 000) and to contain isoleucine as NH_2-terminal residue. After alkaline hydrolysis of the purified material radioactive phosphate was found to be associated to histidine. Identification of the phosphoprotein as glucose-6-phosphatase rested on enzyme assays of the purified fraction and on co-purification of glucose-6-phophatase with the relevant radioactive phosphate. The enzyme was present in all brain regions in association with plasma and other cell membranes except myelin, and appeared to be concentrated in a neuronal perikaryal fraction. As in other organs, its most probable role in brain should be related to the insulin-independent transport of glucose across cell membranes. Phosphorylation of the protein is achieved by carbamyl-phosphate in liver, but the nature of the phosphate donor is unknown in brain. The increased phosphorylation of the brain enzyme during sleep may be causally linked to the higher glucose uptake of the sleeping brain (Van den Noort and Brine, 1970). However, other interpretations based on compartmentation effects are possible and are currently receiving experimental attention.

Glucose-6-phosphatase may not be the only phosphoprotein with an increased phosphate turnover during sleep. As shown by SDS electrophoretic analysis other phosphoproteins with larger molecular weights may become more labelled by ^{32}P-phosphate during the sleep state (Anchors and Karnovsky, 1975).

B. *Proteins*

Using a pharmacological approach to manipulate vigilance states it has been shown that under certain conditions the level of protein synthesis correlates with the amount of SS and PS (Bobillier *et al.*, 1973). Cats with chronic brain electrodes and a ventricular cannula were treated with *p*-chlorophenylalanine (PCPA) which is known to selectively depress the synthesis of serotonin (Pujol *et al.*, 1971). Two days later a group of animals received the serotonin precursor 5-hydroxy-tryptophane (5-HTP), while a control group received saline. Two hours after this treatment a mixture of radioactive amino acids was given intraventricularly for a period of four hours. The animals treated with saline remained largely awake during the period of incorporation, while the cats receiving 5-HTP had almost normal amounts of SS and actually more than twice the amount of PS of control animals, presumably as rebound to the previous sleep-deprivation days. In comparison with untreated (placebo) and PCPA-saline-treated cats, the latter group showed a substantial decrease in the radioactivity of the TCA-soluble fraction in the caudal part of the brain stem and in the cervical spinal cord. No significant difference was present in the remaining brain regions. The specific activity of the protein fraction remained essentially unaffected in all brain regions. In contrast with these negative findings, in the group of animals which had been treated with 5-HTP a positive correlation was detected between the level of protein synthesis in the telencephalon and the amount of PS present during the first hour of incorporation. A similar correlation appeared to exist with the amount of SS. As the initial period of incorporation was likely to correspond to the most active labelling of the protein fraction, more pronounced effects might have been obtained with a shorter incorporation time.

Separation by polyacrylamide gel electrophoresis of the soluble proteins extracted from the telencephalon indicated that a high molecular weight protein band was considerably more labelled in cats treated with PCPA and 5-HTP in comparison with animals receiving PCPA and saline and with untreated controls. This finding should be related to the higher PS time occurring in the former condition. Cats treated with PCPA and 5-HTP were also the only ones to show the presence of PS during the first hour of incorporation.

The rate of cerebral protein synthesis has been reported to increase markedly during PS as compared with SS in bioptic samples taken during the corresponding sleep states (Brodskii *et al.*, 1974). Implan-ted cats were habituated to the experimental conditions for 60–90 min during four consecutive days before the experiment. On the experimental day approximately 50 mg tissue were removed from the parietal cortex of one hemisphere with the help of a special instrument. This was done after 20 min of SS or after 1·5 min of PS. The following day a similar sample was taken from the contralateral hemisphere after 20 min of wakefulness. Protein synthesis was measured by the incorporation of ^{3}H-leucine in the homogenized tissue. The procedure allowed comparison of SS or PS with W in the same animal, thus avoiding individual variability. When both biopsies were obtained after equivalent periods of W the level of protein synthesis was essentially the same in the two hemispheres. Similar rates were also observed when the first bioptic sample was removed after PS. On the other hand, cerebral protein synthesis appeared to be strikingly lower (50%) after a period of SS.

These findings have been recently confirmed and related to the features of neuronal discharges occurring during PS and SS. In particular the rate of protein synthesis in bioptic samples of cat parietal cortex has been reported to increase during PS in comparison with SS in concomitance with a radical improvement in the informational parameters of impulse trains (Kogan et al., 1975).

PS deprivation has been used to study the possible role of this type of sleep in cerebral protein synthesis but with limited success (Bobillier et al., 1971). Adult rats were selectively deprived of PS by the platform method for 54 hours while another group of animals was deprived for 48 hours and allowed to recuperate sleep for six additional hours. After decapitation, tissue slices from the telencephalon and the brain stem were incubated for 45 min with a mixture of ^{3}H-amino acids. In comparison with control rats kept in their home cages the specific activity of the protein fraction remained essentially unaffected in the experimental groups also after correction for the content of radio-activity in the TCA-soluble fraction. The only significant difference was present in the TCA-soluble fraction of the brain stem, whose radioactivity was higher (about 40%) in PS-deprived rats in comparison with control animals and with PS-deprived rats which were allowed to recuperate. As stress appears to increase the uptake of amino acids into cortex slices (Jaboubek et al., 1970) this effect might possibly reflect a generalized stress induced by PS deprivation.

Essentially the same experimental protocol was followed in the analysis of cerebral protein synthesis in vivo (Bobillier et al., 1974). Adult rats were deprived of PS for 48 hours and after i.p. injection of a mixture of ^{3}H-amino acids were kept for six additional hours in the deprived condition or, alternatively, they were allowed to recuperate sleep for the same length of time. Cage controls were similarly treated. In the group of PS-deprived animals there was a slight but general decrease in the specific activity of cerebral proteins which reached significance in the cerebellum and telencephalon and in the nuclear and soluble fractions of the brain stem. In the group of PS-deprived rats which were allowed to recuperate the decrease in protein specific activity was less marked and reached significance only in the nuclear, mitochondrial and soluble fractions of the brain stem. The specific activity of the TCA-soluble fraction remained essentially unchanged in all brain regions of both groups of experimental animals. As consequence, the relative specific activity of the protein fraction was significantly lower in PS-deprived rats in the cerebellum, telencephalon and brain stem. In the group of animals which were allowed a period of recovery sleep the decrease was less pronounced and reached significance only in the telencephalon. In this region maintenance of the deprived state and sleep recovery appeared to have similar negative effects. These results appeared to be specific for brain as in liver the relative specific activity of the protein fraction was not modified by PS deprivation or by PS deprivation followed by sleep recovery. However, the radioactivity of the TCA-soluble fraction in liver was significantly lower in the group of PS-deprived animals. A similar decrease in the specific activity of the protein fraction did not reach significance.

Total sleep deprivation in seven-day-old rats was not accompanied by any major change in brain protein synthesis (Bobillier et al., 1974). However, sleep deprivation was not monitored by EEG techniques and may be more difficult to attain at this age. Rat pups weighing 18 g were injected subcutaneously (s.c.) with ^{3}H-amino acids and placed in individual cages at 34°. One group of animals was allowed to sleep spontaneously, while rats of another group were kept awake by gentle handling. Two hours later the animals were decapitated. The only effect of total sleep deprivation concerned the radioactivity of the TCA-soluble fraction of the telencephalon which decreased slightly (about 10%) but significantly. Slices prepared from the brain stem of sleep-deprived pups were less capable of ^{3}H-amino acid uptake into the TCA-soluble fraction. The specific activity of the protein fraction was also lower, but the relative specific activity was not significantly altered.

A more general decrease in the amino acid uptake of brain slices was produced by total sleep deprivation in 26-day-old rats. After 90 min of sleep deprivation achieved by handling one group of rats was allowed to fall asleep for 90 additional minutes while another group was kept awake. With reference to control animals left in individual cages the uptake of ^{3}H-amino acids by the brain stem was significantly lower (25%) in sleep-deprived rats, and attained higher values in recuperating animals. The specific activity of the protein fraction was also significantly lower (almost 50%) in the former group, but remained essentially the same in the latter group. As consequence, the relative specific activity decreased in deprived rats but was not significantly modified in recuperating animals. Upon subcellular fractionation protein radioactivity was found to be lower in all fractions of sleep-deprived animals and higher in all fractions of recuperating rats. However, significant differences were present only in the microsomal and soluble fractions of deprived rats. A similar pattern of changes was present also in the telencephalon but significance was reached only in the specific activity of the protein fraction which was higher in the group of recuperating animals than in PS-deprived rats.

The possible relationships between sleep and cerebral protein synthesis has been also examined using inhibitors of protein synthesis (Stern et al., 1972). In adult cats implanted with chronic electrodes intraventricular injection of cycloheximide (1 mg every 6 h for a total of 3 mg) induced a significant increase in SS (from 55 to 70%) on the day of administration and a marked increase in PS (from 12 to 20%) during the following nine days. Waking was decreased throughout (from 33– 20%). Cerebral protein synthesis measured by ^{14}C-leucine incorporation in vivo was inhibited 75% on day 1 and was still 50% lower on day 4. In other words, the prolonged increase in PS time was preceded by a previous temporary increase in SS which occurred while cerebral protein synthesis was severely inhibited. A similar experiment carried out with puromycin revealed an insignificant increase in SS and a significant lowering of PS (from 14 to 6%) only during the injection day. Cerebral protein synthesis was inhibited 50% on day 1. The different effect obtained with puromycin might be attributed to the lower inhibition of brain protein synthesis or to the formation of peptidyl-puromycin. The delayed increase in PS time induced by cycloheximide is reminiscent of the prolonged PS rebounds observed after withdrawl from addicting drugs (Oswald, 1969; Haider and Oswald, 1970). This resemblance is further strengthened by the observation that in rats treated with anisomycin the duration of PS was drastically reduced in the period immediately following the injection of the inhibitor (Drucker-Colin et al., 1975a).

Protein concentration has been recently reported to vary in a cyclical fashion in the perfusate obtained from the mesencephalic reticular formation in relation to the sleep–wakefulness cycle (Drucker-Colin et *al.*, 1975b). Freely moving cats implanted with a push–pull cannula were perfused with Ringer solution at a rate of 1 ml/h for periods of 12–21 h. The protein content of the perfusate was found to vary from 26–206 µg/ml and to follow cyclic variations in individual cats with peaks corresponding to periods of PS. In 21 out of 23 animals the protein concentration of the perfusate more than doubled in this state as compared to wakefulness (Drucker-Colin and Spanis, 1975). Similar cyclic changes with a maximum during periods of PS were observed also in perfusates obtained from the hippocampus. The possibility that the protein present in the perfusate might be derived from damaged tissue appeared unlikely in view of the large amount of protein that could be collected per day (about 2 mg). This would have required a far more conspicuous damage (100–200 mg tissue) than it was assumed to occur around the tip of the cannula. In addition, a release of protein from damaged tissue could hardly be expected to undergo cyclic oscillations but would probably show a progressive decrease in time. An origin from serum appeared also to be excluded on the basis of immunoprecipitation analyses which revealed the substantial lack of serum proteins.

C. *Cytochemical Analyses*

Inverse changes in the activity of succinic oxidase have been shown to occur in the neurones of the caudal part of the reticular formation and in their surrounding glia during periods of sleep (presumably SS) and wakefulness (Hyden and Lange, 1965). Rabbits were trained to sleep in individual boxes for five hours a day for 12 days. On the experimental day they were sacrificed 90 min after having been placed in the box. Control animals were kept awake by gentle handling for at least one hour before sacrifice. Neuronal cell-bodies and an equivalent volume of perikaryal glia were dissected from the caudal part of the nucleus reticularis giganto-cellularis and used for the determination of succinic oxidase activity with a microdiver technique. In neurones the level of the enzyme was almost threefold higher during sleep, while in the glia sample it increased significantly during wakefulness. Correspondingly, the ratio of enzyme activity in neurones and glia decreased from 1·46 during sleep to 0·43 during wakefulness. In the oral part of the reticular formation (nucleus reticularis pontis oralis) sleep induced a 60% increase in succinic oxidase activity of the neuronal cell-bodies and no significant change in glia. The effect was specific as no differences were noted in trigeminal and hypoglossal nuclei. The

marked increase in enzyme activity present during sleep in the
neurones of the caudal part of the reticular formation might be related
to their enhanced activity during sleep (Moruzzi, 1963). It is debatable
whether these rhythmic changes reflect a cycle of net protein synthesis
followed by protein degradation or a sequential process of activation
and inactivation of the enzyme. Inverse changes in enzyme activity and

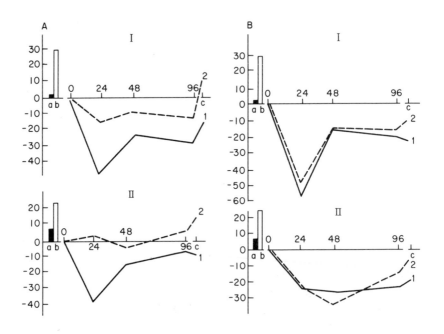

Fig. 4. A. Percentage change in the content of protein (I) and RNA (II) in the neuronal
cytoplasm (a) and in the satellite glia (b) of the supraoptic nucleus of the rat during natural sleep.
The same during PS deprivation in neurones (1) and in glia cells (2). (c) During the period of sleep
subsequent to 96 h of PS deprivation. B. Same as in A except that 1 and 2 refer to the period of
total sleep deprivation induced by phenamine and (c) to the period of sleep subsequent to 96 h of
total phenamine insomnia. (From Demin, 1974.)

RNA content of neurones and glia cells have been generally interpreted as resulting from an interaction of the two partner cells.
Alternatively they might possibly be produced by the movement of
intracellular organelles between dendrites and neuronal cell-bodies
since some dendrites are likely to contaminate the glia sample.
    A depletion of cytoplasmic RNA and protein has been reported to
occur in the neurones of the supraoptic nucleus of adult rats selectively

deprived of PS by the platform technique (Demin and Rubinskaja, 1974). The content of RNA and protein was determined in tissue slices by spectrophotometric techniques after staining with gallocyanin and amido black, respectively. In comparison with awake rats a progressive decrease in RNA and protein was observed in the neuronal cytoplasm depending on the duration of the period of PS deprivation (Fig. 4). The effect was present after three hours and reached a maximum (40–50% decrease) after 24 hours. The loss of protein was in part due to a decrease in protein concentration (15–20% lower), while the loss of RNA reflected merely volume changes. Basic proteins, presumably histones, were found to decrease 15–20% in neurones, but not in glia cells. With longer periods of deprivation the content of RNA tended to return to normal levels (only 10% less after 96 hours) while protein remained approximately 25% lower. No change was present in the RNA content of glia cells and only a moderate decrease occurred in glial protein (10–15%). The above effects might be attributed, at least in part, to the action of unspecific factors, since a group of stressed animals was not included in the analyses. Whatever their origin, the observed changes were found to disappear rapidly after a period of normal sleep.

After a period of deprivation of total sleep induced by phenamine the loss of protein and RNA occurred in neurones as well as in the glia cells of the supraoptic nucleus (Demin, 1974). After one day of deprivation the content of protein decreased 50–60% and that of RNA 25–30% in both cell types (Fig. 4). As in the case of PS deprivation, the effect was due in part to a decrease in protein concentration but reflected only volume changes for RNA. Following the deprivation of total sleep the content of RNA and, in part, of protein returned to normal values after three hours of normal sleep.

While deprivation of PS and of total sleep brought about negative changes in protein and RNA content, the opposite effect was found to prevail during normal sleep (Demin and Rubinskaja, 1974). In comparison with awake controls, the content of RNA and protein increased 25–30% in the satellite glia cells of the supraoptic nucleus but remained essentially unchanged in neuronal perikarya (neuronal RNA increased less than 10%). Basic proteins increased in glia cells (60%) and to a limited extent (20%) also in neurones. No change was noted in the concentration parameters except for a slight decrease in the concentration of neuronal protein.

Somewhat different results were obtained in the nucleus coeruleus (Demin, 1974). During normal sleep there was little or no change in the content and concentration of protein and RNA in glia cells, while in neurones there was a limited fall in protein (14%) and a slight increase in RNA (13%). Deprivation of total sleep or of PS for one day brought about a significant decrease in the content of RNA and protein in both cell types (15–30%). The effect was more marked in glia after deprivation of total sleep. Normal concentrations were attained in neurones after two days of total sleep deprivation, but not after two days of PS deprivation. The content and concentration of neuronal RNA were actually higher than normal after four days of total sleep deprivation. With regard to basic proteins the increase occurring during normal sleep was more pronounced than for total proteins, while the decrease observed during deprivation of PS and of total sleep was lower. All the changes brought about by sleep deprivation were rapidly reversed by a short period of sleep.

Slight variations in the activity of cerebral proteinases have also been described (Glushenko and Demin, 1971). In rats, after a period of normal sleep lasting 30 min, the activity of neutral proteinases increased 10% in the cerebral hemispheres and in the bulb, but remained unchanged in the cerebellum. No change was noted in the activity of acid proteinases. Conversely, the activity of these enzymes appeared to increase in the cerebral hemispheres some time after the beginning of PS deprivation, while neutral proteinases tended to decrease only after prolonged PS deprivation. A period of normal sleep brought about a rapid reversal of these changes. They have been interpreted as suggesting the occurrence of significant variations in the catabolic rate of cerebral proteins.

The involvement of nuclear processes in the transition from sleep to wakefulness is suggested by variations in nuclear diameter detected in neurones of the locus coeruleus (Bubenik and Monnier, 1972). Adult rabbits undergoing extracorporeal dialysis were induced to sleep by thalamic stimulation while a state of arousal was produced by stimulation of the midbrain reticular formation. While the experiments lasted 90 min the values of nuclear diameter were referred to the amount of slow waves present in the EEG pattern during the last 10 or 15 min. In sleeping animals the diameter of neuronal nuclei remained approximately the same as in sham-operated controls while in aroused rabbits it became slightly but significantly larger. As no difference was noted in the neurones of the cerebellar cortex the effect appeared to be specific. A similar increase in nuclear size could be produced in the neurones of the locus coeruleus by hemorrhagic stress. It is uncertain whether the stress effect was mediated by an activation of the ascending reticular system or by a humoral mechanism such as increased ACTH secretion.

D. RNA

Quantitative differences in the types of RNA synthesized in rabbit cerebral cortex have been reported to occur during sleep and wakefulness (Vitale-Neugebauer et al., 1970). Rabbits implanted with dural electrodes were trained to sleep in a box for 1–2 h during five consecutive days in a dimly lighted, soundproof room. Animals to be kept awake were not subjected to this conditioning and remained free to move in a small enclosure at the time of the experiment. They were kept awake by acoustic stimulation and handling. EEG activity was monitored throughout the period of incorporation of ^{14}C-orotic acid given by subarachnoidal injection. The biochemical parameters were expressed as a function of the percentage sleep calculated from the EEG records. After sacrifice by stunning and decapitation total RNA was extracted from the dorsal cortex and analysed by centrifugation in sucrose density gradients. After 60 min of incorporation the ratio of radioactivity between a region of the gradient containing chiefly rRNA precursors (28S to 50S) and a region containing only DNA-like heterogeneous RNA (> 50S) (Vesco and Giuditta, 1967) was found to be consistently higher in animals with a low percentage of EEG synchronization (awake). The difference was larger when the in-corporation time was 105 min. These results were suggestive of a faster rate of synthesis of ribosomal RNA in awake animals in comparison with heterogeneous RNA. This conclusion was in accord with a more formal analysis of the distribution of labelled RNA in the gradients. The values of the moments of the distribution calculated with respect to the position of the 28S RNA component and the median of the distribution showed a regular decrease with increasing percentages of EEG synchronization. Similarly, the values of the moments μ_2–μ_{10} were found to depend consistently on the physiological state of the cortex.

More recently, quantitative differences between sleep and wakeful-ness have been reported to occur in the content of radioactive RNA of a fraction of purified nuclei prepared from rabbit cortex (Giuditta et al., 1974). Rabbits implanted with cortical electrodes and a subdural cannula were left to recover in a large cage in the experimental room. The following day they were connected to the EEG cable and 2–3 h later received a dose of ^{3}H-orotic acid slowly injected by means of a distantly-operated pump. Incorporation time was 60 min. By centri-fugation in a discontinuous sucrose gradient two purified nuclear fractions were obtained from the dorsal cortex which respectively consisted of large nuclei presumably derived from neurones and astroglial cells, and of smaller and darker nuclei presumably of oligodendroglial origin (Giuditta *et al.*, 1972). The content of radioactive RNA per nucleus was found to increase with the percentage of EEG synchronization in the fraction of large nuclei, while no change was present in the fraction of small nuclei. In the former fraction the content of labelled RNA present at 100% synchronization was more than twice as large as in the fully awake condition. The effect was statistically significant and might be interpreted in terms of increased synthesis, reduced degradation and/or reduced cytoplasmic transport of nuclear RNA. Whatever mechanism will be shown to be operative, this result provides an indication of a differential response of cortical cell types to the sleep and wakefulness condition.

VII. Conclusions

Apart from investigations on cerebral neurotransmitters, two main areas of research appear to have attracted the attention of neurochemists interested in the biochemistry of sleep. One concerns intermediary and energy metabolism while the other one deals with macromolecular synthesis and degradation. It appears that the glycolytic flux in brain may change during sleep depending on the previous waking experience of the organism. If the animal is exposed to a novel experience, such as that represented by the experimental condition, in the ensuing sleep period glucose uptake increases and glycolytic reactions accelerate to meet an enhanced energy demand reflected in the lower content of ATP and phosphocreatine. Phosphorylation of the transport enzyme glucose-6-phosphatase may represent a key controlling step of this sequence of reactions. The opposite behaviour, namely a slowing down of glycolytic processes and a moderate accumulation of high energy compounds, prevails when the experimental condition has already become a familiar experience. What is still obscure is the nature of the energy requiring reactions which appear to be activated when sleep follows a novel experience and, in addition, the types of cellular elements which are involved in the process.

A relevant side observation stemming from these studies regards the discrepancy between electrophysiological and neurochemical events in the sleeping brain where similar EEG patterns have been shown to accompany opposite changes in the glycolytic flux. It appears as if during SS the neural machine is set to a special mode corresponding to the well known EEG pattern while the permitted operations are carried out only if relevant perceptual material is available.

Considering brain macromolecules, the picture is still too fragmentary and hazy to allow even tentative generalizations. Prolonged wakefulness appears to enhance catabolic processes while sleep on the whole and PS in particular, are likely to be periods of prevailing synthetic reactions. On this point there is more suggestive evidence regarding proteins than nucleic acids. During PS cerebral protein synthesis may attain levels comparable to those of wakefulness, while according to some reports it may shift to lower rates during SS. The latter finding is at variance with the results of other studies and appears surprising in view of the enhanced release of growth hormone during SS. As to the contribution of the different cellular elements there is evidence of a differential participation of neurones and glia cells in RNA biosynthesis and in the maintenance of the content of protein and RNA in the cell bodies.

What general perspectives can be extracted from this overview of the biochemical events occurring in the sleeping brain? Perhaps the most important conclusion concerns the strict dependence of molecular processes on cellular and organ behaviour, as shown, for instance, by the different biochemical responses which are found in brain according to the previous waking experience, or which accompany neuronal discharge patterns of different informational content. From this point of view it appears simple-minded to maintain *tout court* that the decrement in performance and subjective state brought about by prolonged wakefulness is due to the accumulation of noxious compounds or, in a complementary fashion, to the exhaustion of important substrates. As consequence, one should not expect that sleep restores mental capacities by elimination of toxins or by recovery of biochemical stores. Statements such as these should be qualified by the definition of the cellular and regional sites involved and moreover by the recognition that the processing of information carried out by mammalian brain continues throughout the sleep period with different operations than those prevailing during wakefulness. Understanding the nature of these activities is the main goal of sleep research, to which biochemical investigations can contribute best by remaining tightly linked to structural and physiological considerations.

In this regard the recent association of sleep function with memory processes should prove extremely valuable provided that problems and concepts laid out in the biochemical analysis of memory functions are properly applied in the approach towards a molecular understanding of the sleeping brain. A highly relevant feature of this analysis has stressed the cooperative role of glial and neuronal elements in learning and memory activities. It is likely that elucidation of similar cellular relationships will prove central to the problem of the function of sleep. In addition, a useful distinction which has stemmed from the biochemical investigations of memory processes should also be applied in the analysis of the biochemical behaviour of the sleeping brain. This regards the separation of biochemical data into those related to neuronal activation *per se*, in the strict sense of an increased impulse trade, and into those more specifically connected to memory functions. Although it may not be always possible to keep the borderline sharp, it is clear, for instance, that some of the observations made on brain stem centres should be considered as belonging to the first category of events.

In closing, it will be allowed to a biochemist speculating on the function of sleep to draw attention to the similarities that can be discerned between nutrition and sensory processing. Food and stimuli are essential for life, and to a certain extent coincide in primitive organisms. They both need to undergo a complex sequence of transformations in order to be incorporated into organismal structures and to yield energy which is chemical in one case and motivational in the other. Assuming such a parallelism and taking it to its ultimate consequences, we may hope to define the broad outlines of information processing by analogy with the operations of food uptake and assimilation. In brief, nutritional processes consist of a degradative phase during which chemical bonds are broken, and of a synthetic phase during which chemical bonds are restored according to rules set down by the organism's templates. Complex perceptual inputs obtained from the environment might be assumed to undergo similar operations of bond splitting and bond formation. In the first phase perceptual units of smaller size or lower complexity would be produced, while in the second phase they would be assimilated into larger and more richly connected patterns according to the organism's rules. Perhaps the degradative phase prevails during SS while the synthetic phase prevails during PS. As informational inputs take the form of spatio–temporal patterns of excitation and inhibition going through cellular nets, the rules which the organism uses for their assimilation into its own structures cannot be residing in structures which are less complex than the perceptual units themselves. As consequence, the informational template should be conceived as a larger and more complex pattern of cellular activities. We do not know the code which regulates the synthetic operation of this template, but we are forced to conclude that it must be a cellular code.

Acknowledgements

Thanks are due to Drs A. Hobson, M. Libonati and I. Oswald for reading the manuscript and Drs P. Volpe and A. Neugebauer-Vitale for translating some Russian papers.

References

Agnew, H. W., Webb, W. B. and Williams, R. L. (1967). *Percept. Motor Skills* **24**, 851–858.

Allen, S. R. (1975). *In* "Sleep 1974" (P. Levin and W. P. Koella, eds). Karger, Basel, pp. 373–376.

Anchors, J. M. and Karnovsky, M. L. (1975). *J. Biol. Chem.* **250**, 6408–6416.

Baekeland, F. and Lasky, R. (1966). *Percept. Motor Skills* **23**, 1203–1207.

Bakan, P. (1975). 2nd Intern. Congr. Sleep Res. Abstracts, 17, Edinburgh.

Berger, H. (1929). *Arch. Psychiat.* **87**, 527–570.

Berger, R. J. (1969). *Psychol. Rev.* **76**, 144–164.

Berger, R. J. and Oswald, I. (1962). *J. Ment. Sci.* **108**, 457–465.

Bobillier, P., Sakai, F., Seguin, S. and Jouvet, M. (1971). *Life Sci.* **10**, Part II, 1349–1357.

Bobillier, P., Froment, J.-L., Seguin, S. and Jouvet, M. (1973). *J. Neurochem.* **22**, 3077–3090.

Bobillier, P., Sakai, F., Seguin, S. and Jouvet, M. (1974). *J. Neurochem.* **22**, 23–31.

Bolles, R. C. (1970). *Psychol. Rev.* **77**, 32–48.

Boyar, R. M., Rosenfeld, R. S., Kapen, S., Finkelstein, J. W., Roffwarg, H. P., Weitzman, E. D. and Hellman, L. (1974). *J. Clin. Invest.* **54**, 609–618.

Brodskii, V. Ya., Gusatinskii, V. N., Kogan, A. B. and Nechaeva, N. V. (1974). *Dokl. Akad. Nauk SSSR* **215**, 748–750.

Bryson, D. and Schacher, S. (1969). *Persp. Biol. Med.* **13**, 71–79.

Bubenik, G. and Monnier, M. (1972). *Exp. Neurol.* **35**, 1–12.

Cartwright, R. D. and Ratzel, R. W. (1972). *Arch. Gen. Psychiat.* **27**, 277–282.

Claparède, E. (1905). *Arch. Psychol.* **4**, 246–349.

Cocks, J. A. (1967). *Nature* **215**, 1399–1400.

Cohen, H. B. and Dement, W. C. (1965). *Science* **150**, 1318–1319.

Cohen, H. B. and Dement, W. C. (1966). *Science* **154**, 396–398.

Cohen, H. B., Duncan II, R. F. an Dement, W. C. (1967). *Science* **156**, 1646–1648.

Dement, W. C (1960). *Science* **131**, 1705–1707.

Dement, W. and Greenberg, S. (1966). *EEG Clin. Neurophysiol.* **20**, 523–526.

Demin, N. N. (1974). *In* "Advances in Neurochemistry" (E. M. Kreps *et al.*, eds). Nauka, Leningrad, pp. 29–39.

Demin, N. N. and Rubinskaja, N. L. (1974). *Dokl. Akad. Nauk SSSR* **214**, 940–942.

Desiraju, T. (1972). *J. Neurophysiol.* **35**, 326–332.

Dewan, E. M. (1970). *Int. Psych. Clin.* **7**, 295–307.

Drucker-Colìn, R. R. (1973). *Brain Res.* **56**, 123–134.

Drucker-Colìn, R. R. and Spanis, C. W. (1975). *Experientia* **31**, 551–552.

Drucker-Colìn, R. R., Rojas-Ramirez, J. A., Vera-Trueba, J., Monroy-Ayala, G. and Hernàndez-Peòn, R. (1970). *Brain Res.* **23**, 269–273.

Drucker-Colin, R. R., Spanis, C. W., Cotman, C. W. and McGaugh, J. L. (1975a). *Science* 187, 963–965.

Drucker-Colin, R. R., Spanis, C. W., Huniadi, J., Sassin, J. F. and McGaugh, J. L. (1975b). *Neuroendocrinol.* 18, 1–8.

Empson, J. A. C. and Clarke, P. R. F. (1970). *Nature* 227, 287–288.

Evans, J. I., MacLean, A. W., Ismail, A. A. A. and Love, D. (1971). *Nature* 229, 261–262.

Evarts, E. V. (1964). *J. Neurophysiol.* 27, 152–171.

Evarts, E. V. (1967). *In* "The Neurosciences: A Study Program" (G. C. Quarton, T. Melnechuk, and F. O. Schmitt, eds). Rockefeller Press, pp. 545–556.

Feinberg, I. (1968). *Science* 159, 1256.

Feinberg, I. and Earts, E. V. (1969). *Proc. Amer. Psychopath. Ass.* 58, 334–343.

Fencl, V., Koski, G. and Pappenheimer, J. R. (1971). *J. Physiol.* 216, 565–589.

Fishbein, W., Kastaniotis, C. and Chattman, D. (1974). *Brain Res.* 79, 61–75.

Fishbein, W., McGaugh, J. L. and Schwarz, J. R. (1971). *Science* 172, 80–82.

Fowler, M. J., Sullivan, M. J., and Ekstrand, B. R. (1973). *Science* 179, 302–304.

Giuditta, A., Rutigliano, B., Casola, L. and Romano, M. (1972). *Brain Res.* 46, 313–328.

Giuditta, A., Rutigliano, B., Traverso, R. and Vitale-Neugebauer, A. (1975). *In* "Sleep 1974" (P. Levin and W. P. Koella, eds). Karger, Basel, pp. 326–328.

Giuditta, A., Rutigliano, B., Vitale-Neugebauer, A. and Traverso, R. (1975). *In* "Neurobiology of Sleep and Memory", Proc. Symp. held in Mexico City (J. L. McGaugh and R. R. Drucker-Colin, eds) (in press).

Glushenko, T. S. and Demin, N. N. (1971). *Dokl. Akad. Nauk SSSR* 197, 1222–1225.

Godin, Y. and Mandel, P. (1965). *J. Neurochem.* 12, 455–460.

Greenberg, R. and Dewan, E. (1969). *Nature* 223, 183–184.

Greenberg, R. and Pearlman, C. (1974). *Persp. Biol. Med.* 17, 513–521.

Greenberg, R., Pearlman, C., Fingar, R., Kantrowitz, J. and Kawliche, S. (1970). *Brit. J. Med. Psychol.* 43, 1–11.

Grieser, C., Greenberg, R. and Harrison, R. H. (1972). *J. Abnormal Psychol.* 80, 280–286.

Haider, I. and Oswald, I. (1970). *Brit. Med. J.* 2, 318–322.

Handwerker, M. J. and Fishbein, W. (1975). *Physiol. Psychol.* 3, 137–140.

Hartmann, E. L. (1973a). *Psychosomatics* 14, 95–103.

Hartmann, E. L. (1973b). "The Functions of Sleep". Yale University Press, New Haven, Conn.

Hartmann, E., Baekeland, F. and Zwilling, G. (1972). *Arch. Gen. Psychiatry* 26, 463–468.

Haulică, I., Ababei, L., Teodorescu, C., Roşca, V., Haulică, A., Moisin, M. and Haller, C. (1970). *J. Neurochem.* 17, 823–826.

Heiner, L., Godin, Y., Mark, J. and Mandel, P. (1968). *J. Neurochem.* 15, 150–151.

Hennevin, E. and Leconte, P. (1971). *Anné Psychol.* 71 (2), 489–519.

Hennevin, E., Leconte, P. and Bloch, V. (1974). *Brain Res.* 70, 43–54.

Hobson, J. A. (1968). *Science* 162, 1503–1505.

Horne, J. A. and Porter, J. M. (1975). *Nature* 256, 573–575.

Horne, J. A. and Walmsley, B. (1975). Second Intern. Congr. Sleep Res. Abstracts 254, Edinburgh.

Hyden, H. and Lange, P. W. (1965). *Science* 149, 654–656.

Ingvar, D. H. (1975). *In* "Sleep 1974" (P. Levin and W. P. Koella, eds). Karger, Basel, pp. 164–169.

Jackson, J. H. (1932). *In* "Selected Writings of John Aughlings Jackson" (J. Taylor, ed.), Vols 1 and 2. Hodder and Stoughton, London.

Jakoubek, B., Semiginovsky, B., Kraus, M. and Erdossova, R. (1970). *Life Sci.* **9**, 1169–1179.

Johnson, L. C. (1973). *Amer. Sci.* **61**, 326–338.

Johnson, L. C., Naitoh, P., Moses, J. M. and Lubin, A. (1974). *Psychophysiology* **11**, 147–159.

Jouvet, M. (1967). *Physiol. Rev.* **47**, 117–177.

Jouvet, M. (1972). *Ergb. Physiol.* **64**, 166–307.

Joy, R. M. and Prinz, P. N. (1969). *Physiol. Behav.* **4**, 809–814.

Kales, A., Tan, T.-L., Kollar, E. J., Naitoh, P., Preston, T. A. and Malmstrom, E. J. (1970). *Psychosom. Med.* **32**, 189–200.

Karadžić, V. and Mrśulja, B. (1969). *J. Neurochem.* **16**, 29–34.

Karadžić, V., Mičić, D. and Rakić, Lj. (1971). *Experientia* **27**, 509–511.

King, L. J., Schoepfle, G. M., Lowry, O. H., Passonneau, J. V. and Wilson, S. (1967). *J. Neurochem.* **14**, 613–618.

Kleinschmidt, W. J. (1974). *Perspect. Biol. Med.* **17**, 371–378.

Kogan, A. B., Feldman, G. L. and Gusatinsky, V. N. (1975). 2nd Intern. Congr. Sleep Res., Abstracts, 22, Edinburgh.

Korner, A. (1965). *Rec. Progr. Horm. Res.* **21**, 205–240.

Latash, L. P., Danilin, V. P., Manov, G. A. and Rait, M. L. (1975). *In* "Sleep 1974" (P. Levin and W. P. Koella, eds). Karger, Basel, pp. 356–358.

Leconte, P., Hennevin, E. and Bloch, V. (1974). *Physiol. Behav.* **13**, 675–681.

Legendre, R. et Pieron, H. (1910). *C.R. Soc. Biol. (Paris)* **68**, 1108–1109.

Legendre, R. et Pieron, H. (1913). *Z. Allg. Physiol.* **14**, 235–262.

Lubin, A., Moses, J. M., Johnson, L. C. and Naitoh, P. (1974). *Psychophysiology* **11**, 133–146.

Lucero, M. (1970). *Brain Res.* **20**, 319–322.

MacFadyen, U. M., Oswald, I. and Lewis, S. A. (1973). *J. Appl. Physiol.* **35**, 391–394.

Magnes, J., Allweis, C. and Abeles, M. (1967). *J. Neurochem.* **14**, 859–871.

Mancia, M. (1975). *In* "Sleep 1974" (P. Levin and W. P. Koella, eds). Karger, Basel, pp. 5–13.

Mark, J., Godin, Y. and Mandel, P. (1969). *J. Neurochem.* **16**, 1263–1272.

Matsumoto, J., Nishisho, T., Suto, T., Sadahiro, T. and Miyoshi, M. (1968). *Nature* **218**, 177–178.

Matsumoto, J., Sogabe, K. and Hori-Santiago, Y. (1972). *Experientia* **28**, 1043–1044.

McGaugh, J. L. (1966). *Science* **153**, 1351–1358.

Mendelson, W., Guthrie, R. D., Guynn, R., Harris, R. L. and Wyatt, R. J. (1974). *J. Neurochem.* **22**, 1157–1159.

Mićić, D., Karadžić, V. and Rakić, Lj. M. (1967). *Nature* **215**, 169–170.

Miller, L., Drew, W. G. and Schwartz, I. (1971). *Percept. Motor Skills* **33**, 118.

Monnier, M. and Hatt, A. M. (1971). *Pflügers Arch.* **329**, 231–243.

Monnier, M. and Hösli, L. (1964). *Science* **146**, 796–798.

Monnier, M. and Schoenenberger, G. A. (1972). *Experientia* **28**, 32–33.

Monnier, M., Koller, Th. and Graber, S. (1963). *Exp. Neurol.* **8**, 264–277.

Monnier, M., Hatt, A. M., Cueni, L. B. and Schoenenberger, G. A. (1972). *Pflügers Arch.* **331**, 257–265.

Monnier, M., Dudler, L. and Schoenenberger, G. A. (1973). *Pflügers Arch.* **345**, 23–35.

Moruzzi, G. (1963). *Harvey Lectures, Ser.* **58**, 233–297.

Moruzzi, G. (1969). *Arch. Ital. Biol.* **107**, 175–216.

Moruzzi, G. (1972). *Ergb. Physiol.* **64**, 1–165.

Mršulja, B. B. and Rakić, L. M. (1974). *J. Exp. Mar. Biol. Ecol.* **15**, 43–48.

Nagasaki, H., Iriki, M., Inoué, S. and Uchizono, K. (1974). *Proc. Japan Acad.* **50**, 241–246.

Noda, H. and Ross Adey, W. (1970). *Brain Res.* **19**, 263–275.

Oswald, I. (1969). *Nature* **223**, 893–897.

Pappenheimer, J. R., Miller, T. B. and Goodrich, C. A. (1967). *Proc. Nat. Acad. Sci. USA* **58**, 513–517.

Pappenheimer, J. R., Fencl, V., Karnovsky, M. L. and Koski, G. (1974). *In* "Brain Dysfunction and Metabolic Disorders" (F. Plum, ed.) Res. Publ. Assoc. Nerv. Ment. Dis. 53. Raven Press, New York, pp. 201–210.

Pearlman, C. (1969). *Physiol. Behav.* **4**, 809–814.

Pearlman, C. (1971). *Psychonomic Sci.* **25**, 135–136.

Polzella, D. J. (1975). *J. Exp. Psychol.* **104**, 194–200.

Pujol, J.-F., Bugnet, A., Froment, J. L., Jones, B. and Jouvet, M. (1971). *Brain Res.* **29**, 195–212.

Purpura, P. D. (1956). *Amer. J. Physiol.* **186**, 250–254.

Rechtschaffen, A. (1973). *In* "The Psychophysiology of Thinking" (F. J. McGuigon and R. A. Shoonover, eds). Academic Press, New York and London, pp. 153–205.

Reich, P., Driver, J. K. and Karnovsky, M. L. (1967). *Science* **157**, 336–338.

Reich, P., Geyer, S. J. and Karnovski, M. L. (1972). *J. Neurochem.* **19**, 487–497.

Reich, P., Geyer, S. J., Steinbaum, L., Anchors, M. and Karnovsky, M. L. (1973). *J. Neurochem.* **20**, 1195–1205.

Reivich, M., Isaacs, G., Evarts, E. and Kety, S. (1968). *J. Neurochem.* **15**, 301–306.

Richter, D. and Dawson, R. M. C. (1948). *Amer. J. Physiol.* **154**, 73–79.

Ringle, D. A. and Herndon, B. L. (1968). *Pflügers Arch.* **303**, 344–349.

Ringle, D. A. and Herndon, B. L. (1969). *Pflügers Arch.* **306**, 320–328.

Roffwarg, H. P., Muzio, J. N. and Dement, W. C. (1966). *Science* **152**, 604–619.

Rubin, R. T. (1975). *Progr. Brain Res.* **42**, 73–80.

Rubin, R. T., Kales, A., Adler, R., Fagan, T. and Odell, W. (1972). *Science* **175**, 196–198.

Rubin, R. T., Poland, R. E., Rubin, L. E. and Gouin, P. R. (1974). *Life Sci.* **14**, 1041–1052.

Rubin, R. T., Gouin, P. R., Lubin, A., Poland, R. E. and Pirke, K. M. (1975). *J. Clin. Endocrinol. Metab.* **40**, 1027–1033.

Sassin, J. F., Parker, D. C., Mace, J. W., Gotlin, R. W., Johnson, L. C. and Rossman, L. G. (1969a). *Science* **165**, 513–515.

Sassin, J. F., Parker, D. C., Johnson, L. C., Rossman, L. G., Mace, J. W. and Gotlin, R. W. (1969b). *Life Sci.* **8** (I), 1299–1307.

Sassin, J. F., Grantz, A. G., Weitzman, E. D. and Kapen, S. (1972). *Science* **177**, 1205–1207.

Schnedorf, J. G. and Ivy, A. C. (1939). *Amer. J. Physiol.* **125**, 491–505.

Schoenenberg, G. A. and Monnier, M. (1975). *In* "Sleep 1974" (P. Levin and W. P. Koella, eds). Karger, Basel, pp. 46–55.

Schoenenberger, G. A., Cueni, L. B., Hatt, A. M. and Monnier, M. (1972). *Experientia* **28**, 919–921.

Seligman, M. E. P. (1970). *Psychol. Rev.* **77**, 406–418.

Seylaz, J., Mamo, H., Goas, J. Y., MacLeod, P., Caron, J. P. and Hondart, R. (1971). *Arch. Ital. Biol.* **109**, 1–14.

Shapiro, C. M., Griesel, R. D., Bartel, P. R. and Jooste, T. L. (1975). *J. Appl. Physiol.* **39**, 187–190.

Shimizu, H., Tabushi, K., Hishikawa, Y., Kakimoto, Y. and Kaneko, Z. (1966). *Nature* **212**, 936–937.

Smith, C., Kitahama, K., Valatz, J.-L. and Jouvet, M. (1974). *Brain Res.* **77**, 221–230.

Snyder, F. (1966). *Amer. J. Psych.* **123**, 121–136.

Steriade, M. and Hobson, J. A. (1976). *Progr. Neurobiol.* **6**, 155–376.

Steriade, M., Costantinescu, E. and Apostol, V. (1969). *Brain Res.* **13**, 177–180.

Steriade, M., Deschênes, M. and Oakson, G. (1974). *J. Neurophysiol.* **37**, 1093–1113.

Stern, W. C., Morgane, P. J., Panksepp, J., Zolovick, A. J. and Jalowiec, J. E. (1972). *Brain Res.* **47**, 254–258.

Stern, W. C., Jalowiec, J. E., Shabshclowitz, H. and Morgane, P. J. (1975). *Horm. Behav.* **6**, 189–196.

Tagney, J. (1973). *Brain Res.* **53**, 353–361.

Takahashi, Y., Kipnis, D. M. and Daughaday, W. H. (1968). *J. Clin. Invest.* **47**, 2079–2090.

Tata, J. R. (1968). *Nature* **219**, 331–337.

Tauber, E. S. (1974). "Adv. Sleep Res." (E. D. Witzman, ed.), Vol. 1. Spectrum, pp. 133–172.

Townsend, R. E., Prinz, P. N. and Obrist, W. D. (1973). *J. Appl. Physiol.* **35**, 620–625.

Valatz, J. L., Bugat, R. and Jouvet, M. (1972). *Nature* **238**, 226–227.

Valatz, J. L. and Bugat, R. (1974). *Brain Res.* **69**, 315–330.

Van den Noort, S. and Brine, K. (1970). *Amer. J. Physiol.* **218**, 1434–1439.

Veech, R. L., Harris, R. L., Veloso, D. and Veech, E. H. (1973). *J. Neurochem.* **20**, 183–188.

Vesco, C. and Giuditta, A. (1967). *Biochim. Biophys. Acta* **142**, 385–402.

Vitale-Neugebauer, A., Giuditta, A., Vitale, B. and Giaquinto, S. (1970). *J. Neurochem.* **17**, 1263–1273.

Webb, W. B. (1974). *Percep. Motor Skills* **38**, 1023–1027.

Webb, W. B. and Agnew, H. W. (1965). *Science* **150**, 1745.

Webb, W. B. and Agnew, H. W. (1970). *Science* **168**, 146–147.

Webb, W. B. and Agnew, H. W. (1975). *Psychophysiol.* **12**, 367–370.

Williams, H. L., Lubin, A. and Goodnow, J. J. (1959). *Psychol. Monogr.* **73**, (14, whole no. 484).

Williams, H. L., Hammack, J. T., Daley, R. L., Dement, W. D. and Lubin, N. A. (1964). *EEG Clin. Neurophysiol.* **16**, 269–279.

Williams, H. L., Gieseking, C. F. and Lubin, A. (1966). *Percep. Motor Skills* **23**, 1287–1293.

Zepelin, H. and Recthschaffen, A. (1974). *Brain Behav. Evol.* **10**, 425–470.

Subject Index